Handbook of Essential Tremor and Other Tremor Disorders

Handbook of Essential Tremor and Other Tremor Disorders

edited by
Kelly E. Lyons
Rajesh Pahwa

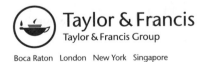

Taylor & Francis
Taylor & Francis Group
Boca Raton   London   New York   Singapore

Published in 2005 by
Taylor & Francis Group
6000 Broken Sound Parkway NW, Suite 300
Boca Raton, FL 33487-2742

© 2005 by Taylor & Francis Group, LLC

No claim to original U.S. Government works
Printed in the United States of America on acid-free paper
10 9 8 7 6 5 4 3 2 1

International Standard Book Number-10: 0-8247-2645-6 (Hardcover)
International Standard Book Number-13: 978-0-8247-2645-6 (Hardcover)

Library of Congress Cataloging-in-Publication Data is also available

---

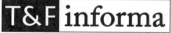

Taylor & Francis Group
is the Academic Division of T&F Informa plc.

Visit the Taylor & Francis Web site at
http://www.taylorandfrancis.com

Foreword

Of all the different types of movement disorders, tremors are probably the most common. These alternating, oscillating, and rhythmical movements are perhaps the most simple and easily recognized abnormal movements; simple in the sense that it is the same pattern or movement over and over again. This is in contrast to how complex abnormal movements can be in other disorders such as tics and dystonia. In dystonia, for example, the type of movement differs depending on what part of the body is affected. With tremor, although all body parts can be affected, the movements are those of rhythmic oscillations. Yet for all the simplicity in the pattern of these alternating movements, their presence under certain conditions—such as when the involved body part is resting in repose, actively engaged in a motor activity such as writing, or just appearing with increased muscle tone such as maintaining a posture against gravity—adds a level of complexity to tremor, resulting in a classification based on what brings on the tremor. Thus, differentiating the types of tremor makes the study of tremor much more complex than one might first appreciate. The same can be said for the causes of tremor—from neurodegenerative disorders, to neurotoxins, to emotional stress or anxiety—there are numerous causes of tremor. Different regions of the brain or peripheral nervous system can give rise to different types of tremor, another factor adding to the complexity of understanding tremor.

This book, organized and edited by two scholars of tremor—Kelly Lyons and Rajesh Pahwa—is very welcome and much needed. It pieces together the entire subject of tremor into one complete monograph. It becomes the source to reach for when one wants to obtain the latest information about tremor. The title places emphasis on the condition known as essential tremor. This is appropriate because essential tremor, as a single entity by itself, is the most common type of movement disorder. Yet genetic studies are showing that there are probably different etiologies causing essential tremor. Although not characterized as a disease by this name until the last century, essential tremor was seen in antiquity, and this type of tremor is mentioned in the bible, although under the general rubric of tremor. Even trembling with fear and strong emotions is described in the bible.

Despite how far back in history tremor has been recognized, new types of tremor continue to be described. These include primary writing tremor, other task specific or posture specific tremors, and tremor occurring while standing and then disappearing on walking or sitting. Identifying the clinical features of these new conditions and making a diagnosis, alone, gives comfort to the physician and patient by placing a name on the particular condition when such a patient is encountered. As more information unfolds, there will be further gains for these patients.

We are witnessing increasing scholarly research on tremors, from epidemiology to physiology to rating scales and to medical and surgical treatments. This activity is indeed fortunate for despite how often tremor is seen, and despite how successful some treatments can be, we are far from conquering these abnormal movements. This book puts this new information, along with older knowledge, into one convenient volume. The clinician, researcher and patient with tremor will welcome this much-needed book.

Stanley Fahn, MD

Preface

Essential tremor is estimated to affect up to 10 million Americans and is one of the most common movement disorders. Although there are multiple types of tremor, essential tremor is the most prevalent. There have been tremendous strides made in the treatment of tremor. In the last few years, clinical trials of the anti-epileptic medication topiramate have shown benefit in essential tremor. Many studies and clinical data have confirmed the safety and efficacy of surgical treatments such as thalamotomy and deep brain stimulation of the thalamus in the treatment medication resistant disabling tremor. However, the management of tremor disorders continues to be a challenge.

The *Handbook of Essential Tremor and Other Tremor Disorders* presents up to date information on the scientific and therapeutic aspects of essential tremor and other tremor disorders in a practical, user-friendly format for easy access for the clinician and academic alike. The book is organized into two primary sections, with the first section specific to essential tremor and the second to the various other tremor disorders. The section on essential tremor contains a comprehensive picture of the disorder including history, epidemiology, etiology, pathophysiology, neurochemistry, neuropathology, clinical characteristics and assessments, and medical and surgical treatment. The second section is dedicated to specific tremor disorders including parkinsonian, dystonic, cerebellar, drug and toxin induced, physiologic, psychogenic and others. Each chapter is a complete review of the particular tremor disorder and its treatment.

We are cognizant of the need for and believe that this book will serve as a valuable resource for neurologists as well as general practitioners, family physicians, and other health care professionals dealing with essential tremor and other tremor disorders. It is a handbook that should thoroughly guide the clinician toward treating the many patients who are afflicted with these often debilitating disorders.

We would like to thank each of the authors for their time and commitment in preparing scholarly reviews of the various aspects of essential tremor and other tremor disorders. We would also like to thank Jinnie Kim other Marcel Dekker, Inc., staff who assisted in the preparation of this book.

Kelly E. Lyons
Rajesh Pahwa

Dedication

*We would like to dedicate this book to Tom and Elaine Lyons
and Anjali, Esha, and Vinay Pahwa
for their continual support*

Contents

Contributors

Jo Ann Antenor, MPH   *Department of Neurology, Washington University in St. Louis, St. Louis, Missouri, USA.*

Yasuhiko Baba, MD   *Department of Neurology, Mayo Clinic, Jacksonville, Florida, USA.*

Peter G. Bain, MA, MD, FRCP   *Department of Neurology, Charing Cross Hospital Campus, Imperial College, London, UK.*

Richard J. Barohn, MD   *Department of Neurology, University of Kansas Medical Center, Kansas City, Kansas, USA.*

Kailash P. Bhatia, MD   *Sobell Department of Movement Neuroscience and Movement Disorders, Institute of Neurology, Queen Square, London, UK.*

Arif Dalvi, MD   *Department of Neurology, University of Chicago, Parkinson's Disease and Movement Disorders Center, Chicago, Illinois, USA.*

Günther Deuschl, MD   *Department of Neurology, University of Kiel, Kiel, Germany.*

Adam S. DiDio, MD   *Department of Neurology, The Mount Sinai Medical Center, New York, New York, USA.*

Rodger J. Elble, MD, PhD   *Department of Neurology, Southern Illinois University School of Medicine, Springfield, Illinois, USA.*

Hubert H. Fernandez, MD   *Department of Neurology, University of Florida, Gainesville, Florida, USA.*

Nestor Galvez-Jimenez, MD, MSc, FACP   *Clinical Associate Professor of Biomedical Science, Department of Biomedical Sciences, The Charles B. Schmidt College of Science, Florida Atlantic University, The Regional Campus* *for the University of Miami School of Medicine, and Chief, Movement Disorders Program, The Cleveland Clinic Florida, Weston, Florida, USA.*

Willibald Gerschlager, MD   *Sobell Department of Motor Neuroscience and Movement Disorders, Institute of Neurology, Queen Square, London, UK.*

Robert A. Hauser, MD   *Departments of Neurology, Pharmacology, and Experimental Therapeutics, University of South Florida and Tampa General Healthcare, Tampa, Florida, USA.*

Neng Huang, MD, PhD   *The Parkinson's Institute, Sunnyvale, California, USA.*

Jennifer S. Hui, MD   *Department of Neurology, University of Southern California, Los Angeles, California, USA.*

Joseph Jankovic, MD   *Parkinson's Disease Center and Movement Disorders Clinic, Department of Neurology, Baylor College of Medicine, Houston, Texas, USA.*

William C. Koller, MD, PhD   *Department of Neurology, University of North Carolina, Chapel Hill, North Carolina, USA.*

Anthony E. Lang, MD, FRCPC   *Department of Neurology, Movement Disorders Center, Toronto Western Hospital, Toronto, Ontario, Canada.*

Mark F. Lew, MD   *Department of Neurology, University of Southern California, Los Angeles, California, USA.*

Elan D. Louis, MD, MS   *Department of Neurology, Columbia University, New York, New York, USA.*

Kelly E. Lyons, PhD   *Department of Neurology, University of Kansas Medical Center, Kansas City, Kansas, USA.*

Nicte I. Mejia, MD   *Parkinson's Disease Center and Movement Disorders Clinic, Department of Neurology, Baylor College of Medicine, Houston, Texas, USA.*

John C. Morgan, MD, PhD   *Department of Neurology, Medical College of Georgia, Augusta, Georgia, USA.*

Michael S. Okun, MD   *Department of Neurology, University of Florida, Gainesville, Florida, USA.*

Anokh Pahwa, BA   *University of Texas Medical Branch, Galveston, Texas, USA.*

Rajesh Pahwa, MD   *Department of Neurology, University of Kansas Medical Center, Kansas City, Kansas, USA.*

Joel S. Perlmutter, MD   *Departments of Radiology, Anatomy, Neurobiology and Program in Physical Therapy, Washington University in St. Louis, St. Louis, Missouri, USA.*

Jan Raethjen, MD *Department of Neurology, University of Kiel, Kiel, Germany.*

Ali Rajput, MD, FAAN *Department of Neurology, Royal University Hospital, Saskatoon, Saskatchewan, Canada.*

Alex Rajput, MD *Department of Medicine, University of Saskatchewan, Saskatoon, Saskatchewan, Canada.*

Jayaraman Rao, MD *Department of Neurology, Professor of Neurology and Neuroscience, Louisiana State University Health Sciences Center, New Orleans, Louisiana, USA.*

David S. Saperstein, MD *Department of Neurology, University of Kansas Medical Center, Kansas City, Kansas, USA.*

Lauren C. Seeberger, MD *Colorado Neurological Institute Movement Disorders Center, Englewood, Colorado, USA.*

Kapil D. Sethi, MD, FRCP *Department of Neurology, Medical College of Georgia, Augusta, Georgia, USA.*

Dee E. Silver, MD *Scripps Memorial Hospital La Jolla, La Jolla, California, USA.*

Tanya Simuni, MD *Department of Neurology, Northwestern University Feinberg School of Medicine, Chicago, Illinois, USA.*

Natividad P. Stover, MD *Assistant Professor of Neurology, University of Alabama at Birmingham, Birmingham, Alabama, USA.*

James Tetrud, MD *The Parkinson's Institute, Sunnyvale, California, USA.*

Michele Tinazzi, MD *Sobell Department of Motor Neuroscience and Movement Disorders, Institute of Neurology, Queen Square, London, UK and Neurology Unit, Azienda Ospedasliera di Verona, Italy.*

Alexander I. Tröster, PhD *Department of Neurology, University of North Carolina School of Medicine, Chapel Hill, North Carolina, USA.*

Karen A. Tucker, PhD *Department of Neurology, University of North Carolina School of Medicine, Chapel Hill, North Carolina, USA.*

Ryan J. Uitti, MD *Department of Neurology, Mayo Clinic, Jacksonville, Florida, USA.*

Ray L. Watts, MD *Department of Neurology, University of Alabama at Birmingham, Birmingham, Alabama, USA.*

Cindy Zadikoff, MD *Department of Neurology, Toronto Western Hospital, Toronto, Ontario, Canada.*

Part I: Essential Tremor

1

The History of Essential Tremor

Adam S. DiDio

The Mount Sinai Medical Center, New York, New York, USA

William C. Koller

University of North Carolina, Chapel Hill, North Carolina, USA

I. INTRODUCTION

Essential tremor is one of the most prevalent movement disorders and has affected people from the beginning of modern human existence. As far back as history has been recorded, references are made to medical diseases, including general descriptions of tremor. The distinct entity of essential tremor, however, was not fully described until the end of the 19th century, and the term "essential

3

tremor" was not routinely used by neurologists until the second half of the 20th century (1). Advancements have been made in the treatment of essential tremor, and we continue to look for new medications and modalities to treat this disease.

II. ANCIENT HISTORY—THE ACKNOWLEDGMENT OF TREMOR

If one traces modern human civilization back to its earliest roots, evidence of tremor can be found. In Egypt, during the 7th century BC, hieroglyphics were used as one of the first forms of written and recorded language. One particular hieroglyph has been consistently interpreted to represent "trembling" or "shuddering." This hieroglyph was usually used in the setting of trauma, and may have actually meant "seizure," but in at least a few instances it appears to have indicated a disease-induced state. Written language at that time was less explicit, and it may be that this symbol represented a few conditions where trembling, shaking, or shuddering were known to occur (1).

Documentation of tremor became somewhat more precise in India, from 5000 to 3000 BC. The *Ayurveda*, which was the literature system of that time, makes many references to tremor. Physicians recognized that in certain circumstances humans developed repetitive, oscillating movements that appeared involuntary. The term *kampa* was used to indicate "tremor," and *kampavata*, to mean imbalance due to tremor (2).

In Greece from the 300s to 400s BC, Hippocrates made certain references to tremors in his Aphorisms. He quoted, "Quibus in febre ardente tremores fiunt, delirium solvit," which translates as "when tremors occur in ardent fevers, they are terminated by delirium" (3).

In later ancient history, around 200 BC, a passage written in the Book of Ecclesiastes makes use of the concept of tremor. One passage roughly translates as "the keepers of the house shall tremble" or "the guardians of the house became unsteady" (4). Again, specific reference or description of essential tremor was not documented in these ancient times, but physicians appeared to be aware of different conditions that cause or result in tremor.

III. EARLY HISTORY—DISTINCTION BETWEEN REST AND ACTION TREMOR

It was not until the times Anno Domini that physicians became more illustrative when describing tremor. Between 130 and 200 AD, Claudius Galen of Pergamon, a Turkish physician who treated the gladiators, was the first to describe tremor as an involuntary up-and-down motion. Later in his life, he wrote a treatise on tremor, and coined the terms "tremor" and "palpitation" to distinguish between action tremor and rest tremor, respectively. In one passage he wrote, "No one trembles who does not choose to move his limb." This unquestionably equates his term "tremor" to what we routinely today call action tremor (5).

IV. EARLY MODERN HISTORY—IDENTIFICATION OF "ESSENTIAL TREMOR"

During the 17th century, further distinction was made between action and rest tremor. In 1680, a neurologist from Holland named Franciscus de la Boe, better known as Sylvius de la Boe, differentiated between tremor during volitional movement (*motus tremulous*) versus tremor at rest (*tremor coactus*) (6). Later, in the 1700s, a Dutch physician named Gerhard Van Swieten also differentiated between rest tremor and intention tremor (7). In 1817, the famous English general practitioner, James Parkinson, distinguished essential tremor from all other tremors, including the resting tremor found in the disease that carries his namesake (8). In 1888, the French neurologist, Jean-Martin Charcot, concurred with this distinction (9).

Also in the 17th century, clinicians began recognizing that certain types of tremor seemed to run in families. They noticed that patients in these families shared a "general clinical resemblance," having action tremors that differed from those of known causes, such as tremors from toxic ingestion. Therefore, they began using the term "familial tremor" to describe such cases. Other than being passed down from one generation to the next, these familial tremors had no obvious cause (10). A French neurologist, Francois Boissier de Sauvages de la Croix, wrote specifically of the familial tremor in 1768. Later, in compliance with the latest Parisian fashions, Charcot demonstrated the presence of a head tremor in female patients with "familial tremor" during his clinical lessons. He let them wear a hat with large ostrich feathers, and visualized the exaggerated tremulous movement of the feathers (9).

In the 19th century, the term "essential" was applied to many disease entities of unknown cause. For example, "essential" convulsions, "essential" paralysis, and "essential" vertigo were new terms in circulation. The term "essential tremor" was used to describe the hereditary tremor, even though for years it was still more widely known as "familial tremor." In 1836, a neurologist named Most described several patients with a familial form of essential tremor (11). By the second half of the 19th century, the term "essential tremor" was widely used in neurology textbooks (12).

In 1887, a New York neurologist named Charles Dana described the clinical characteristics of a case of familial tremor (10):

> It [the tremor] affects his arms most, but also his lower limbs. The tremor affects the two sides about equally .... It is slightly apparent with handwriting .... He controls the tremor better and writes more smoothly with a lead pencil .... When excited the tremor affects his head, which oscillates, and also his muscles of articulation, so that speech is indistinct. The upper extremities are most noticeably affected, but it may involve the head [and] neck .... It ceases during sleep. Everything that produces excitement or nervousness increases the tremor .... It neither stops nor increases during volitional movements; in this respect differing from the tremors of paralysis agitans .... It is entirely distinct

from paralysis agitans, in the fact of its hereditary, non-progressiveness, and absence of any other neuromotor or vasomotor symptoms.

In the 1920s, a Russian neurologist, Minor, reviewed the clinical features of essential tremor. He claimed that patients with essential tremor had higher intelligence, longer life-spans, and were more fertile. His assertions were not supported by subsequent investigations (13). In 1949, Critchley provided the most detailed description of the natural history and phenomenology of essential tremor. He recognized that conditions known as "congenital tremor," "infantile tremor," "juvenile tremor," "presenile tremor," and "senile tremor" were all simply manifestations of essential tremor, at different stages of life, and were not distinct disorders (14).

V. PEOPLE IN HISTORY WITH ESSENTIAL TREMOR

Throughout history, there were undoubtedly many famous people who suffered with essential tremor. Many, however, remained undiagnosed or were mislabeled as having another movement disorder (i.e., Parkinson's disease). In addition, some famous figures were never in the public eye long enough for the tremor to be noticed. Perhaps one of the best-documented cases of essential tremor in a famous person is the case of Samuel Adams (1722–1803). Adams, the American Revolutionist and beer brewer, is thought to have suffered from essential tremor. To verify this, his old personal and political letters, as well as his speeches which were initially handwritten by Adams, were studied. After reviewing old reports, it seems that Adams had a tremor that affected his hands, head, and voice. The tremor had surfaced by his early 40s, although it was reportedly mild at first. Adams experienced progressive difficulty with his ability to write while in his 50s and early 60s. He made frequent references to his tremor in personal letters, and a review of his letters shows that his handwriting deteriorated over time. By age 71, he was no longer able to write, and was forced to dictate all of his letters and speeches. His tremor was also familial, as it affected his daughter and her children (15).

VI. MILESTONES IN THE TREATMENT OF ESSENTIAL TREMOR

Essential tremor, even when accurately recognized and described, was not readily treated. Initially, essential tremor was not thought to be treatable. In 1968, Marshall suggested the use of beta-adrenergic blockers in essential tremor. He stated, "As the tremor is exacerbated by adrenaline, beta-adrenergic blockers are worthy of a trial though, as yet, extensive clinical experience with these substances is lacking" (16). Evidence of the efficacy of beta-adrenergic blockade, was confirmed in 1971 by Winkler and Young (17) who noticed that a patient being treated with propranolol for a cardiac condition, who also had co-morbid essential tremor, had a dramatic reduction in tremor after starting the medication. They stated,

Recently, one of us (GW) made the serendipitous observation that a severe essential tremor disappeared when a patient with a cardiac arrhythmia was treated with propranolol. This particular patient reported that, for the first time in five years, she could sign her name.

Also, in 1971, Sevitt (18) described 4 patients aged 60–84 with essential tremor, with marked improvement of symptoms while being treated with propranolol.

The effect of propranolol on tremor was first brought to my notice by the first patient in this series .... [The patient] is a managing director and the tremor in his hands is severe enough to prevent his signing cheques. This was probably a senile tremor. He was put on propranolol, 10 mg. thrice daily, because he was unable to take enough digoxin to control his atrial fibrillation. Soon after starting propranolol he reported that his tremor had disappeared completely.

Since these reports, there have been numerous placebo-controlled, double-blind studies confirming the efficacy of beta-adrenergic blockers, particularly propranolol. Overall, 40–50% of patients experience symptomatic relief, especially in controlling tremor of the hands (19).

Many patients with essential tremor quickly learn that after ingesting alcohol, the severity of their tremor dramatically decreases. Critchley himself noted the excessive use of alcohol in patients with essential tremor, and suggested that it was likely an attempt at self-medication (14). Growdon et al. (20) reported in 1975 that alcohol works orally, but not intra-arterially, to reduce the symptoms of essential tremor. Koller and Biary (21) showed that alcohol is one of the most potent suppressants of essential tremor. With alcohol, however, there has always been the concern of addiction, tolerance, and danger of use. In 1982, Schroeder and Nasrallah (22) reported alcohol abuse in 67% of patients with essential tremor. In contrast, Koller (23) found that alcohol use is not more common in patients with essential tremor than in patients with other neurological diseases. Other alcohols have also been explored for the treatment of essential tremor. Teravainen et al. (24) found that methylpentynol, a six carbon alcohol, did not reduce the severity of essential tremor. Other alcohols, such as octanol, still need to be further studied.

In 1981, O'Brien et al. (25) reported that when primidone was given to a patient with co-morbid epilepsy and essential tremor, the severity of his tremor was dramatically reduced. Following this observation, they administered primidone to twenty other patients with essential tremor, and found that sixty percent had good responses. In 1982, Findley and Calzetti (26) reported primidone to be effective in treating essential tremor, based on a double-blind, controlled trial. In 1986, Koller and Royse (27) reported that primidone was 40–50% efficacious in treating essential tremor. Since that time, other clinical trials have shown primidone to be effective in symptomatically treating essential tremor of the hands. These studies, however, have shown that primidone works poorly on symptomatically treating tremor involving the head or voice. The mechanism of the anti-tremor effect remains unknown (19).

Various other medications have been experimented with to treat essential tremor. Since the early 1980s, benzodiazepines have been used in essential tremor. In a double-blinded controlled study, gabapentin was found to be no more efficacious than placebo (28). Over the past 20–30 years, numerous medications, including carbonic anhydrase inhibitors, calcium channel blockers, typical and atypical neuroleptics, methylxanthines, and centrally acting anti-hypertensive medications, such as clonidine, have been studied for the treatment of essential tremor. Although initial reports suggested efficacy with some medications, these medications were not found to be significantly efficacious when studied in a blinded, controlled fashion (19). In 2002, Connor (29) found topiramate to improve functional measures of essential tremor in a double-blind, placebo-controlled trial. Presently, propranolol and primidone remain the mainstay pharmacological treatment of essential tremor.

Botulinum toxin injections are another modality known to be useful for treating essential tremor. In 1998, Modugno et al. (30) studied the effect of botulinum toxin type A injections in 10 patients with essential tremor. Botulinum toxin produced a 20% functional improvement in tremor, and it was hypothesized that botulinum toxin could be used effectively in essential tremor. In 1996, Jankovic et al. (31) conducted a randomized, double-blind, placebo-controlled trial of botulinum toxin type A in essential hand tremor. The subjects experienced only modest improvement, and many patients noted some degree of finger weakness. Brin et al. (32) conducted a randomized, double-blind, placebo-controlled trial of botulinum toxin type A in essential tremor, which showed a significant improvement of postural hand tremor, but not kinetic tremor. Overall, botulinum toxin appears to be only minimally effective for tremor of the hands, with a possible adverse side effect of hand weakness. Botulinum toxin is, however, more successful in treating head and voice tremors (19).

Thalamotomy was the first surgical approach to treating essential tremor. As early as 1950, doctors performed surgical lesions in the thalamus and basal ganglia, to observe the effects it had upon involuntary movements (33). In 1983, 51 patients with various kinds of tremor, received stereotaxic ventralis intermedius (VIM) thalamotomies. In all cases but one, a small thalamic lesion immediately eradicated the tremor. In the only unsuccessful case, the lesion was estimated to be too small. The effect persisted for over ten years in some cases (34).

Thalamic stimulation is also a widely recognized treatment for essential tremor. The original concept of stimulating the thalamus dates back as far as 1952, when Baird et al. (35), while performing experiments on cats, stimulated the anterior thalamic nuclei and noted a response in motor control. Later, in 1956, the inhibitory effect of thalamic stimulation on neuronal activity in the motor cortex was studied (36). The first organized study to evaluate the long-term suppression of tremor by thalamic stimulation was in France in 1991 (37). Of 43 patients receiving thalamic stimulation, 27 patients had complete relief from tremor and 11 patients showed major improvement in severity of tremor which results in 88% of patients obtaining some degree of benefit (37). Many studies have since reported the long-term efficacy of thalamic stimulation (19). In 2003, Rehncrona et al. (38) studied the efficacy of deep brain stimulation after electrode implantations in the ventralis intermedius nucleus of the thalamus in 39 patients with severe tremor. They concluded that thalamic stimulation can efficiently suppress severe tremor in essential tremor and Parkinson's disease >6 years after implantation. Thalamic stimulation is commonly used today, and is preferred over surgical lesions.

VII. PATHOPHYSIOLOGY OF ESSENTIAL TREMOR

The pathophysiological mechanism of essential tremor is unknown. Various positron emission tomography (PET) studies over the years have inconsistently implicated the cerebellum, inferior olives, and other structures with cerebellar connections. In 1993, Jenkins et al. (39) used PET studies to demonstrate that essential tremor involves the cerebellum. In 1993, Hallett and Dubinsky (40), using PET with [18F] fluoro-2-deoxyglucose, showed significant glucose hypermetabolism of the medulla, particularly the inferior olivary nuclei, and thalami, but not of the cerebellar cortex, in patients with essential tremor. In 1994, Wills et al. (41), using PET with radioactive water [H2(15)O], demonstrated increased blood flow in the cerebellum and red nucleus, but not the inferior olive. Repeated studies using PET to measure cerebral blood flow have shown increased cerebellar blood flow in all types of tremor (42). In animal studies, harmaline and serotonergic drugs enhance olivary rhythmicity, and produce an action tremor similar to that in essential tremor (42). Gross, microscopic, and magnetic resonance imaging (MRI) evaluations have failed to show conclusive evidence of structural damage in the cerebellum in patients with essential tremor, and it is possible that there are no distinct pathological changes in essential tremor. We have yet to pinpoint exactly which central nervous system structures are involved, and what the patho-physiological mechanism is in essential tremor.

VIII. CONCLUSION

Essential tremor has been observed since the beginning of modern human existence. Over many centuries, the cumulative study and research of physicians across the globe has resulted in accurate identification and practical treatments for this condition. Although we have effective treatments for some patients, future research will hopefully produce more powerful tools to understand the patho-physiological mechanisms and aid the discovery of better treatments for essential tremor.

REFERENCES

1. Louis ED. Essential tremor. Arch Neurol 2000; 57(10):1522–1524.
2. Gourie-Devi M, Ramu MG, Venkataram BS. Treatment of Parkinson's disease in "Ayurveda" (ancient Indian system of medicine): discussion paper. JR Soc Med 1991; 84:491–492.
3. Hippocrates. The Aphorisms of Hippocrates. Birmingham AL, ed. The Classics of Medicine Library, 1982.
4. The Revised English Bible. Ecclesiastes 12:3. Oxford, England: Oxford University Press, 1989.
5. Galen. De Tremore, palpitatione, convulsione et rigore. In: Kuhn CG, ed. Opera Omnia Knobloch. Germany: Lipsiae, 1824.
6. De la Boe SF. Opera Medica (Editio Altera Correctior and Emendatior). Amsterdam, The Netherlands: Danielem Elsevirium and Abrahamum Wolfgang, 1690.
7. Van Swieten G. Commentaria in Hermanni Boerhaave Aphorismos de Cognoscendis et Curandis Morbis. Lugduni Batavorum, The Netherlands: Verbeek, 1742.
8. Parkinson J. Essay on the Shaking Palsy. London: Whittingham and Rowland for Sherwood, Neely and Jones, 1817.
9. Charcot JM. Lecons sur les Maladies du Systeme Nerveux Faites a la Salpetriere. 4th ed. Paris: Delahaye et Le Cronsnier, 1880:155–188.
10. Dana CL. Hereditary tremor: a hitherto undescribed form of motor neurosis. Am J Med Sci 1887; 94:386–393.
11. Most GF. End de Med Praxis. 1836; 2:555.
12. Reynolds RJ. A System of Medicine. Philadelphia, PA: Henry C Lea, 1879.
13. Minor L. Uber das erbliche zittern zblges. Neurol Psychiatry 1925; 99:586–633.
14. Critchley M. Observations on essential (heredo familial) tremor. Brain 1949; 72:113–139.
15. Louis ED. Samuel Adams' tremor. Neurology 2001; 56(9):1201–1205.
16. Marshall J. Tremor. In: Vinken PJ, Bruyn GW, eds. Handbook of Clinical Neurology. Vol. 6. Amsterdam, The Netherlands: North-Holland, 1968.
17. Winkler GF, Young RR. The control of essential tremor by propranolol. Trans Am Neurol Assoc 1971; 96:66–68.
18. Sevitt I. The effect of adrenergic beta-receptor blocking drugs on tremor. Practitioner 1971; 207:677–678.
19. Lyons KE, Pahwa R, Comella CL et al. Benefits and risks of pharmacological treatments for essential tremor. Drug Saf 2003; 26:461–481.
20. Growdon JH, Shahani BT, Young RR. The effect of alcohol on essential tremor. Neurology 1975; 25:259–262.
21. Koller WC, Biary N. Effect of alcohol on tremors:comparison with propranolol. Neurology 1984; 34:221–222.
22. Schroeder D, Nasrallah HA. High alcoholism rate in patients with essential tremor. Am J Psychiatry 1982; 139:1471–1473.
23. Koller WC. Alcoholism in essential tremor. Neurology 1983; 33:1074–1076.
24. Teravainen H, Huttunen J, Lewitt P. Ineffective treatment of essential tremor with an alcohol, methylpentynol. J Neurol Neurosurg Psychiatry 1986; 49:198–199.
25. O'Brien MD, Upton AR, Toseland PA. Benign familial tremor treated with primidone. Br Med J 1981; 282:178–180.
26. Findley LJ, Calzetti S. Double-blind, controlled study of primidone in essential tremor: preliminary results. Br Med J (Clin Res Ed) 1982; 285:608.

27. Koller WC, Royse VL. Efficacy of primidone in essential tremor. Neurology 1986; 36:121–124.
28. Pahwa R, Lyons K, Hubble J et al. Double-blind, controlled trial of gabapentin in essential tremor. Mov Disord 1998; 13:465–467.
29. Connor GS. A randomized double-blind placebo controlled trial of topiramate treatment for essential tremor. Neurology 2002; 59:132–134.
30. Modugno N, Priori A, Berardelli A, Vacca L, Mercuri B, Manfredi M. Botulinum toxin restores presynaptic inhibition of group Ia afferents in patients with essential tremor. Muscle Nerve 1998; 21(12):1701–1705.
31. Jankovic J, Schwartz K, Clemence W et al. A randomized double-blind, placebo-controlled study to evaluate botulinum toxin type A in essential hand tremor. Mov Disord 1996; 11:120–256.
32. Brin MF, Lyons KE, Doucette J et al. A randomized, double masked, controlled trial of botulinum toxin type A in essential hand tremor. Neurology 2001; 56(11):1523–1528.
33. Wycis HT, Spiegel EA. The effect of thalamotomy and pallidotomy upon involuntary movements in chorea and athetosis. Surg Forum 1950; 92:329–332.
34. Hirai T, Miyazaki M, Nakajima H, Shibazaki T, Ohye C. The correlation between tremor characteristics and the predicted volume of effective lesions in stereotaxic nucleus ventralis intermedius thalamotomy. Brain 1983; 106:1001–1018.
35. Baird HW, Guidetti B, Reyes V, Wycis HT, Spiegel EA. Stimulation and elimination of the anterior thalamic nuclei in man and cat. Pflugers Arch 1952; 255(1):58–67.
36. Li CL. The inhibitory effect of stimulation of a thalamic nucleus on neuronal activity in the motor cortex. J Physiol 1956; 133(1):40–53.
37. Benabid AL, Pollak P, Gervason C, Hoffmann D, Gao DM, Hommel M, Perret JE, de Rougemont J. Long-term suppression of tremor by chronic stimulation of the ventral intermediate thalamic nucleus. Lancet 1991; 337(8738):403–406.
38. Rehncrona S, Johnels B, Widner H, Tornqvist AL, Hariz M, Sydow O. Long-term efficacy of thalamic deep brain stimulation for tremor: double-blind assessments. Mov Disord 2003; 18(2):163–170.
39. Jenkins IH, Bain PG, Colebatch JG, Thompson PD, Findley LJ, Frackowiak RSJ, Marsden CD, Brooks DJ. A positron emission tomography study of essential tremor: Evidence for overactivity of cerebellar connections. Ann Neurol 1993; 34:82–90.
40. Hallett M, Dubinsky RM. Glucose metabolism in the brain of patients with essential tremor. J Neurol Sci 1993; 114(1):45–48.
41. Wills AJ, Jenkins IH, Thompson PD, Findley LJ, Brooks DJ. Red nuclear and cerebellar but no olivary activation associated with essential tremor: a positron emission tomographic study. Ann Neurol 1994; 36(4):636–642.
42. Deuschl G, Elble RJ. The pathophysiology of essential tremor. Neurology 2000; 54(suppl 4):S14–S20.

2

Epidemiology and Etiology of Essential Tremor

Elan D. Louis

Columbia University, New York, New York, USA

I. INTRODUCTION

Essential tremor is a chronic, progressive neurological disease. The motor feature that is the hallmark of the illness is a 4–12 Hz kinetic tremor that may involve several regions of the body, including the arms and head but rarely the legs (1–6). The pathophysiology of this disorder is poorly understood. As with other progressive neurological disorders of later life (e.g., motor neuron disease, parkinsonism), essential tremor may represent a family of related diseases rather than a single disease, and neurological manifestations as exhibited in any one patient may be dependent upon the localization of the disease pathology or pathologies within the nervous system. Thus, while the kinetic tremor in essential tremor may be the result of an abnormality in an olivo-cerebellar-thalamic pathway, often patients with essential tremor have signs of more widespread cerebellar involvement (e.g., intention tremor, ataxia, eye movement abnormalities) (7–10), abnormalities of the basal ganglia (e.g., rest tremor and subtle bradykinesia) (11,12), and cognitive-neuropsychiatric manifestations that may be the result of abnormalities in cerebellar, subcortical, or cortical centers (13,14). In addition, involvement of the cerebellar-thalamic pathway and possibly other pathways in other progressive neurological diseases (e.g., Parkinson's disease) can result in an action tremor, further increasing the clinical similarity between essential tremor and these diseases.

An understanding of the epidemiology of essential tremor is important for several reasons. First, it will help to identify the causes (etiologies) of the disorder, leading to measures to prevent the disease and second, it will provide clues about the underlying disease processes (pathophysiology), which are vital to the conception and development of effective protective and symptomatic therapies. This chapter will serve as an introduction and review of the epidemiology of essential tremor.

II. CASE DEFINITION AND DIAGNOSIS

The prime issue that needs to be addressed when examining the epidemiology of a disorder is case definition. How does one define a case? Case definition in essential tremor is problematic for a variety of reasons. The first is that the clinical manifestations of the disease, as currently understood, are relatively restricted, with a kinetic tremor being the major feature (2–4,6). This contrasts with Parkinson's disease, which is characterized by four hallmark features (tremor at rest, bradykinesia, rigidity, and postural instability). Recent research has expanded the clinical characterization of patients with essential tremor, with nonmotor manifestations becoming apparent, but further work is needed to fully characterize these. Second, the hallmark clinical feature of essential tremor, kinetic tremor, may be a feature of a myriad of disorders of the central and peripheral nervous system (6); it is not specific to essential tremor. Third, kinetic tremor of the arms can be seen as a normal finding in the population and particularly in the elderly, among whom essential tremor is also most prevalent (15,16). This blurs the boundary between the disease state and normalcy. Fourth, there is no diagnostic test (serological, imaging, physiological, or pathological) that may be used to validate a clinical diagnosis of essential tremor (6).

Attempts at case definition have been heavily influenced by the source of the cases; consensus definitions (17), while useful because they reflect the opinions and experience of many of the leaders in the field, have fallen short in essential tremor because they have not been designed from an epidemiological perspective but rather from the perspective of the neurology clinic (18,19). While it is important to consider Parkinson's disease and other movement disorders in the exclusionary criteria, from the population perspective, these are rare diseases and enhanced physiological tremor is far more common (20). It is important for diagnostic criteria to attempt to exclude individuals with enhanced physiological tremor. This means that the criteria must specify, in detail, the extent of tremor that must be present to qualify for a diagnosis of essential tremor. Present consensus criteria note that bilateral action tremor must be present but do not specify the extent of tremor that must be present (17). This is problematic for population-based studies and for genetic studies because the prevalence of kinetic tremor is high in the normal population. The Washington Heights-Inwood Genetic Study of Essential Tremor criteria specify the number and types of activities during which kinetic tremor must be present in order to qualify for a diagnosis of essential tremor (18,21–23). In this regard, the criteria are particularly useful for population-based, familial aggregation, and epidemiological studies. Leaving this issue aside, all current criteria for essential tremor specify that action tremor of the arms must be present or isolated head tremor may be present in the absence of signs of dystonia. Other neurological diseases such as Parkinson's disease must be absent and the tremor cannot be due to drugs.

III. SPECIFIC METHODOLOGICAL CONSIDERATIONS

Case definition in essential tremor is clinical rather than laboratory-based. There are a number of other important methodological considerations that influence the study of the epidemiology of essential tremor. First, tremor may be mild, particularly when observed in cases who were ascertained from the population rather than from treatment settings and the prevalence of asymptomatic essential tremor is high (18,24). As a result, screening questionnaires for essential tremor lack sensitivity (21), particularly for mild cases, resulting in many false negatives and an under-ascertainment of cases (25). Second, because the large majority of essential tremor cases do not seek treatment (26–28), clinic-based series reflect a small proportion of essential tremor cases whose selection is prone to bias, resulting, for example, in increased prevalence of familial forms of the disease (29) and increased ascertainment of young onset forms of the disease (30). Therefore, careful distinction must be drawn between population-based and clinic-based studies of essential tremor. Finally, if cognitive deficits are indeed present in patients with essential tremor (13,31–34), then the validity of self-reported information must take this into account.

IV. PREVALENCE

There have been more than twenty studies of the prevalence of essential tremor, including studies in North America, South America, Europe, Asia, and Africa (35). Estimates of the crude prevalence of this disorder have varied considerably from study to study, with the range in prevalence estimates spanning three orders of magnitude (0.008–22%). Factors that have contributed to this variability include differences in study design and in the characteristics of the study populations (35). Many of the studies did not define the entity or specify how the diagnosis was made and many were not population-based. If one limits the studies to those that specified how they defined the disease, were population-based, and that provided age-stratified data, the prevalence in the population among those ≥60 years of age ranges from 1.3% to 5.1% (35). A problem with these studies, however, is that cases were ascertained using a two-phase approach in which the initial phase was a screening questionnaire. Given the low sensitivity of screening questionnaires for mild cases of essential tremor, this strategy is likely to have resulted in an underestimate of the prevalence of essential tremor. In a recent population-based study in Turkey, in which all individuals were examined by a study neurologist regardless of the screening questionnaire results, the prevalence of essential tremor was 4.0% among individuals age ≥40 years and was 6.3% among individuals ≥60 years of age (25). In another population-based study in Finland (26) that used similar methods, the authors examined participants who screened positive to a tremor questionnaire and a sub-sample who screened negative, allowing them to estimate the proportion of false negatives. The prevalence of essential tremor in individuals ≥40 years was 5.6% and was 9.0% among individuals ≥60 years of age. Taking these prevalence estimates (4–5.6% among individuals ≥40 years and 6.3–9.0% among those age ≥60), one can begin to estimate the number of individuals with essential tremor in the United States, using United States Census data from the year 2000. The number of individuals age ≥40 years with essential tremor in the United States in 2000 would have been 4.8–6.7 million and the number age ≥60 would have been 2.9–4.1 million. This makes essential tremor the most common tremor disorder and one of the most common movement disorders.

V. INCIDENCE

There is one study of the incidence of essential tremor (36). This study was a 45-year retrospective study of essential tremor based on a medical record review using data from the Rochester Epidemiology Project (36). While the records linkage system is designed to capture all health encounters of individuals living in Olmstead County Minnesota, entry into the record as essential tremor would have required, in most instances, that the problem be important enough to be recognized by the patient and deemed important enough by the treating general medical doctor to require a medical entry. Hence, mild cases of essential tremor or cases in individuals with other more pressing medical issues are not likely to have been entered, resulting in low estimates of disease prevalence and incidence. In fact, the estimated prevalence in this study was very low at 0.3%. The age and sex adjusted incidence was 23.7 per 100,000 US Caucasian population. This did not differ in men and women. There is a need for additional, more comprehensive incidence data.

VI. PROGRESSION

Despite the fact that essential tremor is a progressive disorder, there are few longitudinal studies in patients with essential tremor. Most data on disease progression are anecdotal information from clinicians who have followed patients over time (37) or based on examination of cross-sectional data of patients with disease of different durations (38). In one study (39), 44 patients were followed prospectively for a four year period and accelerometry and surface electromyography (EMG) were used to measure hand tremor and motor unit entrainment in the extensor carpi radialis brevis every two years. The frequency of action tremor decreased by ∼0.06–0.08 Hz per year. The 29% increase in tremor amplitude over the four year period (∼7% per year) narrowly missed statistical significance which may have been related to the small sample size. These data confirm and quantify the clinical anecdotal sense that the action tremor of essential tremor worsens over time.

It is not only the action tremor of essential tremor that worsens over time. Patients with essential tremor can also develop rest tremor. This rest tremor typically occurs in individuals with disease of longer duration and greater severity (12). In addition, head tremor occurs in 35–50% of patients with essential tremor. While isolated head tremor can occur, it is rare. Head tremor generally develops in essential tremor cases who have had arm tremor for a number of years. In one study that examined this issue (40), arm tremor severity was associated with an increased risk of head tremor (i.e., individuals with severe arm tremor were more likely to have head tremor). This suggests that the underlying pathology might begin in the arm representation region of the cerebellum or its outflow pathways and then progress by increasing within the arm region and by extending to the head region. These data suggest that essential tremor may be a progressive disorder. The progressive nature of this disorder implies that the underlying pathogenesis of the disease, could be neurodegenerative.

VII. MORTALITY

Although it is presumed that mortality in essential tremor cases and control subjects is similar, there are few data on which to base this statement and this is an area of research that requires attention. Several investigators have proposed that essential tremor promotes longevity. In the early 1900s (41), Minor promoted the idea of status macrobioticus multiparus, characterized by tremor, longevity, and fecundity in individuals with tremor and their relatives. He observed a dispropor- tionately large number of elderly persons in tremor families as compared to the general population of France. One in every 14.5 of his essential tremor cases was ≥80 years of age, compared to one in every 116 people in the general population of France according to the 1876 census records. Three (0.4%) of the 683 relatives of his essential tremor cases were ≥100 years of age, while the total number of citizens of this age in France was only 150 (0.0004%) out of 40 million. More recently, Jankovic et al. (42) examined data on parents of essential tremor cases. The parents who were reported to have had tremor lived a median of 8 years longer than did parents who did not have tremor. While one interpretation is that tremor confers a longevity factor, the authors noted that an alternative explanation is that the risk of essential tremor increases markedly with age, and older relatives are more likely to manifest tremor than are younger relatives. In other words, living to an older age may increase the likelihood of developing essential tremor rather than the converse.

Others have suggested that essential tremor does not alter life span. More than a century ago, based on a single family with essential tremor, Dana (43) concluded that essential tremor did not alter life span because individuals in the family lived to "advanced old age." Dana did not provide the actual ages of these individuals. In more recent times, in a longitudinal retrospective study of essential tremor patients in Rochester, Minnesota (36), 266 patients were selected and their medical records abstracted. The authors used a group of historical control subjects. The survival after diagnosis of essential tremor was comparable to the expected survival for persons of similar age and sex from the west north central region of the United States. In that study, the mean age at diagnosis was 58 years, and the mean length of follow up after diagnosis was 9.7 years, suggesting that some of the cases may not have been followed into advanced age. It is possible that at these ages the risk of mortality in essential tremor rises.

There has not been a prospective study of mortality in essential tremor nor has there been a study in which risk of mortality was assessed in essential tremor cases in comparison with a contemporaneously-enrolled (rather than historical) group of control subjects. The often-repeated statement in the literature that the disease is not associated with an increased risk of mortality is not based on very much data. Given the possibility that essential tremor may be a neurodegen- erative disease, the issue of mortality needs to be assessed.

VIII. RISK FACTORS

Age is clearly a risk factor for essential tremor. The one incidence study (36) clearly showed an age-associated rise in the incidence of this disorder, with the most dramatic rise beginning to occur in those who were entering their 50s. Prevalence studies consistently have shown a similar increase in the prevalence of essential tremor with age (25,35). Age is not only a risk factor for disease onset but also, for disease progression.

Besides age, ethnicity may be a risk factor for essential tremor. A trend toward higher prevalence in Caucasians than in African-Americans has been reported in two community-based studies (44,45), one in northern Manhattan, New York (44) and one in Copiah County, Mississippi (45). The study in Manhattan also showed that the prevalence in Hispanics was intermediate between Caucasians and African-Americans (44). In a third study, individuals from four communities in different regions of the United States answered a standardized screening questionnaire for essential tremor that included the question "has a doctor diagnosed you as having familial tremor or benign essential tremor?" (46). When this standardized screening question was used, the proportion of participants with physician-diagnosed essential tremor was similar across four communities, suggesting that the prevalence of this condition may be less variable than is often reported. However, Caucasians were 5 times more likely to have physician-diagnosed essential tremor than were African-Americans. A family history of essential tremor is a risk factor for essential tremor, as the disease is in some cases familial. These data will be reviewed in the next section.

IX. ETIOLOGY

A. Genetic vs. Nongenetic Etiologies

The etiologies of essential tremor are both genetic and nongenetic (47,48). One important question is the magnitude of a genetic contribution to the etiology of this disease. It is commonly stated in the literature that 50% of essential tremor cases are attributed to genetic causes. This estimate appears to be based on the proportion of cases who report a family history. However, estimates of the proportion with a family history range from as low as 17% to as high as 100% (49). Furthermore, the proportion with a positive family history does not accurately reflect the proportion with a genetic etiology. Most of the studies examining this question have not enrolled control subjects. Many of the positive family histories could be explained by chance co-occurrence of a highly prevalent disorder rather than a genetic predisposition for tremor (18,49). Studies suggest that as many as 18% of families may contain an affected individual, even if ascertained through an unaffected control subject (23). Additional methodological problems with previous studies raise further doubt about the proportion of genetic cases. Most studies have reported the percentage of probands with a family history rather than the proportion of at-risk relatives who are affected with essential tremor, making it impossible to test consistency with genetic models or to control for characteristics of the relatives (18). Most studies have selected probands from clinical care settings (hospitals, doctors' offices, clinics) rather than from the community. Essential tremor cases who are seen in clinics and doctors' offices probably represent a very small proportion of all essential tremor cases in the population (as few as 0.5%) (28), and these cases are 5 times more likely to report a positive family history than are those who never make it to clinics (29). Clinic populations might be self-selected to over-represent familial and genetic forms of essential tremor, and possibly autosomal dominant forms as well. Finally, most studies have obtained family history information by interviewing the probands rather than by examining the relatives themselves, and the sensitivity of probands' reports may be as low as 16% (50).

In the Washington Heights-Inwood Genetic Study of Essential Tremor, a population-based family study of essential tremor that enrolled relatives of essential tremor cases and relatives of control subjects, we found that a first-degree relative of an essential tremor case was 4.7 times more likely to have essential tremor than was a first-degree relative of a control subject (23). If essential tremor were a completely genetic disease, and we assumed an autosomal dominant model of inheritance, a disease prevalence of 1%, and a penetrance of 100%, then the relative risk should be ~50 rather than 4.7 (51). Even if we were to assume:

(1) autosomal recessive inheritance, the relative risk should be closer to 15;
(2) a higher disease prevalence (5%), the relative risk should be greater than 20;
(3) a penetrance of only 50%, the relative risk should be closer to 25;
(4) the proportion of sporadic cases was 50%, the relative risk should be closer to 25 (48,51).

These data suggest that a sizeable proportion of essential tremor cases do not occur on a simple Mendelian genetic basis. Nongenetic (environmental) risk factors may be contributing partially or entirely to the etiology and/or expression of many cases of essential tremor (48). Alternative explanations include a polygenic or mitochondrial cause in some cases. In a twin study (47), 3 of 5 (60%) monozygotic twins were concordant for essential tremor, compared with only 3 of 8 (27%) dizygotic twins. Although concordance in monozygotic twins was approximately two times that in dizygotic twins, the monozygotic concordance was not 100%, also supporting the notion that environmental factors could be contributing to the etiology of essential tremor. Overall, these data support the notion that both genetic and environmental factors make important contributions to the etiology of essential tremor. Further, the interaction between genetic and environmental causes may be important.

B. Genetic Etiologies

Specific genes for essential tremor have not yet been identified. Given the high prevalence of this disorder, one would expect that multiple genetic loci may contribute to essential tremor. Linkage has been reported on two different chromosomes (3q13 and 2p22) (52,53).

Gulcher et al. (52) reported the results of a genome scan for familial essential tremor (FET) genes in 16 Icelandic families containing 75 affected individuals.

The average age of family members was ~50 years. The scan revealed significant evidence for linkage to chromosome 3q13 under an autosomal dominant model assuming 1% disease prevalence and 90% penetrance. In that same year, Higgins et al. (23) reported the results of a linkage analysis in a large American family of Czech descent. Data were available on 67 family members, among whom 18 were affected. Evidence was obtained for linkage to chromosome 2p22-25. For this study, they assumed a disease prevalence of 1%, an autosomal dominant model of inheritance, and a penetrance of 100%. Other investigators have demonstrated the absence of linkage in essential tremor families to either of these two loci, suggesting that there is further genetic heterogeneity (54).

C. Environmental Etiologies

The entity of nonfamilial essential tremor or "sporadic" essential tremor is well recognized by most clinicians, who distinguish this form of essential tremor from "hereditary" essential tremor (55,56). In fact, in most series, the majority (>50%) of essential tremor cases have not reported affected relatives (48), and despite the high prevalence of the disease, families that are informative for genetic linkage studies have been difficult to locate. The existence of intra-familial differences in age of onset and severity of tremor (23,28) also suggests that environmental (or perhaps other genetic) factors may serve as modifiers of an underlying susceptibility genotype. Therefore, the environmental epidemiology of essential tremor is an important area of study. Two recent studies (57,58) have implicated β-carboline alkaloids and lead as possible environmental toxicants that may be involved in the etiology of essential tremor.

The β-carboline alkaloids, including harmine and harmane, are a group of highly tremorogenic chemicals. Laboratory animals injected with large doses of these chemicals acutely exhibit an action tremor that resembles essential tremor (57). Human volunteers acutely exposed to large doses display a reversible coarse tremor (57). Sources of β-carboline alkaloids both exogenous and endogenous to the body exist. β-carboline alkaloids are naturally present in the food chain, especially when meats are cooked at high temperatures for long periods of time, and these chemicals are normal body constituents that are produced *in vivo* by the cyclization of indole-alkylamines with aldeydes, occurring in most tissues in animals and humans (57). The specificity of individual β-carboline alkaloids for different brain receptors suggests that they probably have normal biological functions (57). To explore the hypothesis that high concentrations of β-carboline alkaloids are associated with essential tremor, blood concentrations of harmane and harmine, which are among the most tremorogenic and most well studied β-carbolines, were measured in essential tremor cases and control subjects and their concentrations were elevated in essential tremor. The study did not provide an explanation for the case-control difference, but possibilities include increased exogenous (dietary) exposure or increased endogenous production or impaired metabolism in essential tremor cases.

In a second study (58), lead was examined as a possible environmental toxicant in essential tremor. Lead is a ubiquitous toxicant and laboratory animals and humans who are exposed to high levels of either inorganic or organic forms of lead develop neurological disorders in which action tremor is prominent (58). Destruction of cerebellar Purkinje cells is a major feature of the pathology of lead toxicity (58). To test the hypothesis that essential tremor is associated with lead exposure blood lead concentrations were measured in essential tremor patients and in control subjects who were enrolled in a study of the environmental epidemiology of essential tremor. Blood lead concentration was higher in essential tremor patients than in controls. Whether this association was due to increased exposure to lead or a difference in lead kinetics in essential tremor patients requires further investigation. These two studies provide an initial glimpse of the potential role of environmental toxicants in the etiology of essential tremor. Clearly further studies are needed.

X. SUMMARY

Essential tremor is one of the most common adult onset movement disorders. The disorder is progressive and the clinical features are more heterogeneous and widespread than appreciated in the past. The disease is associated with functional disability. The attendant morbidity and mortality associated with this disorder have not been well-studied. In addition, we are now on the verge of uncovering the genetic and environmental causes of this disorder. This knowledge, along with insights into the basic disease mechanisms of essential tremor that will come about with clinical-pathological studies, will allow for the development of preventative measures and additional symptomatic treatments in the future.

REFERENCES

1. Louis ED, Barnes L, Albert SM et al. Correlates of functional disability in essential tremor. Mov Disord 2001; 16:914–920.
2. Louis ED, Greene P. Essential tremor. In: Rowland LP, ed. Merritt Textbook of Neurology, 10th ed. Philadelphia: Lea & Febiger, 2000:678–679.
3. Hubble JP, Busenbark KL, Koller WC. Essential tremor. Clin Neuropharm 1989; 12:453–482.
4. Findley LJ, Koller WC. Essential tremor: a review. Neurology 1987; 37:1194–1197.
5. Critchley M. Observations on essential tremor (heredofamilial tremor). Brain 1949; 72:113–139.
6. Louis ED. Essential tremor. N Engl J Med 2001; 345:887–891.
7. Stolze H, Petersen G, Raethjen J, Wenzelburger R, Deuschl G. Gait analysis in essential tremor- further evidence for a cerebellar dysfunction. Mov Disord 2000; 15(suppl 3):87.
8. Deuschl G, Wenzelburger R, Loffler K, Raethjen J, Stolze H. Essential tremor and cerebellar dysfunction. Clinical and kinematic analysis of intention tremor. Brain 2000; 123:1568–1580.

9. Singer C, Sanchez-Ramos J, Weiner WJ. Gait abnormality in essential tremor. Mov Dis 1994; 9:193–196.

10. Helmchen C, Hagenow A, Miesner J et al. Eye movement abnormalities in essential tremor may indicate cerebellar dysfunction. Brain. 2003; 126:1319–1332.

11. Rajput AH, Rozdilsky B, Ang L, Rajput A. Significance of Parkinsonian manifestations in essential tremor. Can J Neurol Sci 1993; 20:114–117.

12. Cohen O, Pullman S, Jurewicz E, Watner D, Louis ED. Rest tremor in essential tremor patients: Prevalence, clinical correlates, and electrophysiological characteristics. Arch Neurol 2003; 60:405–410.

13. Gasparini M, Bonifati V, Fabrizio E et al. Frontal lobe dysfunction in essential tremor. A preliminary study. J Neurol 2001; 248:399–402.

14. Chatterjee A, Jurewicz EC, Applegate LM, Louis ED. Personality in essential tremor. Mov Disord (Under Revision).

15. Louis ED, Ford B, Pullman S, Baron K. How normal is "normal"? Mild tremor in a multi-ethnic cohort of normal subjects. Arch Neurol 1998; 55:222–227.

16. Louis ED, Wendt KJ, Ford B. "Senile tremor": What is the prevalence and severity of tremor in older adults? Gerontology 2000; 46:7–11.

17. Bain P, Brin M, Deuschl G et al. Criteria for the diagnosis of essential tremor. Neurology 2000; 54(suppl 4):S7.

18. Louis ED, Ottman RA, Ford B, Pullman S, Martinez M, Fahn S, Hauser WA. The Washington heights essential tremor study: methodologic issues in essential-tremor research. Neuroepidemiology 1997; 16:124–133.

19. Louis ED. Olfactory dysfunction in essential tremor: A deficit unrelated to disease duration or severity. Neurology 2003; 61:872.

20. Louis ED, Ford B, Wendt KJ, Lee H, Andrews H. A comparison of different bedside tests for essential tremor. Mov Disord 1999; 14:462–467.

21. Louis ED, Ford B, Lee H, Andrews H. Does a screening questionnaire for essential tremor agree with the physicians' examination? Neurology 1998; 50:1351–1357.

22. Louis ED, Ford B, Lee H, Andrews H, Cameron G. Diagnostic criteria for essential tremor: A population perspective. Arch Neurol 1998; 55:823–828.

23. Louis ED, Ford B, Frucht S, Barnes LF, Tang M-X, Ottman R. Risk of tremor and impairment from tremor in relatives of patients with essential tremor: a community-based family study. Ann Neurol 2001; 49:761–769.

24. Louis ED, Ford B, Pullman S. Prevalence of asymptomatic tremor in relatives of patients with essential tremor. Arch Neurol 1997; 54:197–200.

25. Dogu O, Sevim S, Camdeviren H, Sasmaz T, Bugdayci R, Aral M, Kaleagasi H, Un S, Louis ED. Prevalence of essential tremor: Door-to-door neurological exams in Mersin Province, Turkey. Neurology 2003; 61:1804–1807.

26. Rautakorpi I, Takala J, Martilla RJ, Sievers K, Rinne UK. Essential tremor in a Finnish population. Acta Neurol Scandinav 1982; 66:58–67.

27. Rautakorpi I. Essential tremor. An epidemiological, clinical and genetic study. Research Reports from the Department of Neurology, No. 12, University of Turku, Finland, 1978.

28. Larsson T, Sjogren T. Essential tremor: a clinical and genetic population study. Acta Psychiatrica Et Neurologica Scandinavica 1960; 36(suppl 144):1–176.

29. Louis ED, Barnes LF, Ford B, Ottman R. Family history information on essential tremor: Potential biases related to the source of the cases. Mov Disord 2001; 16:320–324.

30. Louis ED, Ford B, Wendt KJ, Cameron G. Clinical characteristics of essential tremor: data from a population-based cohort. Mov Disord 1998; 13:803–808.
31. Lombardi WJ, Woolston DJ, Roberts JW, Gross RE. Cognitive deficits in patients with essential tremor. Neurology 2001; 57:785–790.
32. Lacritz LH, Dewey R Jr, Giller C, Cullum CM. Cognitive functioning in individuals with "benign" essential tremor. J Int Neuropsych Soc 2002; 8:125–129.
33. Duane DD, Vermilion KJ. Cognitive deficits in patients with essential tremor. Neurology 2002; 58:1706.
34. Vermilion K, Stone A, Duane D. Cognition and affect in idiopathic essential tremor. Mov Disord 2001; 16:S30.
35. Louis ED, Ottman R, Hauser WA. How common is the most common adult movement disorder?: estimates of the prevalence of essential tremor throughout the world. Mov Disord 1998; 13:5–10.
36. Rajput AH, Offord KP, Beard CM, Kurkland LT. Essential tremor in Rochester, Minnesota: a 45-Year Study. J Neurol Neurosurg Psychiatry 1984; 466–470.
37. Critchley M. Observations on essential (heredofamilial tremor). Brain 1949; 72:113–139.
38. Louis ED, Jurewicz EC, Watner D. Community-based data on associations of disease duration and age with severity of essential tremor: Implications for disease pathophysiology. Mov Disord 2003; 18:90–93.
39. Elble RJ. Essential tremor frequency decreases with time. Neurology 2000; 55:1547–1551.
40. Louis ED, Ford B, Frucht S. Factors associated with increased risk of head tremor in essential tremor: A community-based study in northern manhattan. Mov Disord 2003; 18:432–436.
41. Minor L. Uber hereditaren temor. Abl ges Neurol Psychiat. 1922; 28:514–516.
42. Jankovic J, Beach J, Schwartz PA, Contant C. Tremor and longevity in relatives of patients with Parkinsons disease, essential tremor, and control subjects. Neurology 1995; 45:645–648.
43. Dana CL. Hereditary tremor, a hitherto undescribed form of motor neurosis. Amer J Med Sci 1887; 94:386–389.
44. Louis ED, Marder K, Cote L et al. Differences in the prevalence of essential tremor among elderly African-Americans, Whites and Hispanics in Northern Manhattan, NY. Arch Neurol 1995; 52:1201–1205.
45. Haerer AF, Anderson DW, Schoenberg BS. Prevalence of essential tremor. Results from the Copiah county study. Arch Neurol 1992; 39:750–751.
46. Louis ED, Fried LP, Fitzpatrick AL, Longstreth WT, Newman AB. Regional and racial differences in the prevalence of physician-diagnosed essential tremor in the United States. Mov Disord 2003; 18:1035–1040.
47. Tanner CM, Goldman SM, Lyons KE et al. Essential tremor in twins: An assessment of genetic vs. environmental determinants of etiology. Neurology 2001; 57:1389–1391.
48. Louis ED. Etiology of essential tremor: Should we be searching for environmental causes? Mov Disord 2001; 16:822–829.
49. Louis ED, Ottman R. How familial is familial tremor?: genetic epidemiology of essential tremor. Neurology 1996; 46:1200–1205.
50. Louis ED, Ford B, Ottman R, Wendt KJ. Validity of family history data in essential tremor. Mov Disord 1999; 14:456–461.

51. Weiss KM, Chakraborty R, Majumder PP. Problems in the assessment of relative risk of chronic disease among biological relatives of affected individuals. J Chron Dis 1982; 35:539–551.
52. Gulcher JR, Jonsson P, Kong A et al. Mapping of a familial essential tremor gene, FET1, to chromosome 3q13. Nature Genetics 1997; 17:84–87.
53. Higgins JJ, Loveless JM, Jankovic J, Patel PI. Evidence that a gene for essential tremor maps to chromosome 2p in four families. Mov Disord 1998; 13:972–977.
54. Kovach MJ, Ruiz J, Kimonis K. Genetic heterogeneity in autosomal dominant essential tremor. Genet Med 2001; 3:197–199.
55. Herskovitz E, Blackwood W. Essential (familial, hereditary) tremor: a case report. J Neurology Neurosurg Psychiatry 1969; 32:509–511.
56. Bain PG, Findley LJ, Thompson PD, Gresty MA, Rothwell JC, Harding AE, Marsden CD. A study of heredity of essential tremor. Brain 1994; 117:805–824.
57. Louis ED, Zheng W, Jurewicz EC, Watner D, Chen J, Factor-Litvak P, Parides M. Elevation of blood β-carboline alkaloids in essential tremor. Neurology 2002; 59:1940–1944.
58. Louis ED, Jurewicz EC, Applegate L, Factor-Litvak P, Parides M, Andrews L, Slavkovich V, Graziano JH, Carroll S, Todd A. Association between essential tremor and blood lead concentration. Environ Health Perspect 2003; 111:1707–1711.

3

Pathophysiology of Essential Tremor

Jan Raethjen and Günther Deuschl

University of Kiel, Kiel, Germany

I. INTRODUCTION

The understanding of the physiology of essential tremor is dependent on the methodological tools which are available at a given time. Early attempts to understand tremor go back to researchers such as Pelnar, Altenholz, and Jung (1–4). These were mainly based on recordings of muscle volume and dealt with the analysis of tremor rhythms in different muscles. New tools to study the positive and negative symptoms of tremor have led to a better understanding of the mechanisms of these rhythmic involuntary movements.

Two main streams of research have significantly contributed to our knowledge of the pathophysiology and possible origin of essential tremor. The first are animal models of tremor. The most relevant one to essential tremor is the tremor induced by harmaline. It shares many of the clinical characteristics of essential tremor and has been shown to arise from abnormal synchronized rhythmic activity of the inferior olive (5). Experiments indicate that the olivocerebellar oscillations seem to be maintained independently of input from the periphery or other central structures (6). Deficits in cerebellar functions as indicated by an impaired conditioning learning in rabbits seems to go along with these oscillations. These observations have lead to a number of new hypotheses on the origin of essential tremor. The second line of research includes patient studies targeting the physiological characteristics of the tremor, abnormalities of movement performance or tests of physiologic functions. These aspects will be covered in detail in the present paper.

A third approach to explain the pathophysiology of essential tremor is through epidemiology and genetics. On the basis of epidemiological studies a strong influence of genetic factors has been demonstrated in the study of Larssen and Sjögren (7) and subsequent epidemiological studies in various countries (8). It is obvious, that essential tremor is not a unique entity (9). Heterogeneity is likely and sporadic cases do occur (10). Moreover, environmental factors are likely to explain some of the variance found in essential tremor (11,12). There are two twin studies showing a strong influence (13) of genetic factors or even an almost complete explanation by heredity (14). So far linkage has been found for three genes in different cohorts of patients (15–18).

II. PHYSIOLOGICAL CHARACTERISTICS OF PERIPHERAL TREMOR

The current standard for tremor recordings includes accelerometric recordings of the tremor excursions in parallel to surface electromyographic (EMG) recordings from the driving muscles (19–22) of the tremulous limb. Modern computer technology encouraged a broad application of the Fourier transform and its extensions (spectral and cross-spectral analysis) to tremor time series (23,24). Spectral analysis transforms the time series into the frequency domain. It is very sensitive to rhythmic activity which will show up as a peak at the respective frequency even when it is covered by observational noise and is therefore not detectable by visual inspection. Cross-spectral methods like cross-correlation or coherence can detect correlations between two simultaneously recorded tremor time series (23,25).

A. Tremor Analysis

The results of spectral analyses of accelerometrically recorded oscillations and the EMG of the driving muscles allow important conclusions on the origin of the tremor. Theoretically tremor oscillations can emerge from two basic mechanisms. Any movable limb can be regarded as a pendulum with the capability to swing rhythmically, that is to oscillate. These oscillations will automatically assume the resonant frequency of this limb which is dependent on its mechanical properties; the greater its weight the lower its resonant frequency and the greater the joint stiffness the higher this frequency (26). Any mechanical perturbation can activate such an oscillation. In the hands which are most often affected by tremors the main and most direct mechanical influence comes from the forearm muscles. Indeed, it has been shown that the tremor measured in normal subjects during muscle activation mainly emerges from an amplification of the muscles' effect on the hand at its resonant frequency (25,27). Thus although the muscles show normal non-rhythmic isometric activity they contribute to these resonant oscillations which account for most of the tremor seen in the physiologic situation (28). Spectral analysis of the accelerometrically measured tremor will show a peak at the tremor frequency and the activity of the muscles typically is flat without a distinct peak at this frequency [Fig. 3.1(a)]. Such a pure resonant phenomenon does not produce pathologic tremors as its amplitude is typically quite low. However, as this low amplitude oscillation leads to rhythmic activation of muscle receptors it activates segmental (spinal) or long (e.g., transcortical) reflex loops which can greatly enhance this oscillation.

In case of a relevant reflex enhancement of the oscillation, the muscle spectrum will not remain flat as in pure resonance but it will show a peak at the tremor frequency driven by the oscillating reflex loop [Fig. 3.1(b)]. As the limb mechanics and possibly reflex loops play a role in these oscillations they are termed "*mechanical-reflex oscillations.*" The second basic mechanism of tremor is a transmission of oscillatory activity within the central nervous system (CNS) to the peripheral muscles. The rhythmic activity of the muscles then leads to tremor. Spectral analysis will again show a peak at the tremor frequency in the accelerometer spectrum as well as the muscle spectrum [Fig. 3.1(c)]. These oscillations are called "*central oscillations.*" In contrast to the mechanical-reflex oscillations, central oscillations occur at the centrally determined frequency and are independent of the limbs' mechanics (29,30). This crucial difference between the two basic mechanisms can be utilized to distinguish them. The limb mechanics can easily be influenced by putting additional weight on the limb under study. As we know that increasing weight leads to a decrease in resonant frequency, the tremor frequency should become lower with additional

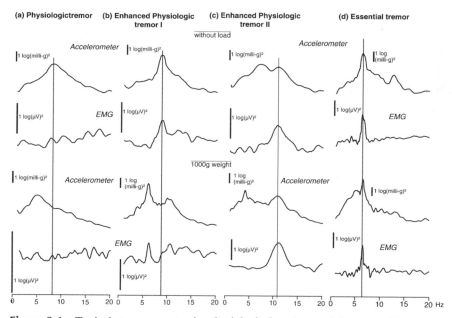

Figure 3.1 Typical power spectra in physiological and essential tremor. The power, spectra of accelerometric recordings of postural tremor from the dorsum of the hand and from the forearm extensor muscles with and without 1000 g weight added to the hand. (a–c) display different forms and mechanisms of physiologic tremor. In (a) there is a broad accelerometric peak around 7–8 Hz which drops to 4–5 Hz under 1000 g weight and the EMG spectrum is flat without any visible tremor activity. This is the typical mechanical resonant oscillation without any reflex enhancement. When these oscillations become stronger they can activate reflex loops that will lead to rhythmic EMG activation at the tremor frequency. As this EMG activity is driven by the resonant oscillation its frequency drops under weight together with the accelerometrically measured tremor frequency (b). (c) displays an example of an additional central component in physiological tremor. There is one peak in the accelerometer spectrum that corresponds to the driving EMG rhythm. Both the accelerometer and EMG peaks remain constant under weight load indicating independence from the peripheral resonance. The same is true in an essential tremor patient displayed in (d) also indicating a centrally driven tremor.

weight in the case of mechanical-reflex oscillations while it should remain unchanged in the case of central oscillations. Loading the limb in purely mechanical and reflex enhanced physiological tremor indeed lowers the tremor frequency markedly (22,25,27,31) [Fig. 3.1(a) and (b)].

In essential tremor, however, the tremor frequency remains constant under weight load (32–34) leading to the conclusion that essential tremor is a central tremor emerging from a central oscillator. However, the mechanical loading approach to distinguish the two types of oscillations has its limitations. The greater the involvement of reflex pathways in mechanical-reflex oscillations the less dependent is the frequency upon limb mechanics. In these cases it is more dependent upon reflex arc length (latency) (35–37). As this differs between distal and proximal muscles, the frequency should also differ between different muscle groups in the case of reflex involvement. All studies dealing with essential tremor in different muscles have found remarkably uniform frequencies throughout the body (34,38,39), being another argument for a central oscillator involved in the generation of essential tremor.

In early stage low amplitude essential tremor one can often see the physiological mechanical-reflex oscillation with a decreasing frequency under weight load coexisting with a central oscillation with a constant frequency and corresponding EMG peaks at the same frequency. This situation resembles the weak central component of physiological tremor which is present in some normal subjects (21,28,40) [Fig. 3.1(c)]. In the course of the disease the central oscillatory drive increases and the mechanical-reflex component becomes less clear and cannot be detected in the spectrum [Fig. 3.1(d)]. This observation has lead to the hypothesis that essential tremor and the central component of physiologic tremor may share similar mechanisms which are pathologically enhanced in essential tremor (32).

Another characteristic of the peripheral tremor recordings is the timing between the antagonistic muscle bursts. While this has been regarded typical for different forms of pathological tremors, it has been recently suggested in larger studies and long term tremor recordings that there is a continuum between reciprocal alternating and simultaneous activation of antagonistic muscles in essential tremor even within the same patient (19,41).

B. Correlation between Tremor in Different Limbs

The findings described in the previous paragraph have lead to the concept of one central oscillator that transmits its oscillatory activity to all the muscles involved in the tremor. This was supported by the remarkably uniform tremor frequency in all the affected limbs in patients with central tremors (42). However, equal frequencies do not necessarily mean that the rhythms measured in the periphery originate from the same central source. Cross spectral methods have to be applied to test this hypothesis. Coherence analysis is the method of choice, as it gives the degree to which two time series are related at a particular frequency. It is a normalized linear measure, taking on a value of one in the case of a perfect linear dependence and zero in the case of complete independence between the two processes. The statistical significance of coherence is assessed by the 95% confidence limit, which is derived under the hypothesis of linear independence. Estimated values of coherency lying below this confidence limit can be taken as an indication of a lacking linear dependence between the two processes (23,25). If the tremor in all the peripheral muscles originates from the same central oscillator one would expect a significant coherence between all the rhythmically active muscles at the tremor frequency. However, it has been shown in two studies that the tremor activity is not coherent between different limbs in essential tremor patients, while it is highly coherent between the muscles within the same limb (38,39). Therefore the concept of one single oscillator distributing its oscillatory activity to all the muscles in the periphery is questionable. The independence of the oscillations in different limbs indicates that there are several independent oscillators for each of the limbs involved in the tremor (39). One possible structural basis for this may be somatotopically separated oscillating loops in the CNS.

III. OTHER NEUROPHYSIOLOGIC TESTS IN ESSENTIAL TREMOR

Apart from the measurement of the tremor itself, a number of other neurophysiologic techniques have been applied to essential tremor patients. The vast majority of these studies examined responses to different stimuli (43–63).

A. Resetting the Tremor Rhythm by Peripheral and Central Stimuli

The most interesting studies in this field looked at the tremor rhythm itself after application of different stimuli to the peripheral or central nervous system. They have demonstrated that the phase of essential tremor can be reset by peripheral perturbations (mechanical) and peripheral nerve stimuli to the trembling hand. In patients with high amplitude essential tremor the perturbations had to be much stronger to cause a phase reset than in less affected individuals (43–45). When sinusoidal forces were applied to the wrists of essential tremor patients the tremor frequency could be entrained within a small frequency band (46). These results seem to cast some doubt on the postulated central oscillator in essential tremor. However, no matter where this oscillator may be situated within the CNS it will most likely have not only efferent but also afferent connections through which such peripheral perturbations can influence the central oscillation. Thus these results point out that peripheral influences must not be neglected even when dealing with central tremors, but they do not argue against a central origin of essential tremor. An interaction between central oscillations and peripheral mechanical reflex oscillations most likely occurs at least intermittently in all central tremors (46) and may account for some of the spontaneous fluctuations in tremor frequency (47) and its dependence on limb positioning (31,34,48).

Studies using magnetic stimulation of the motor cortex have shown that the tremor rhythm in essential tremor can also be interrupted and its phase reset by stimuli to the CNS (49–51). This seems to confirm the important role of central oscillations in essential tremor. In parkinsonian tremor not only the phase was reset but the tremor period (frequency) transiently changed (49). One possible conclusion is that transcortical pathways may be more intricately involved in the pathogenesis of parkinsonian tremor than in essential tremor. However, just as the peripheral stimuli may influence central pacemakers, a centrally evoked motor potential may influence mechanical-reflex oscillations through descending volleys to elements of the spinal reflex arcs, that is the spinal motor neurons and possibly interneurons.

Thus, wherever the resetting stimulus is delivered to the motor system it will most likely get access to both the peripheral and the central components that may be responsible for the tremor oscillations. Therefore the resetting studies emphasize that pathological tremors like essential tremor are not unalterable fixed rhythms but indirectly underlie varying influences from the periphery and the CNS that can introduce variability. However, they can not be interpreted in terms of a central vs. peripheral origin of the tremor. Examples from a peripheral and central resetting study are displayed in Fig. 3.2.

B. Evoked Potentials and Reflex Studies

There are several smaller H-reflex studies in essential tremor. The basic characteristics of the H-reflex (latency, amplitude, H/M ratio, H-reflex recovery curves) are not significantly different from normal controls (52). It was shown, however, that the late presynaptic phase of reciprocal inhibition is reduced (53,54) and can be normalized by botulinum toxin injections (55). Another study demonstrated a reduced reflex inhibition following electrical stimulation of tendon afferents (56). The early component of the long latency reflex (*LLR I*) is frequently enhanced in essential tremor patients (57). In a study on

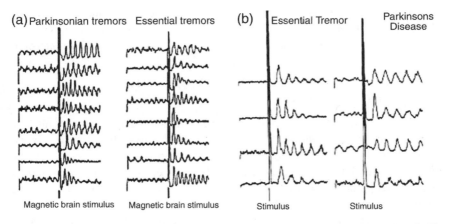

Figure 3.2 Resetting of the tremor rhythm after peripheral and cortical stimuli. The resetting of the essential tremor and parkinsonian tremor rhythm after suprathreshold magnetic stimulation over the primary motor cortex (a) and supramaximal electrical median nerve stimuli (b) are displayed. The traces show the rectified flexor EMG averaged across 50 stimulations. It is evident that in all the displayed patients and for the peripheral as well as the central stimuli the tremor rhythm becomes time-locked to the stimulus indicating a clear reset in phase. [From Refs. (45) and (49)].

essential head tremor an increased brainstem interneuronal excitability was found as indicated by an abnormal recovery curve of the blink reflex and an abnormal masseteric inhibitory reflex (58). All the abnormalities found in these reflex studies seem to hint to reduced inhibitory mechanisms in the spinal or brainstem circuitry. It has been postulated that this arises from defective central control (53). However, the rhythmic overactivity of the spinal and brainstem motor neurons in essential tremor that will inevitably be superimposed on such reflex recordings makes the interpretation of the results difficult. There is one study that analyzed cortical excitability in essential tremor using cortical magnetic stimulation. The threshold for eliciting motor evoked potentials, the effects of paired stimuli and the subsequent silent period were all normal, indicating a normal cortical excitability in essential tremor (59).

Two recent studies looked at the effects of magnetic stimulation over the cerebellum. One applied single stimuli that did not reset the tremor rhythm and the time-locked effects on the cortically evoked motor potentials was not different from normal controls (60). However, the other study employed low-frequency repetitive magnetic stimulation (rTMS) which lead to a relatively short lived but clear reduction in tremor severity (61). This suggests the involvement of the cerebellum and potential for the therapeutic use of rTMS in essential tremor; however, more work is clearly needed here.

Sensory evoked potentials (SEP) after median nerve stimulation have been analyzed in essential tremor patients. The effect of movement and the SEP was found to be abnormal for only a single cortical component of the SEP in essential tremor patients (N30) (62). This is a very subtle abnormality but it may reflect the involvement of the sensorimotor cortex in essential tremor. In another study the P300 component of the visually evoked potential was found to be elevated at certain recording sites in essential tremor (63). This result is difficult to interpret.

IV. INTERACTION OF ESSENTIAL TREMOR WITH VOLUNTARY MOVEMENTS

It is a long-standing hypothesis that essential tremor pathophysiology may be connected to the cerebellar system. One basis for this hypothesis is the clinical observation that a lesion of the cerebellum or its outflow tracts can abolish the tremor in essential tremor patients almost completely (64–66). Many animal studies have pointed to the neurons in the inferior olive to be especially prone to produce synchronized oscillatory activity (6,67,68). As the olive is tightly connected to the cerebellum, the olivo-cerebellar system has been hypothesized to contribute to the oscillatory activity in essential tremor (69). This notion was much enhanced by the study of the rare condition of *symptomatic palatal tremor*, the pathophysiology of which is probably one of the best understood among all tremor disorders. In these patients, a lesion of the cerebellum or its outflow tract and a marked ipsilateral hypertrophy of the inferior olive is typically found. As there was a variable time interval between the cerebellar or brainstem damage and the occurrence of olivar hypertrophy and palatal tremor it was postulated that the tremor was due to damage of the inhibitory cerebellar outflow to the inferior olive leading to uninhibited synchronized oscillatory activity and olivar hypertrophy. This putative oscillatory activity is the likely cause of the low frequency palatal oscillations seen clinically. All patients also suffered from some cerebellar symptoms. The fact that there were rhythmical phenomena time-locked to the palatal tremor bursts also in other muscles of the body lead to the hypothesis that a similar mechanism in the olivocerebellar system may also be responsible for pathological tremor of the extremities, notably essential tremor (70,71). Functional imaging studies have in parallel shown hyperactivity of the cerebellum and its connections (72–74). Although the interpretation of this finding is difficult it is certainly in line with the assumption that the cerebellar system plays a role in the pathophysiology of essential tremor. If the cerebellar system is involved in essential tremor generation at least some subtle clinical cerebellar abnormalities should be present in essential tremor patients. This was the starting point for a number of studies taking a closer look at the execution of different voluntary movements in essential tremor patients.

A. The Muscle Activation Pattern

The first approach to the study of the influence of essential tremor on voluntary movements was the analysis of muscle activation during simple ballistic single joint movements. During these movements a typical triphasic EMG burst pattern occurs. It starts with an activation of the agonist initiating and accelerating the movement which is followed by an antagonist activation decelerating movement. This antagonist burst is then followed by a slightly weaker second agonist activation to stabilize the final position after the movement (75). The timing of the different bursts in relation to the preceding one is critical to prevent the limb from oscillating before reaching its final position. It is not simply related to peripheral feed back in reponse to the movement but seems to be centrally programmed as it is similarly present in deafferented subjects (76). In cerebellar disease the triphasic pattern shows typical delays in muscle activation leading to an oscillation in the final phase of the movement (intention tremor) (77–79). Britton et al. (80) were the first to report EMG burst patterns during ballistic movements in essential tremor patients. Indeed they found a delay of the second agonist burst accompanied by some oscillations after the movement which were correlated with the delay of this burst in a proportion of their patients. They concluded that this was a sign of mild cerebellar dysfunction and at least contributes to the kinetic tremor seen in essential tremor. A later study looked at two groups of essential tremor patients, one with clinical signs of intention tremor and one with only postural tremor (81). They could show that in the group with clinically visible intention tremor the changes in the EMG burst pattern was almost indistinguishable from the changes in cerebellar disease with a marked delay not only of the second agonist activation but also the antagonist burst. Thus the changes in the triphasic EMG pattern during ballistic movements correlate with the presence of intention tremor in essential tremor supporting a deficit of cerebellar functions.

B. Goal-Directed Movements

It has been accepted that essential tremor is a monosymptomatic disorder without any other disabilities apart from the tremor being characterized as a mainly postural tremor which does not become strikingly worse during action (9,33). However, most clinicians regularly dealing with essential tremor patients have seen an enhancement of tremor during movement in a considerable proportion (82,83). In fact, this kinetic tremor often increases markedly in the final phase of goal-directed movements similar to intention tremor which is characteristic of cerebellar disease (84). These phenomena were analysed clinically and physiologically in a group of 79 patients with clinically definite essential tremor (85). In 52% of these patients clinical signs of an intentional component were present (ET_{IT}) while the rest presented with pure postural tremor (ET_{PT}). These two groups showed some characteristic clinical differences. ET_{IT} patients on average were older than those with ET_{PT}, their cranial muscles and the trunk were more often involved and the tremor amplitudes were significantly higher in ET_{IT}. In 28 of the ET_{IT} patients the onset of their postural tremor and intention tremor could be assessed retrospectively in detailed interviews. In all patients, the intention tremor had not been present initially but gradually developed during the course of the disease. The time interval between the onset of essential tremor and the onset of intention tremor seemed to be dependent on age. Older patients developing essential tremor reported symptoms of intention tremor after a few years while in younger patients it took up to 30–40 years until an intention tremor component appeared and contributed to disability. The data of this clinical survey show that ET_{PT} and ET_{IT} can be regarded as a continuum of the same disease rather than two separate disease entities. In addition, a natural multijoint goal directed movement was analyzed in a subgroup of these essential tremor patients and was compared with the movement execution in patients with cerebellar disease and normal controls. The movement trajectories during a reach to grasp movement showed a few low frequency irregular oscillations just before the target was reached in the ET_{IT} patients while ET_{PT} patients approached the goal on a direct path with hardly any corrective movements (Fig. 3.3). Apart from these oscillations which correspond to the clinically visible intention tremor there was an overall slowing of the movement especially of the final phase and a clear "overshoot" of the target (the wrist is moved above the target before finally approaching it). These abnormalities in the ET_{IT} patients were almost indistinguishable from those in patients with cerebellar disease (Fig. 3.3).

C. Gait

There has been evidence from clinical studies (86–88) that gait can be abnormal in essential tremor. Clinically abnormal tandem gait was described in almost

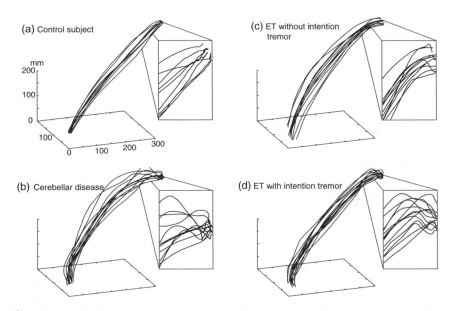

Figure 3.3 Hand trajectories during a natural reach to grasp movement. Representative examples of the hand trajectories in space are displayed for a normal control subject, a patient with cerebellar disease and two patients with essential tremor, one showing clinical signs of an intentional component and one without intention tremor. The normal subject and the essential tremor patient without intention tremor (a and c) approach the target directly on slightly curved trajectories. The insets displaying the final phase before reaching the target in more detail do not show any overshoot or oscillations. The patient with essential tremor with intention tremor (d) shows a typical overshoot above the target and 2–3 low frequency irregular oscillations before it is reached. The trajectory of the patient with cerebellar disease (b) is almost indistinguishable from this. [From Ref. (85).]

50% of the patients. These clinical results again cast doubt on essential tremor being a purely monosymptomatic disorder. In combination with the finding of a cerebellar-like intentional component these findings stimulated a more detailed quantitative study of gait in essential tremor (89). In this study the gait of 25 essential tremor patients, 10 with predominantly postural tremor and 15 with a clear intentional component, was analyzed quantitatively by means of a three-dimensional motion analysis system and again compared to a group of healthy controls and cerebellar disease patients. In normal free speed treadmill loco-motion the only abnormality found in the essential tremor patients was a slightly increased step width. All the other gait parameters were not significantly different from the control group. When examining tandem gait on the treadmill more abnormalities could be detected being in line with the previous qualitative clini-cal reports (87). The step width was markedly increased compared to normal treadmill locomotion. Only a small minority of the ET_{IT} patients managed to walk on a straight line putting one foot exactly in front of the other. The tandem gait trajectories showed variable and irregular deviations from the ideal path as if the leg movements were overshooting intermittently (Fig. 3.4). These abnormalities were very similar to those in the patients with cerebellar disease. In ET_{PT}, tandem gait was not significantly different from the normal controls (Fig. 3.4). One of the questions is whether these deficits in gait control could be simply due to kinetic leg tremor superimposed on the gait movements. However, the abnormal gait parameters were not correlated with the presence or severity of action tremor in the legs while they were closely correlated with the severity of intention tremor in the arms. It can therefore be concluded that the gait disorder in ET_{IT} is most likely due to an impaired cerebellar function and is part of the mild to moderate cerebellar syndrome that accompanies advanced essential tremor.

D. Oculomotor Function

Given the evidence for functional impairment of the cerebellum in advanced essential tremor one may expect that oculomotor control, which is another prominent cerebellar function, is also disturbed in ET_{IT} patients. However, there have not been any reports on clinically visible abnormalities of eye movements in essential tremor. Only in a study applying quantitative eye movement analysis (scleral search-coil technique and electro-oculography) has it been possible to demonstrate a selective impairment of specific oculomotor functions (90). The two main abnormalities were a reduced initial eye acceleration in smooth pursuit movements and a pathological suppression of the vestibulo-ocular reflex time constants by head tilts. Other oculomotor functions like saccades and gaze-holding were normal.

E. Cerebellar Involvement

The abnormalities of three different kinds of movements resembling the motor deficits in cerebellar disease are evidence for an involvement of the cerebellum in essential tremor. While the overshoot and intention tremor during goal-directed movements most likely indicate malfunctioning cerebellar hemispheres, the gait disorders would be compatible with a disturbance in the paravermal region and the oculomotor deficits could indicate an impairment of the caudal vermis. Thus the cerebellar involvement seems to be generalized rather than focal. The nature of reduced cerebellar function remains unclear. One possibility would be a primary abnormality in the cerebellum making the olivocerebellar system more prone to oscillations, as the disturbance progresses the cerebellar symptoms and the tremor would worsen. The tremor oscillations of essential tremor possibly emerging from the olivocerebellar system could also be the primary abnormality which in turn alters the function of the cerebellum. The

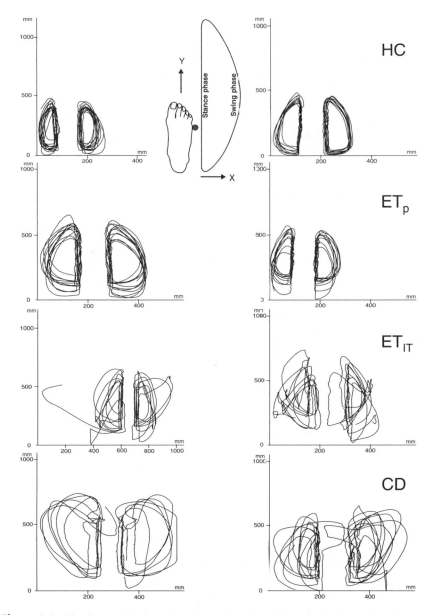

Figure 3.4 Tandem gait trajectories. The trajectories of both feet in the horizontal plane are displayed for tandem gait on the treadmill. Both feet show the stereotyped well reproducible trajectory in a normal control (HC) and in an essential tremor patient without intention tremor (ET_{PT}). In the essential tremor patient with intention tremor of the hands (ET_{IT}) this trajectory was highly variable with the feet often missing the midline at the end of the step. This profile was very similar in the patient with cerebellar disease (CD). [From Ref. (89).]

stronger the oscillations (tremor) the more they may alter cerebellar function. Thus both of these speculations would be compatible with the observed relation between tremor amplitude and cerebellar signs and are currently under debate. In this context two recent studies using magnetic resonance spectroscopy of the cerebellum are of note. Both showed a clear reduction in the neuronal marker N-acetyl-aspartate (NAA) in relation to the other typical peaks in the magnetic resonance spectrum (91,92). This may reflect a neuronal loss in the cerebellum of essential tremor patients possibly indicating neurodegeneration, that is a primary cerebellar abnormality.

V. REPRESENTATION OF ESSENTIAL TREMOR RHYTHM IN THE CENTRAL NERVOUS SYSTEM

Having shown that the cerebellum most likely is involved in the generation of essential tremor, the question remains as to how oscillatory activity from the olivocerebellar system may reach the peripheral muscles. One of the main output channels of the cerebellum reaches the motor cortex and secondary frontal cortical areas via the thalamus. Thus the oscillatory signal could be transmitted to the cortex and then travel down the corticospinal tract to the motor neurons of the affected limbs. However, the cerebellum also has other efferent connections to the spinal cord (e.g., via bulbospinal pathways) bypassing the thalamocortical pathway. Following these theoretical considerations a number of studies have sought to test for thalamic and cortical involvement in essential tremor generation or oscillation.

A. Tremor Related Activity in the Thalamus

The involvement of the thalamus in essential tremor pathophysiology has been discussed following the observation that lesions of the thalamus are a very effective therapy for essential tremor (93). This effect has been used increasingly for severely disabled essential tremor patients with the renaissance of stereotactic surgical treatment of movement disorders in the past decade. Apart from the lesional approach, it has been shown that chronic stimulation through electrodes implanted in the nucleus ventralis intermedius (VIM) of the thalamus is equally effective (94,95). This approach allows for recording from deep brain structures in the process of targeting and implanting the electrodes. Using this approach, a number of groups have looked for oscillatory activity in the thalamus of severely affected essential tremor patients. Single cells in the area of the VIM that showed rhythmic bursting discharges at the peripheral tremor frequency have been found (96–100). Coherence analyses between these rhythmic thalamic discharges and the peripheral tremor activity often revealed a significant correlation (coherence) (97). Thus the tremor rhythm of essential tremor seems to be represented in the thalamus. An example of a thalamic tremor cell discharging in a bursting mode coherently to the peripherally recorded tremor is displayed in Fig. 3.5. The mechanism or role of this rhythmic activity with respect to the peripheral tremor remains unclear. This finding may be an indication of the thalamus as part of the generating network of essential tremor but it may only be a sign of rhythmic feedback from the periphery. Only a measure of the direction of information flow from the thalamus to the periphery or vice versa and the time delay between the central and the peripheral signal could solve this problem. As the common mathematical methods for time delay estimation require relatively broad band signals (23,101) they could not be applied to the narrow band tremor activity, and new mathematical methods are being evaluated for biological data (102).

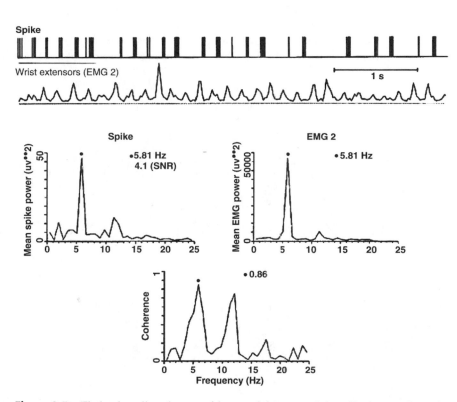

Figure 3.5 Thalamic cells coherent with essential tremor. A bursting neuron from the nucleus VIM of the thalamus in an essential tremor patient is displayed in the top row. In the next row the rectified and demodulated forearm extensor EMG of the same patient is displayed. Below this the power spectra of the spike train and the EMG are given. Both show a clear peak at the same frequency around 6 Hz indicating rhythmic activity at both recording sites. The coherence spectrum at the bottom shows very high values at this frequency indicating that the burst activity in the thalamic neurons is correlated to the tremor in the periphery. [From Ref. (97).]

B.   Tremor Related Activity in the Cortex

If the thalamus is part of the tremor-generating network in essential tremor, it would be very likely that the primary motor cortex or secondary cortical areas are part of this network as well. As cortical activity can be measured non-invasively by electro-encephalography (EEG) or magnetoencephalography (MEG) the study of the role of the cortex in tremor production attracts increasing attention. Halliday et al. (103) were the first to record cortical MEG in parallel to peripheral tremor in essential tremor. They found the typical physiological corticomuscular coherence ~20 Hz (104–106) but no coherence at the tremor frequency of 5–7 Hz. The tremor in their essential tremor patients seemed to be unrelated to cortical activity. They concluded that whatever the central source of essential tremor may be, it must be subcortical and seems to bypass the cortex on its way to the periphery. However, another group recently found corticomuscular coherence at the tremor frequency in some of their essential tremor patients (107). As displayed in Fig. 3.6 the coherent cortical areas corresponded well to the primary sensorimotor cortex.

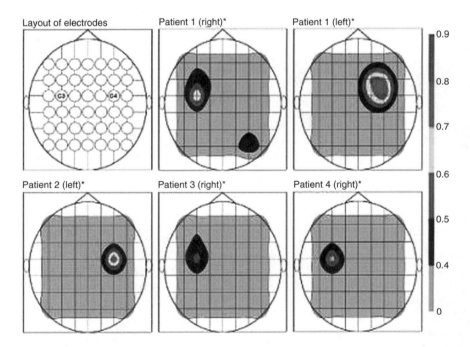

Figure 3.6 Corticomuscular coherence at the tremor frequency of essential tremor. Isocoherence lines for the essential tremor-related cortical activity recorded by EEG are displayed for 5 different patients. It is evident that the tremor-related cortical activity that is the corticomuscular coherence at the tremor frequency is centered around the contralateral primary sensorimotor cortex. The muscle recorded was the forearm extensor muscle of the more affected arm. [From Ref. (107).]

They justified the difference from previous results and between their own patients by differences in tremor intensity. They showed that tremor-related cortical activity was only present in patients with high amplitude tremor, while in patients with weak tremor there was no corticomuscular coherence. It is not possible to determine whether the oscillations are transmitted from the cortex to the periphery or whether it is merely feedback from the tremulous limbs to the cortex. We have recently looked for corticomuscular coherence in nine essential tremor patients and were able to detect coherence in single recordings in all the patients (108). However, analyzing corticomuscular coherence over time, the tremor-related cortical activity vanishes intermittently although the tremor remains unchanged. Like Halliday et al. (103), coherence in the physiological 20 Hz range was found in the majority of the essential tremor patients. In Parkinson's disease, cortical activity related to tremor has been shown in the vast majority of patients (109–111). This cortical involvement seems to be less clear in essential tremor. However, the data from deep brain recordings of the thalamus and cortical recordings indicate that the thalamocortical connections at least intermittently take part in the oscillations of essential tremor. Thus oscillations within the cerebello-thalamo-cortical loop may at least intermittently contribute to the generation of essential tremor. The possibility to record the peripheral tremor, cortical (EEG) activity and thalamic activity simultaneously in the context of the implantation of deep brain stimulation electrodes is a new and promising approach to this problem. Marsden et al. (112), who have used this setting in a small group of essential tremor patients, have obtained interesting results concerning the physiologic interaction between these three recording sites, but the conclusions on the thalamic and cortical role in tremor production were very limited, as most of their patients did not exhibit strong tremor at the time of recording because of a strong lesional effect from the electrode implantation. More data from specifically selected patients and the application of advanced multivariate mathematical analyses of those data are clearly needed.

VI. GENERAL CONCLUSIONS

Power spectral analysis of the peripheral tremor in essential tremor under different conditions has shown that the oscillation is forced upon the extremities from a central oscillator. Extending these analyses using coherence as a measure of the correlation between the tremor in different limbs has lead to the concept of multiple central oscillators causing essential tremor. Although the tremor frequency is remarkably uniform throughout the body in most patients, the oscillations in different limbs are unrelated (noncoherent) and therefore indicate several independent oscillators for each limb. The long-standing hypothesis that the cerebellum is involved in the central generation of essential tremor has recently received strong support from analyses of reach-to-grasp movements, gait, and eye movements, all of which have shown clear cerebellar-like deficits. Combining these results with the finding of at least intermittent tremor-related activity in the thalamus and primary sensorimotor cortex may be an indication of oscillations in cerebello-thalamo-cortical loops being at least one origin of essential tremor. The somatotopy of those loops which is obviously preserved may constitute the postulated multiple oscillators for different limbs. However, recent data seem to support the notion derived from earlier cortical resetting experiments that the thalamocortical loops are less intricately involved in the pathogenesis of essential tremor than in parkinsonian tremor. One speculative interpretation of the presently available data could be that the cortex is only intermittently involved in essential tremor generation, and subcortical loops or mechanisms, involving the olivocerebellar system, may maintain the tremor oscillations. However, more work is needed to corroborate this hypothesis.

REFERENCES

1. Pelnár J. Das Zittern. Seine Erscheinungsformen, seine Pathogenese und klinische Bedeutung. In: Alzheimer ALM, ed. Berlin: Julius Springer, 1913.
2. Altenburger H. Elektrodiagnostik. In: Bumke OFO, ed. Handbuch der Neurologie. Vol. Band III. Berlin: Julius Springer, 1937:1036–1086.
3. Hassler R. Zur pathologischen Anatomie des senilen und des parkinsonistischen Tremor. J für Psychol und Neur 1939; 49:193–230.
4. Jung R. Physiologische Untersuchungen über den Parkinsontremor und andere Zitterformen beim Menschen. Zsch ges Neurol und Psychiat 1941; 173:263–332.
5. Llinas R. Rebound excitation as the physiological basis for tremor: a biophysical study of the oscillatory properties of mammalian central neurons *in vitro*. In: Findley LJ, Capildeo R, eds. Movement Disorders, Tremor. London: Macmillan, 1984:339–351.
6. Wilms H, Sievers J, Deuschl G. Animal models of tremor. Mov Disord 1999; 14:557–571.
7. Larssen T, Sjögren T. Essential tremor: a clinical and genetic population study. Acta Psychiatrica Scandinavica 1960; 36:1–176.
8. Louis ED, Ottman R. How familial is familial tremor? The genetic epidemiology of essential tremor. Neurology 1996; 46:1200–1205.
9. Marsden CD. Origins of normal and pathologic tremor. In: Findley LJ, Capildeo R, eds. Movement Disorders: Tremor. London: Macmillan Press, 1984:37–84.
10. Louis ED, Wendt KJ, Ford B. Senile tremor. What is the prevalence and severity of tremor in older adults? Gerontology 2000; 46:12–16.
11. Louis ED, Jurewicz EC, Applegate L et al. Association between essential tremor and blood lead concentration. Environ Health Perspect 2003; 111:1707–1711.
12. Louis ED, Marder K, Cote L et al. Prevalence of a history of shaking in persons 65 years of age and older: diagnostic and functional correlates. Mov Disord 1996; 11:63–69.
13. Tanner CM, Goldman SM, Lyons KE et al. Essential tremor in twins: an assessment of genetic vs environmental determinants of etiology. Neurology 2001; 57:1389–1391.
14. Lorenz D, Frederiksen H, Moises H, Kopper F, Deuschl G, Christensen K. High concordance for essential tremor in monozygotic twins of old age. Neurology 2004; 62:208–211.

15. Higgins JJ, Pho LT, Nee LE. A gene (ETM) for essential tremor maps to chromosome 2p22-p25. Mov Disord 1997; 12:859–864.
16. Higgins JJ, Lombardi RQ, Pucilowska J, Ruszczyk MU. Integrated physical map of the human essential tremor gene region (ETM2) on chromosome 2p24.3-p24.2. Am J Med Genet 2004; 127B:128–130.
17. Farrer M, Gwinn-Hardy K, Muenter M et al. A chromosome 4p haplotype segregating with Parkinson's disease and postural tremor. Hum Mol Genet 1999; 8:81–85.
18. Gulcher JR, Jonsson P, Kong A et al. Mapping of a familial essential tremor gene, FET1, to chromosome 3q13. Nat Genet 1997; 17:84–87.
19. Deuschl G, Krack P, Lauk M, Timmer J. Clinical neurophysiology of tremor. J Clin Neurophysiol 1996; 13:110–121.
20. Hallett M. Overview of human tremor physiology. Mov Disord 1998; 13(suppl 3):43–48.
21. Elble RJ. Characteristics of physiologic tremor in young and elderly adults. Clin Neurophysiol 2003; 114:624–635.
22. Raethjen J, Lauk M, Koster B et al. Tremor analysis in two normal cohorts. Clin Neurophysiol 2004; 115:2151–2156.
23. Halliday DM, Rosenberg JR, Amjad AM, Breeze P, Conway BA, Farmer SF. A framework for the analysis of mixed time series/point process data–theory and application to the study of physiological tremor, single motor unit discharges and electromyograms. Prog Biophys Mol Biol 1995; 64:237–278.
24. Timmer J, Lauk M, Deuschl G. Quantitative analysis of tremor time series. Electroencephalogr Clin Neurophysiol 1996; 101:461–468.
25. Timmer J, Lauk M, Pfleger W, Deuschl G. Cross-spectral analysis of physiological tremor and muscle activity. I. Theory and application to unsynchronized electromyogram. Biol Cybern 1998; 78:349–357.
26. Lakie M, Walsh EG, Wright GW. Passive mechanical properties of the wrist and physiological tremor. J Neurol Neurosurg Psychiatry 1986; 49:669–676.
27. Elble RJ, Randall JE. Mechanistic components of normal hand tremor. Electroencephalogr Clin Neurophysiol 1978; 44:72–82.
28. Raethjen J, Pawlas F, Lindemann M, Wenzelburger R, Deuschl G. Determinants of physiologic tremor in a large normal population. Clin Neurophysiol 2000; 111:1825–1837.
29. Elble RJ, Brilliant M, Leffler K, Higgins C. Quantification of essential tremor in writing and drawing. Mov Disord 1996; 11:70–78.
30. Deuschl G, Raethjen J, Lindemann M, Krack P. The pathophysiology of tremor. Muscle Nerve 2001; 24:716–735.
31. Homberg V, Hefter H, Reiners K, Freund HJ. Differential effects of changes in mechanical limb properties on physiological and pathological tremor. J Neurol Neurosurg Psychiatry 1987; 50:568–579.
32. Elble RJ. Physiologic and essential tremor. Neurology 1986; 36:225–231.
33. Findley LJ, Koller WC. Essential tremor: a review. Neurology 1987; 37:1194–1197.
34. Elble RJ, Higgins C, Leffler K, Hughes L. Factors influencing the amplitude and frequency of essential tremor. Mov Disord 1994; 9:589–596.
35. Stiles RN. Mechanical and neural feedback factors in postural hand tremor of normal subjects. J Neurophysiol 1980; 44:40–59.
36. Elble RJ, Schieber MH, Thach WT Jr. Activity of muscle spindles, motor cortex and cerebellar nuclei during action tremor. Brain Res 1984; 323:330–334.

37. Bock O, Wenderoth N. Dependence of peripheral tremor on mechanical perturbations: a modeling study. Biol Cybern 1999; 80:103–108.
38. Lauk M, Koster B, Timmer J, Guschlbauer B, Deuschl G, Lucking CH. Side-to-side correlation of muscle activity in physiological and pathological human tremors. Clin Neurophysiol 1999; 110:1774–1783.
39. Raethjen J, Lindemann M, Schmaljohann H, Wenzelburger R, Pfister G, Deuschl G. Multiple oscillators are causing parkinsonian and essential tremor. Mov Disord 2000; 15:84–94.
40. Elble RJ, Randall JE. Motor-unit activity responsible for 8- to 12-Hz component of human physiological finger tremor. J Neurophysiol 1976; 39:370–383.
41. Boose A, Spieker S, Jentgens C, Dichgans J. Wrist tremor: investigation of agonist-antagonist interaction by means of long-term EMG recording and cross-spectral analysis. Electroencephalogr Clin Neurophysiol 1996; 101:355–363.
42. Hunker CJ, Abbs JH. Uniform frequency of parkinsonian resting tremor in the lips, jaw, tongue, and index finger. Mov Disord 1990; 5:71–77.
43. Lee RG, Stein RB. Resetting of tremor by mechanical perturbations: a comparison of essential tremor and parkinsonian tremor. Ann Neurol 1981; 10:523–531.
44. Britton TC, Thompson PD, Day BL, Rothwell JC, Findley LJ, Marsden CD. "Resetting" of postural tremors at the wrist with mechanical stretches in Parkinson's disease, essential tremor, and normal subjects mimicking tremor. Ann Neurol 1992; 31:507–514.
45. Britton TC, Thompson PD, Day BL, Rothwell JC, Findley LJ, Marsden CD. Modulation of postural tremors at the wrist by supramaximal electrical median nerve shocks in essential tremor, Parkinson's disease and normal subjects mimicking tremor. J Neurol Neurosurg Psychiatry 1993; 56:1085–1089.
46. Elble RJ, Higgins C, Hughes L. Phase resetting and frequency entrainment of essential tremor. Exp Neurol 1992; 116:355–361.
47. O'Suilleabhain PE, Matsumoto JY. Time-frequency analysis of tremors. Brain 1998; 121(pt 11):2127–2134.
48. Sanes JN, Hallett M. Limb positioning and magnitude of essential tremor and other pathological tremors. Mov Disord 1990; 5:304–309.
49. Britton TC, Thompson PD, Day BL, Rothwell JC, Findley LJ, Marsden CD. Modulation of postural wrist tremors by magnetic stimulation of the motor cortex in patients with Parkinson's disease or essential tremor and in normal subjects mimicking tremor. Ann Neurol 1993; 33:473–479.
50. Pascual-Leone A, Valls-Sole J, Toro C, Wassermann EM, Hallett M. Resetting of essential tremor and postural tremor in Parkinson's disease with transcranial magnetic stimulation. Muscle Nerve 1994; 17:800–807.
51. Yu HY, Chen JT, Lee YC et al. Single-pulse transcranial magnetic stimulation reset the rhythm of essential tremor but not heart beat. Zhonghua Yi Xue Za Zhi (Taipei) 2001; 64:271–276.
52. Sabbahi M, Etnyre B, Al-Jawayed I, Jankovic J. H-reflex recovery curves differentiate essential tremor, Parkinson's disease, and the combination of essential tremor and Parkinson's disease. J Clin Neurophysiol 2002; 19:245–251.
53. Mercuri B, Berardelli A, Modugno N, Vacca L, Ruggieri S, Manfredi M. Reciprocal inhibition in forearm muscles in patients with essential tremor. Muscle Nerve 1998; 21:796–799.

54. Munchau A, Schrag A, Chuang C et al. Arm tremor in cervical dystonia differs from essential tremor and can be classified by onset age and spread of symptoms. Brain 2001; 124:1765–1776.
55. Modugno N, Priori A, Berardelli A, Vacca L. Mercuri B, Manfredi M. Botulinum toxin restores presynaptic inhibition of group Ia afferents in patients with essential tremor. Muscle Nerve 1998; 21:1701–1705.
56. Burne JA, Blanche T, Morris JG. Loss of reflex inhibition following muscle tendon stimulation in essential tremor. Muscle Nerve 2002; 25:58–64.
57. Deuschl G, Lucking CH. Physiology and clinical applications of hand muscle reflexes. Electroencephalogr Clin Neurophysiol Suppl 1990; 41:84–101.
58. Valls-Sole J, Tolosa ES, Nobbe F et al. Neurophysiological investigations in patients with head tremor. Mov Disord 1997; 12:576–584.
59. Romeo S, Berardelli A, Pedace F, Inghilleri M, Giovannelli M, Manfredi M. Cortical excitability in patients with essential tremor. Muscle Nerve 1998; 21:1304–1308.
60. Pinto AD, Lang AE, Chen R. The cerebellothalamocortical pathway in essential tremor. Neurology 2003; 60:1985–1987.
61. Gironell A, Kulisevsky J, Lorenzo J, Barbanoj M, Pascual-Sedano B, Otermin P. Transcranial magnetic stimulation of the cerebellum in essential tremor: a controlled study. Arch Neurol 2002; 59:413–417.
62. Restuccia D, Valeriani M, Barba C et al. Abnormal gating of somatosensory inputs in essential tremor. Clin Neurophysiol 2003; 114:120–129.
63. Antal A, Dibo G, Keri S et al. P300 component of visual event-related potentials distinguishes patients with idiopathic Parkinson's disease from patients with essential tremor. J Neural Transm 2000; 107:787–797.
64. Duncan R, Bone I, Melville ID. Essential tremor cured by infarction adjacent to the thalamus. J Neurol Neurosurg Psychiatry 1988; 51:591–592.
65. Dupuis MJ, Delwaide PJ, Boucquey D, Gonsette RE. Homolateral disappearance of essential tremor after cerebellar stroke. Mov Disord 1989; 4:183–187.
66. Nagaratnam N, Kalasabail G. Contralateral abolition of essential tremor following a pontine stroke. J Neurol Sci 1997; 149:195–196.
67. Llinas R, Volkind RA. The olivo-cerebellar system: functional properties as revealed by harmaline-induced tremor. Exp Brain Res 1973; 18:69–87.
68. Elble RJ. Animal models of action tremor. Mov Disord 1998; 13(suppl 3):35–39.
69. Elble RJ. Central mechanisms of tremor. J Clin Neurophysiol 1996; 13:133–144.
70. Elble RJ. Inhibition of forearm EMG by palatal myoclonus. Mov Disord 1991; 6:324–329.
71. Deuschl G, Toro C, Valls-Sole J, Zeffiro T, Zee DS, Hallett M. Symptomatic and essential palatal tremor. 1. Clinical, physiological and MRI analysis. Brain 1994; 117(pt 4):775–788.
72. Colebatch JG, Findley LJ, Frackowiak RS, Marsden CD, Brooks DJ. Preliminary report: activation of the cerebellum in essential tremor. Lancet 1990; 336:1028–1030.
73. Jenkins IH, Bain PG, Colebatch JG et al. A positron emission tomography study of essential tremor: evidence for overactivity of cerebellar connections. Ann Neurol 1993; 34:82–90.
74. Bucher SF, Seelos KC, Dodel RC, Reiser M, Oertel WH. Activation mapping in essential tremor with functional magnetic resonance imaging. Ann Neurol 1997; 41:32–40.

75. Hallett M, Shahani BT, Young RR. EMG analysis of patients with cerebellar deficits. J Neurol Neurosurg Psychiatry 1975; 38:1163–1169.
76. Rothwell JC, Traub MM, Day BL, Obeso JA, Thomas PK, Marsden CD. Manual motor performance in a deafferented man. Brain 1982; 105(pt 3):515–542.
77. Flament D, Hore J. Movement and electromyographic disorders associated with cerebellar dysmetria. J Neurophysiol 1986; 55:1221–1233.
78. Hore J, Wild B, Diener HC. Cerebellar dysmetria at the elbow, wrist, and fingers. J Neurophysiol 1991; 65:563–571.
79. Hallett M, Berardelli A, Matheson J, Rothwell J, Marsden CD. Physiological analysis of simple rapid movements in patients with cerebellar deficits. J Neurol Neurosurg Psychiatry 1991; 54:124–133.
80. Britton TC, Thompson PD, Day BL, Rothwell JC, Findley LJ, Marsden CD. Rapid wrist movements in patients with essential tremor. The critical role of the second agonist burst. Brain 1994; 117(pt 1):39–47.
81. Koster B, Deuschl G, Lauk M, Timmer J, Guschlbauer B, Lucking CH. Essential tremor and cerebellar dysfunction: abnormal ballistic movements. J Neurol Neurosurg Psychiatry 2002; 73:400–405.
82. Biary N, Koller W. Kinetic predominant essential tremor: successful treatment with clonazepam. Neurology 1987; 37:471–474.
83. Louis ED, Ford B, Wendt KJ, Cameron G. Clinical characteristics of essential tremor: data from a community-based study. Mov Disord 1998; 13:803–808.
84. Holmes G. The cerebellum of man. Brain 1939; 62:1–30.
85. Deuschl G, Wenzelburger R, Loffler K, Raethjen J, Stolze H. Essential tremor and cerebellar dysfunction clinical and kinematic analysis of intention tremor. Brain 2000; 123(pt 8):1568–1580.
86. Critchley E. Clinical manifestations of essential tremor. J Neurol Neurosurg Psychiatry 1972; 35:365–372.
87. Singer C, Sanchez-Ramos J, Weiner WJ. Gait abnormality in essential tremor. Mov Disord 1994; 9:193–196.
88. Hubble JP, Busenbark KL, Pahwa R, Lyons K, Koller WC. Clinical expression of essential tremor: effects of gender and age. Mov Disord 1997; 12:969–972.
89. Stolze H, Petersen G, Raethjen J, Wenzelburger R, Deuschl G. The gait disorder of advanced essential tremor. Brain 2001; 124:2278–2286.
90. Helmchen C, Hagenow A, Miesner J et al. Eye movement abnormalities in essential tremor may indicate cerebellar dysfunction. Brain 2003; 126:1319–1332.
91. Pagan FL, Butman JA, Dambrosia JM, Hallett M. Evaluation of essential tremor with multi-voxel magnetic resonance spectroscopy. Neurology 2003; 60:1344–1347.
92. Louis ED, Shungu DC, Mao X, Chan S, Jurewicz EC. Cerebellar metabolic symmetry in essential tremor studied with 1H magnetic resonance spectroscopic imaging: implications for disease pathology. Mov Disord 2004; 19:672–677.
93. Hassler R, Reichert T. Indikation und Lokalisationsmethode der gezielten Hirnoperationen. Nervenarzt 1954; 25:441–447.
94. Benabid AL, Pollak P, Seigneuret E, Hoffmann D, Gay E, Perret J. Chronic VIM thalamic stimulation in Parkinson's disease, essential tremor and extra-pyramidal dyskinesias. Acta Neurochir Suppl (Wien) 1993; 58:39–44.
95. Schuurman PR, Bosch DA, Bossuyt PM et al. A comparison of continuous thalamic stimulation and thalamotomy for suppression of severe tremor. N Engl J Med 2000; 342:461–468.

96. Ohye C, Shibazaki T, Hirai T, Wada H, Hirato M, Kawashima Y. Further physiological observations on the ventralis intermedius neurons in the human thalamus. J Neurophysiol 1989; 61:488–500.
97. Hua SE, Lenz FA, Zirh TA, Reich SG, Dougherty PM. Thalamic neuronal activity correlated with essential tremor. J Neurol Neurosurg Psychiatry 1998; 64:273–276.
98. Nandi D, Chir M, Liu X et al. Electrophysiological confirmation of the zona incerta as a target for surgical treatment of disabling involuntary arm movements in multiple sclerosis: use of local field potentials. J Clin Neurosci 2002; 9:64–68.
99. Lee BH, Lee KH, Chung SS, Chang JW. Neurophysiological identification and characterization of thalamic neurons with single unit recording in essential tremor patients. Acta Neurochir Suppl 2003; 87:133–136.
100. Brodkey JA, Tasker RR, Hamani C, McAndrews MP, Dostrovsky JO, Lozano AM. Tremor cells in the human thalamus: differences among neurological disorders. J Neurosurg 2004; 101:43–47.
101. Lindemann M, Raethjen J, Timmer J, Deuschl G, Pfister G. Delay estimation for cortico-peripheral relations. J Neurosci Methods 2001; 111:127–139.
102. Muller T, Lauk M, Reinhard M, Hetzel A, Lucking CH, Timmer J. Estimation of delay times in biological systems. Ann Biomed Eng 2003; 31:1423–1439.
103. Halliday DM, Conway BA, Farmer SF, Shahani U, Russell AJ, Rosenberg JR. Coherence between low-frequency activation of the motor cortex and tremor in patients with essential tremor. Lancet 2000; 355:1149–1153.
104. Conway BA, Halliday DM, Farmer SF et al. Synchronization between motor cortex and spinal motoneuronal pool during the performance of a maintained motor task in man. J Physiol 1995; 489(pt 3):917–924.
105. Salenius S, Portin K, Kajola M, Salmelin R, Hari R. Cortical control of human motoneuron firing during isometric contraction. J Neurophysiol 1997; 77:3401–3405.
106. Brown P, Salenius S, Rothwell JC, Hari R. Cortical correlate of the Piper rhythm in humans. J Neurophysiol 1998; 80:2911–2917.
107. Hellwig B, Haussler S, Schelter B et al. Tremor-correlated cortical activity in essential tremor. Lancet 2001; 357:519–523.
108. Raethjen J, Kopper F, Govindan RB, Deushl G. Motor cortex involvement in the generation of essential tremor. Mov Disord 2004; 19(suppl 9):S455, 1335.
109. Volkmann J, Joliot M, Mogilner A et al. Central motor loop oscillations in parkinsonian resting tremor revealed by magnetoencephalography. Neurology 1996; 46:1359–1370.
110. Hellwig B, Haussler S, Lauk M et al. Tremor-correlated cortical activity detected by electroencephalography. Clin Neurophysiol 2000; 111:806–809.
111. Timmermann L, Gross J, Dirks M, Volkmann J, Freund HJ, Schnitzler A. The cerebral oscillatory network of parkinsonian resting tremor. Brain 2003; 126:199–212.
112. Marsden JF, Ashby P, Limousin-Dowsey P, Rothwell JC, Brown P. Coherence between cerebellar thalamus, cortex and muscle in man: cerebellar thalamus interactions. Brain 2000; 123(pt 7):1459–1470.

4

Animal Models of Essential Tremor

Jayaraman Rao

Louisiana State University Health Sciences Center,
New Orleans, Louisiana, USA

I. INTRODUCTION

Essential tremor is one of the most common movement disorders. The major manifestation of essential tremor is a postural or kinetic tremor affecting predominantly the hands, head, and the voice at a frequency of 4–12 Hz. A significant number of patients report a positive family history of essential tremor, but many sporadic cases are also seen (1). Despite the use of a wide variety of drugs to control these tremors, medical treatment has been far less satisfactory (1,2) than deep brain stimulation (DBS) of the nucleus ventralis intermedialis (VIM) of the thalamus which provides remarkable improvement in tremor and the disabilities associated with essential tremor in almost all patients (3).

II. ANIMAL MODELS AND HUMAN NEUROLOGICAL DISORDERS

The etiology and the pathogenesis of essential tremor are not known. Efforts to create animal models of parkinsonian and other types of tremors by making lesions in the ventromedial tegmentum and other areas were unsuccessful in creating a model that exhibited features of essential tremor (4). Among the numerous drugs that can induce tremor (5), harmaline-induced tremor appears to exhibit several features that are similar to that of essential tremor. In different species of animals, harmaline induces a tremor of 8–12 Hz within 2–4 min after acute injections, and the tremors are prominent in the head, proximal muscles of the extremities and trunk and are exacerbated with movements (5,6). In rare cases of harmine and harmaline poisoning, animals and humans exhibit significant tremor, autonomic dysfunction and many other features similar to that of serotonin syndrome (5,7,8). It is important to point out that harmaline tremors are induced in animals after acute injections, which is in contrast to the signs and symptoms of essential tremor which develop over many years. This chapter will discuss the neuroanatomical substrate and mechanisms of harmaline-induced tremor in cats and rats and will speculate on its implications to essential tremor.

III. ANATOMICAL ORGANIZATION OF THE OLIVO-CEREBELLAR SYSTEM

The inferior olivary nuclear complex (ION) is the main site of genesis of harmaline-induced tremor. The details of the connectivity of the ION with the cerebellar cortex and the cerebellar nuclei have been defined mostly in cats and rats. The connectivity pattern in primates has not been established in great detail, and positron emission tomography (PET) scans and functional magnetic resonance imaging (fMRI) are facilitating the understanding of the functional organization of the human cerebellum. The following discussion will focus mostly on the organization of the olivocerebellar system in cats and rats, and refer to findings in primate and humans when pertinent.

A. Cerebellar Cortical Output is Organized into Specific "Modules" or "Zones"

The seminal concept in the understanding of the anatomical, physiological and functional organization of the cerebellum, is that the cerebellar cortical output system, on the basis of the arrangement of Purkinje cells and their afferent and efferent systems, is organized into longitudinal and parallel "modules" or "zones" (9–11). Each longitudinal module is a basic unit of function of the cerebellar output system and appears to be so important that this pattern is established even during very early stages of embryogenesis (12). The genesis of these bands is initiated by the migration of chemically specific Purkinje cells from the midline which are then connected with specific afferents and efferents (13–15). Most of the understanding of the anatomical organization of these cerebellar cortical zones is derived from studies in cats; however, the same general principles of organization may be present in rats and other animals. The presence of such a modular organization has not been established in human cerebellum.

B. Cerebellar Cortical Modules Project to Specific Regions of the Cerebellar and Thalamic Nuclei and Cerebral Cortical Areas

There are 13 "Voogd" zones and of these, eight zones have been studied extensively. In fact, each one of these zones may contain several "microzones" (9,16). Among the eight different well recognized modules, modules A, X, and B are in the vermal regions of the cerebellum and have intricate connectivity with the medial cerebellar (fastigial) nucleus. Modules C1, C3, and C2 are in the paramedian regions of the cerebellum and are predominantly connected with the anterior and posterior divisions of the nucleus interpositus, and the D1 and D2 bands in the lateral regions of the cerebellar hemispheres are connected with the lateral cerebellar (dentate) nucleus [Fig. 4.1(a) and (b)].

On the basis of currently available data of cerebello-thalamo-cortical studies in primates, Voogd (10) has proposed that the information from the vermal A module ultimately reaches the medial regions of the VIM nucleus and prefrontal cortex, frontal eye field, premotor and motor cortex, supplementary motor cortex, and area 7b of the parietal lobe. The paravermal modules C1, C3, and C2 project to the anterior and posterior divisions of the nucleus interpositus. These cerebellar nuclei send their efferents to the lateral VIM, the thalamic target for DBS procedures, and the lateral VIM projects to the motor and supplementary motor cortical regions. The output of the lateral "cognitive regions" of the cerebellar hemispheres is mediated by the D1 and D2 zones and the lateral cerebellar nucleus. The lateral cerebellar nucleus projects to the lateral subdivision of the VIM, the motor cortex, and the supplementary motor area.

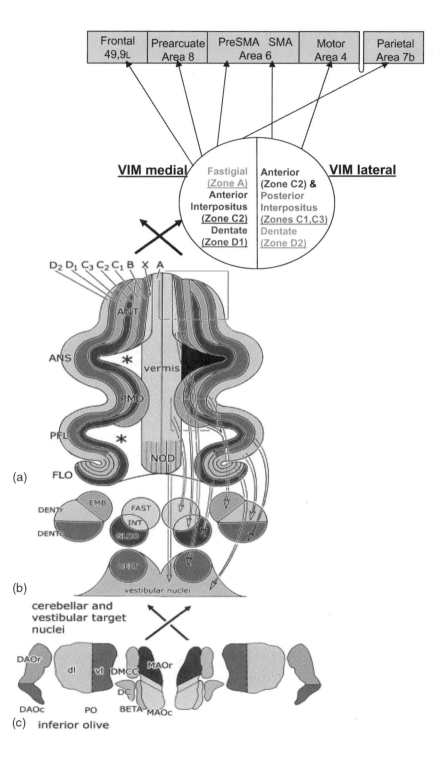

C. Somatotopy in the Cerebellum

Another important concept for understanding of cerebellar functions is that the homunculi of the motor and sensory systems are organized in a somatotopic fashion (animalculi) in the cerebellar cortex of rats, cats, primates, and humans. Early studies to define the functions of the cerebellum and the existence of a somatotopic organization within the cerebellar cortex have generated significant discussion over the last 200 years (17). Studies in primates and cats in the late 1930s and early 1940s showed that the exteroceptive and interoceptive inputs from the spinal cord as well as projections from the cerebral motor cortex converge somatotopically in three different areas of the cerebellum. [Fig. 4.2(a)]. In monkeys, in the anterior lobe of the cerebellum, the face region is represented in the vermal and paravermal regions in the lobulus simplex, the arm in lateral regions of the culmen, the leg in the lobulus centralis, and the trunk in the pyramis. Since voice tremor is very common in essential tremor, the area of localization of vocal cords is of interest. By stimulating the superior laryngeal nerve, the major sensory nerve supply to the larynx, evoked potentials have been localized to the medial third of the adjacent lips of folia 3 and 4 of the paramedian lobule bilaterally. Laryngeal response was also recorded anteriorly in Crus I of the ansiform lobes adjacent to the vermis in cats (18). In primates, laryngeal response was evoked in the lobulus simplex, but not in the paramedian lobules (19). In all of these sites, the laryngeal response appears to be localized in a small region of 0.5–1.5 mm between the areas representing the face and upper extremities. Auditory and visual information are represented in an overlapping fashion in the vermis regions of folium, tuber, and the lobulus simplex. The two other areas of

---

Figure 4.1 The diagram [adapted from Ref. (9; Fig. 4) and Ref. (10; Fig. 11.22)] shows that the different subnuclei of the inferior olivary complex (c) project to specific regions of longitudinally organized cerebellar cortical modules (zones) (a). The projections from these cerebellar modules terminate in specific areas of the cerebellar nuclei (b). This composite drawing is derived mostly from studies in cats. The efferent projections from these cerebellar nuclei terminate in the medial and lateral divisions of VIM, which in turn terminate in the frontal, premotor, motor, and parietal cortex. The segment of the diagram that depicts the cerebello-rubro-thalamo-cortical projection pattern is based on studies in primates and humans. Abbreviations: PreSMA: Presupplementary motor area; SMA: Supplementary motor area; VIM: Nucleus ventral intermedialis; A, X, B, C1, C2, C3, D1, D2: Longitudinal modules of cerebellar cortex; ANT: Anterior lobule; ANS: Ansiform lobule; PMD: Paramedian lobule; PFL: Paraflocculus lobule; FLO: Flocculus; NOD: Nodulus; Fast: Fastigial nucleus; INT and EMB: Nucleus interpositus anterior (Emboliform nucleus); GLOB: Nucleus interpositus posterior; DENTr and c: Rostral and caudal divisions of the dentate nucleus; DEIT: Deiter's (lateral vestibular) nucleus; DAOr and DAOc: Rostral and caudal divisions of dorsal accessory olivary nucleus; dl and vl of PO: Dorsal and ventral lamellae of principal olivary nucleus; DMCC: Dorsomedial cell column; DC: Dorsal cap of Kooy; Beta: Group beta of medial accessory nucleus; MAOr and MAOc: Rostral and caudal divisions of medial accessory olivary nucleus.

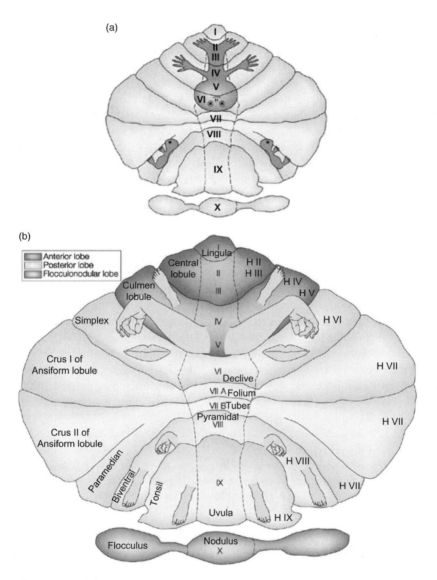

Figure 4.2 This diagram [adapted from Ref. (17; Figs. 2 and 5)] shows the significant similarities between the somatotopic organization of the cerebellar cortex in monkeys (a) and humans (b). Compare the anatomical connectivity pattern in Fig. 4.1 with that of the somatotopic organization of the monkey and human cerebellar cortex shown in this figure.

somatotopic organization in the paramedian lobule of the posterior cerebellum have not been explored in detail. Neuroimaging techniques of fMRI and PET (20) appear to confirm that in the anterior lobe, the face, limb, and trunk areas are represented somatotopically in the vermis and the intermediolateral parts of the cerebellar cortex in a fashion that is significantly similar to the pattern described in primates and cats [Fig. 4.2(b)]. Movements of the arm and elbow have a representation in the medial regions of vermis of lobule V, the wrist and the fingers are represented in the intermediolateral zones of HV and HVI regions. The foot is represented in HIV and HIII. PET and fMRI studies have identified a second somatotopically organized area in the posterior cerebellum in HVIII and HIX (20). The details of organization within these regions remain to be explored further.

D. Different Subdivisions of the ION Project to Specific Areas of Somatotopically Defined Areas of Cerebellar Cortical Modules

The inferior olive provides a major source of afferent information from the spinal cord and brainstem to the cerebellum by sending climbing fibers to Purkinje cells and the cerebellar nuclei. Even though the ION contains cell types that are similar throughout the entire ION complex, they are divided, on the basis of their cerebellar, brainstem, vestibular and spinal cord connections into the medial accessory olivary nucleus (MAO), the dorsal accessory olivary nucleus (DAO) and the principal olivary nucleus (PO). The MAO has been further divided into a caudal MAO with a, b, c, and β subdivisions, a dorsomedial cell complex and a rostral complex. Of these, the caudal MAO projects to the cerebellar cortical module A and the medial cerebellar (fastigial) nucleus. The rostral MAO projects to the C2 module and the posterior division of the nucleus interpositus. The dorsal cap of Kooy and the ventrolateral outgrowth of the principal PO project to the vestibulocerebellum and the lateral vestibular nucleus. The ventral and dorsal lamellae of PO send their efferents to the D1 and D2 column and the caudal and rostral lateral cerebellar nuclei (dentate in primates and humans). The caudally located dorsal fold of DAO projects to the lateral vestibular nucleus. The ventral fold sends its efferents to C1 and C3 modules of the cerebellar cortex and the anterior division of the nucleus interpositus (9,10,21,22). To summarize, the fastigial nucleus receives projections from somatotopically organized cerebellar cortical regions in which the trunk and head are represented, the interpositus receives projections from areas in which the feet and the hands are represented and the dentate nucleus receives projections from the lateral regions of the cerebellar hemispheres.

IV. HARMALINE-INDUCED TREMOR MAY BE MEDIATED BY THE VENTRAL FOLD OF DAO AND CAUDAL MAO OF THE ION AND THEIR CEREBELLAR CORTICAL MODULES

A. Anatomical and Neuroimaging Evidence for Olivary Involvement in Harmaline-Induced Tremor

Harmaline is a beta carboline and has been used by Native Americans for medicinal and religious purposes. It inhibits monoamino oxidase A $10,000\times$ more than monoamino oxidase B and also has significant binding affinity to 5HT2A and 5HT2C receptors, sharing several serotonergic actions of other hallucinogens (23–25).

Despite an earlier opinion that harmaline-induced tremors originate in the basal ganglia (26), current evidence strongly supports the concept that harmaline-induced tremors originate in the inferior olivary nucleus (26–31). Harmaline results in an increased, sustained, synchronized rhythmic activity of the olivary neurons. Local microinjections of harmaline in the caudal aspects of the dorsal and medial accessory olivary neurons provide the best response (28). Destruction of the olivary neurons and their climbing fibers with 3-acetylpyridine completely resolves harmaline-induced tremor (32,33).

Experimental manipulation of the expression of the immediate early gene c-fos has been used to identify the individual areas of the brain as well as the circuitry that respond to many physiological, pharmacological, and neurochemical stimuli (34). Acute injections of harmaline induce c-fos diffusely in the entire olivary complex, but more prominently in the dorsal and medial accessory olivary nuclei than the principal olivary nucleus (35,36). The areas of MAO and DAO which get intensely labeled with Fos are identical to the areas of MAO and DAO wherein Fos gets activated after rats have been walking on a rotating drum for 75 minutes, thereby suggesting that active ongoing movements influence the same regions of ION as harmaline (37). Within 15 minutes after harmaline injections, Fos immunoreactivity is noted in the olivary nucleus, in 30 minutes in the cerebellar nuclei, 1 hour in the Purkinje cells and in 2–6 hours in the vermal and paravermal regions of the cerebellar cortex in a longitudinal modular fashion (38), but the lateral regions of the cerebellar hemispheres were relatively unlabeled. This pattern of labeling of cerebellar cortex by Fos is quite consistent with the established pattern of projections of ION to the cerebellar nuclei and cerebellar cortex in cats and rats. The areas of Fos expression also correspond well with the somatotopically organized areas in the vermis and the intermediolateral regions of the cerebellar cortex. Unlike another tremorogenic agent, oxotremorine, which induces c-fos in the basal ganglia and related regions by interacting with muscarinic cholinergic receptors, the induction of c-fos in the olivary nucleus and related regions in the cerebellum, is specific to harmaline (36). The pattern of expression of Fos is also consistent with the areas of intense labeling of ION by 2-deoxyglucose (DG) and PET. The ION is labeled intensely with 2-[14C] deoxyglucose especially in the caudal two thirds of MAO and the caudolateral half of DAO corresponding to an area of increased synchronous discharges of ION neurons in cats (39,40) and rats (41). These anatomical and neuroimaging studies suggest that harmaline induces its neurobiological effects through activating the olivocerebellar and olivonuclear pathways.

B.   Electrophysiological Evidence for Olivary Involvement in Tremor

Electrophysiological mapping of harmaline-responsive areas of ION in rats and cats clearly point to MAO and DAO as the only regions involved in the genesis of the rhythmic bursts [Fig. 4.2(c)]. The continuous, synchronous, and rhythmic activity of ION were not abolished by transection of the midbrain, caudal to red nucleus, or by the removal of superior, middle, and inferior cerebellar peduncles thereby deafferenting the cerebellum completely from all of its proprioceptive and other afferent inputs or by total cerebellectomy suggesting that the tremorogenic actions originate within the brain stem and possibly in the ION (31,41). In rats paralyzed with flexedil, a drug that causes paralysis and thereby reduces all proprioceptive inputs to the cerebellum and brainstem, the rhythmic discharges could still be recorded in the ION, but not in the adjacent neurons of the lateral reticular nucleus or the medullary subdivisions of the raphe nucleus (41).

Harmaline-induced rhythmic activity could also be recorded in wide areas of the cerebellar cortex. Electrophysiological recording of a single Purkinje cell elicits two types of spikes, viz., simple spikes and complex spikes. The simple spikes are generated by the parallel fibers and the complex spikes by the climbing fibers from the inferior olivary neurons. The excitatory amino acids, glutamate and aspartate, are the neurotransmitters released by the climbing fibers (38). After harmaline, spikes can be recorded at a rate of 5–10 Hz predominantly in the vermal zones of lobule I–VIII of rat cerebellar cortex, and the intermediate zones of paravermis, but not in the lateral regions of the cerebellar hemispheres [Fig. 4.3(b)]. Regions corresponding to the vestibulocerebellum were not affected by harmaline (41). Horseradish peroxidase, a neuronal tracer, injected in complex spike responsive areas of the cerebellar cortex clearly identified neurons in specific areas of MAO and DAO as the source of afferent projections to these somatotopically organized areas of the cerebellar cortex (41).

In addition to the ION and the cerebellar cortex, rhythmic synchronous activity was also noted in the cerebellar output nuclei (42). The most prominent recording was in the posterior and anterior subdivisions of the nucleus interpositus and in significant regions of the fastigial nucleus, but not in the dentate nucleus. These anatomical, electrophysiological, and neuroimaging studies indicate that harmaline induces a synchronous rhythmic discharge and an 8–12 Hz tremor generated by specific regions of MAO and DAO.

V. HARMALINE-INDUCED TREMOR AND SEROTONIN

In cats, injections of harmaline induce a strong, synchronous, and rhythmic activity of the climbing fibers originating in caudal MAO and caudolateral DAO as well as the Purkinje cells (43). The unique aspect of the neurochemical organization of these two subnuclei of the ION is that MAO and DAO are more densely innervated with serotonergic terminals than the PO and the rest of the ION (43,44) suggesting a role for serotonin in harmaline-induced tremor. The raphe pallidus and the raphe obscurus divisions of the serotonergic system, which are highly responsive to specific motor tasks in freely moving cats (45,46), are the principal source of serotonergic innervation to the ION (44,47). Microinjections of 5HT into the ION increased the firing rate of the ION neurons and the degree of synchrony of the complex spikes of the Purkinje

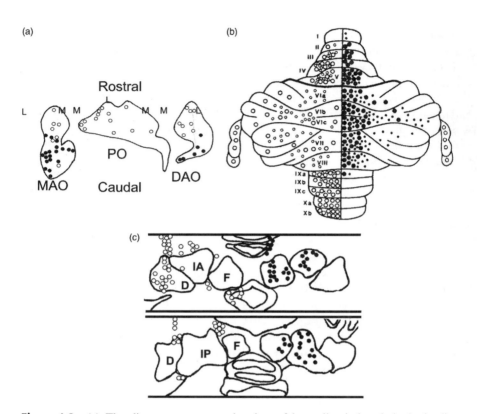

Figure 4.3 (a) The diagram represents the sites of harmaline-induced rhythmic discharges in the MAO and DAO, but not in the principal olivary nucleus (PO) in cats. [Adapted from Ref. (28; Fig. 3).] Abbreviations: L: Lateral; M: medial. (b) The diagram shows the site of recording of harmaline-induced complex spikes from Purkinje cells in the entire cerebellar cortex of rats. Note that the cells with complex spikes were located in the vermis and the intermediolateral zones, but not the lateral zone. [Adapted from Ref. (42; Fig. 1E).] (c) This diagram shows that the harmaline-induced rhythmic activity was recorded in the anterior, posterior interpositus and the fastigial nuclei, but not in the lateral cerebellar nucleus in cats. [Adapted from Ref. (41; Fig. 5A).] Abbreviations: F: Fastigial nucleus; IA and IP: Anterior and posterior divisions of nucleus interpositus; D: Dentate nucleus. In all of these figures closed circles denote cells that demonstrated harmaline-induced synchronous discharges and the open circles denote harmaline unresponsive neurons.

cells in the cerebellar cortex in rats (48). In mice, intraperitoneal injections of 20 mg/kg of harmaline initiated a tremor within 3–4 minutes and the intensity of the tremor peaked at 25 minutes. The drug effect and the tremor lasted for 4 hours. The highest intensity of tremors coincided with the highest levels (2.5 fold compared with control) of serotonin in the olivary nucleus and the cerebellum, a decreased level of dopamine and no alteration in levels of norepinephrine (49). Increased levels of serotonin induced by the antidepressant citalopram, a selective serotonin reuptake inhibitor (50), 5HT receptor agonist 5-methoxy-*N,N*-dimethyltryptamine, and MAO A inhibition (51) increased harmaline tremors.

Lesioning of the dorsal and medial raphe (52) and reserpine, a compound that decreases presynaptic and synaptic levels of monoamines, decreased harmaline-induced tremors (53). Parachlorophenylalanine (PCPA), a tryptophan hydroxylase inhibitor that decreases 5HT levels, reduced the intensity of the tremor (43,49). 5,6-Dihydroxytryptamine and 5,7-dihydroxytryptamine, drugs that destroy the 5HT terminals, and not 6-hydroxydopamine, which reduces levels of dopamine, decreased harmaline-induced tremors (43,51). These results indicate that factors that increase serotonin levels in the ION result in an increased rhythmic synchronous activity of the ION complex and tremor, and factors that decrease serotonin may attenuate harmaline-induced tremor. However, serotonin, mediating its actions by stimulating the 5HT2 receptors in the ION, may actually improve harmaline-induced tremor as well as tremors (and myoclonus) in other conditions of serotonin deficiency (54,55). Microinjections of harmaline in the ION resulted in an increased synchronous rhythmic activity and only 5HT reversed the increased activity but not acetylcholine, GABA, norepinephrine, dopamine, or even some of the 5HT receptor antagonists (54). Serotonin may play the important role of maintaining the membrane conductance and functions of calcium and potassium channels of the neurons of the ION, especially that of low threshold calcium channels (56,57).

VI. HARMALINE-INDUCED TREMOR IN ANIMALS AND ESSENTIAL TREMOR

The harmaline animal model of tremor suggests that the circuit that is involved predominantly, if not exclusively, is the ventral lamella of the DAO that receives cuneo-cerebellar projections from the upper limb and neck regions. The ventral fold of DAO projects to the Purkinje cells in the foot and arm areas of the C1 and C3 modules of the cerebellar cortex and the anterior division of the nucleus interpositus, which in turn projects to the lateral regions of the VIM of the thalamus and motor and premotor cortex ultimately. The animal model also suggests that the dysfunctions of the DAO and MAO neurons might be triggered by an altered serotonergic transmission of these olivary neurons.

In patients with essential tremor, the tremors are most prominent in the hands, followed by the head, voice, and legs. In rare cases the tremors may also be observed in the trunk, chin, and tongue. Oculomotor abnormalities have been reported in monkeys (59) and in essential tremor (60), but not in harmaline models of rats (61) and cats (42). Gait dysfunctions are also rare in essential tremor (62,63). These observations suggest that the vestibulocerebellum may be involved only rarely in essential tremor. The clinical features of essential tremor suggest that the areas of the cerebellar cortex in which the hand, elbow, arm, and vocal cords are represented are the primary areas affected. These different body regions are represented in the longitudinal C1 and C3 modules of the intermediate and lateral regions of lobule V, HV, IV, and HIV regions of the cerebellum.

Neuroimaging studies in humans support the involvement of the olivo-cerebello-rubro-thalamo-cortical pathway in essential tremor. One of the earliest PET studies using 18F fluoro-2-deoxyglucose in essential tremor patients showed glucose hypermetabolism of the medulla and thalami, but not the cerebellar cortex, leading the authors to conclude that brain circuits of the inferior olivary nuclei in the medulla and thalami may be involved in the genesis of essential tremor (64). A study using H_2 ^{15}O concluded that an overactivity of the cerebello-rubral pathway, but not the olivary nuclei, may be involved in the generation of essential tremor (65). In a follow-up study, using H_2 ^{15}O as a marker, it was concluded that essential tremor involves bilateral cerebellar cortex including the vermis, and suppression of essential tremor by alcohol was mediated by the olivo-cerebellar-olivary projections (66).

VII. CONCLUSIONS

On the basis of information from harmaline animal models of tremor and the somatotopic organization of the cerebellar cortex in animals, it can be hypothesized that serotonin-mediated, low threshold calcium channel activity of neurons of the ventral fold of DAO and caudal MAO may be responsible for harmaline-induced tremor. Neuroimaging techniques suggest that the olivocerebellar pathway may be the principal region involved in essential tremor. The dramatic and almost complete and sustained disappearance of essential tremor after the control of VIM output to the cerebral cortex with DBS procedures suggest that the thalamic, motor, and prefrontal cortex play an important role, probably in the expression of the tremor if not the primary site of genesis of the tremor.

Existing evidence suggests a major role for serotonin and its receptors, but not dopamine, in the genesis or improvement of harmaline-induced tremors in rats and cats. The role played by GABA, glutamate, and acetylcholine, traditional neurotransmitters that might regulate neurons of the ION, remains to be explored. Drugs that act on the different serotonergic receptors in the olivary nucleus as well as different calcium channels should be carefully examined in essential tremor. In this context, isomers of octanol, especially 1-octanol, an alcohol that blocks the low threshold calcium channels very effectively, inhibits harmaline-induced tremors (67). Early open-label clinical trials of 1-octanol have been shown to be effective in the treatment of essential tremor (68,69). The beneficial response to 1-octanol may actually be a pharmacological confirmation of the hypothesis that dysfunction of the calcium channel in the olivary neurons may be involved in essential tremor. The ventral fold of DAO as the principal site of pathology in essential tremor may be further explored with improved resolution of fMRI.

ACKNOWLEDGMENT

Supported by Grace Benson Memorial Fund for Parkinson's disease.

REFERENCES

1. Chen JJ, Swope DM. Essential tremor: diagnosis and treatment. Pharmacotherapy 2003; 23(9):1105–1122.
2. Lyons KE, Pahwa R, Comella CL et al. Benefits and risks of pharmacological treatments for essential tremor. Drug Saf 2003; 26(7):461–481.
3. Lyons KE, Pahwa R. Deep brain stimulation and essential tremor. J Clin Neurophysiol 2004; 21(1):2–5.
4. Elble RJ. Animal models of action tremor. Mov Disord 1998; 13(suppl 3):35–39.
5. Wilms H, Sievers J, Deuschl G. Animal models of tremor. Mov Disord 1999; 14(4):557–571.
6. Deuschl G, Elble RJ. The pathophysiology of essential tremor. Neurology 2000; 54(11 suppl 4):S14–S20.
7. Pennes HH, Hoch PH. Psychomimetics, clinical and theoretical considerations: harmine, Win-2299 and Nalline. Am J Psychiat 1957; 113:885–892.
8. Mahmoudian M, Jalilpour H, Salehian P. Toxicity of Peganum harmala: review and a case report. Iranian J Pharmacol Ther 2002; 1(1):1–4.
9. Voogd J. The Human cerebellum. J Chem Neuroanat 2003; 26:243–252.
10. Voogd J. Cerebellum and precerebellar nuclei. In: Paxinos G, Mai JK, eds. The Human Nervous System. San Diego: Elsevier Academic Press, 2004:321–392.
11. Voogd J, Ruigrok TJ. Transverse and longitudinal patterns in the mammalian cerebellum. Prog Brain Res 1997; 114:21–37.
12. Hawkes R. An anatomical model of cerebellar modules. Prog Brain Res 1997; 114:39–52.
13. Ozol K, Hayden JM, Oberdick J, Hawkes R. Transverse zones in the vermis of the mouse cerebellum. J Comp Neurol 1999; 412(1):95–111.
14. Sanlioglu-Crisman S, Oberdick J. Functional cloning of candidate genes that regulate Purkinje cell-specific gene expression. Prog Brain Res 1997; 114:3–19.
15. Goldowitz D, Hamre K. The cells and molecules that make a cerebellum. Trends Neurosci 1998; 21(9):375–382.
16. Garwicz M. Micro-organisation of cerebellar modules controlling forelimb movements. Prog Brain Res 2000; 124:187–199.
17. Manni E, Petrosini L. A century of cerebellar somatotopy: a debated representation. Nat Rev Neurosci 2004; 5(3):241–249.
18. Lam RL, Ogura JH. An afferent representation of the larynx in the cerebellum. Laryngoscope 1952; 62:486–495.
19. Larson CR, Sutton D, Lindeman RC. Cerebellar regulation of phonation in rhesus monkey (Macaca mulatta). Exp Brain Res 1978; 33(1):1–18.
20. Grodd W, Hulsmann E, Lotze M, Wildgruber D, Erb M. Sensorimotor mapping of the human cerebellum: fMRI evidence of somatotopic organization. Hum Brain Mapp 2001; 13(2):55–73.
21. Ruigrok TJ, Voogd J. Organization of projections from the inferior olive to the cerebellar nuclei in the rat. J Comp Neurol 2000; 426(2):209–228.

22. Ruigrok TJ. Cerebellar nuclei: the olivary connection. Prog Brain Res 1997; 114:167–192.
23. McKenna DJ, Towers GH, Abbott F. Monoamine oxidase inhibitors in South American hallucinogenic plants: tryptamine and beta-carboline constituents of ayahuasca. J Ethnopharmacol 1984; 10(2):195–223.
24. Grella B, Dukat M, Young R et al. Investigation of hallucinogenic and related beta-carbolines. Drug Alcohol Depend 1998; 50(2):99–107.
25. Riba J, Valle M, Urbano G, Yritia M, Morte A, Barbanoj MJ. Human pharmacology of ayahuasca: subjective and cardiovascular effects, monoamine metabolite excretion and pharmacokinetics. J Pharmacol Exp Ther 2003; 306(1):73–83.
26. Lamarre Y, Mercier LA. Neurophysiological studies of harmaline-induced tremor in the cat. Can J Physiol Pharmacol 1971; 49(12):1049–1058.
27. Lamarre Y, de Montigny C, Dumont M, Weiss M. Harmaline-induced rhythmic activity of cerebellar and lower brain stem neurons. Brain Res 1971; 32(1):246–250.
28. De Montigny C, Lamarre Y. Rhythmic activity induced by harmaline in the olivo-cerebello-bulbar system of the cat. Brain Res 1973; 53(1):81–95.
29. Lamarre Y, Joffroy AJ, Dumont M, De Montigny C, Grou F, Lund JP. Central mechanisms of tremor in some feline and primate models. Can J Neurol Sci 1975; 2(3):227–233.
30. Lamarre Y, Puil E. Induction of rhythmic activity by harmaline. Can J Physiol Pharmacol 1974; 52(4):905–908.
31. De Montigny C, Lamarre Y. Effects produced by local applications of harmaline in the inferior olive. Can J Physiol Pharmacol 1975; 53(5):845–849.
32. Guidotti A, Biggio G, Costa E. 3-Acetylpyridine: a tool to inhibit the tremor and the increase of cGMP content in cerebellar cortex elicited by harmaline. Brain Res 1975; 96(1):201–205.
33. Simantov R, Snyder SH, Oster-Granite ML. Harmaline-induced tremor in the rat: abolition by 3-acetylpyridine destruction of cerebellar climbing fibers. Brain Res 1976; 114(1):144–151.
34. Kiba H, Jayaraman A. Nicotine induced c-fos expression in the striatum is mediated mostly by dopamine D1 receptor and is dependent on NMDA stimulation. Brain Res Mol Brain Res 1994; 23(1–2):1–13.
35. Oldenbeuving AW, Eisenman LM, De Zeeuw CI, Ruigrok TJ. Inferior olivary-induced expression of Fos-like immunoreactivity in the cerebellar nuclei of wild-type and Lurcher mice. Eur J Neurosci 1999; 11(11):3809–3822.
36. Miwa H, Nishi K, Fuwa T, Mizuno Y. Differential expression of c-fos following administration of two tremorgenic agents: harmaline and oxotremorine. Neuroreport 2000; 11(11):2385–2390.
37. Ruigrok TJ, van der Burg H, Sabel-Goedknegt E. Locomotion coincides with c-Fos expression in related areas of inferior olive and cerebellar nuclei in the rat. Neurosci Lett 1996; 214(2–3):119–122.
38. Beitz AJ, Saxon D. Harmaline-induced climbing fiber activation causes amino acid and peptide release in the rodent cerebellar cortex and a unique temporal pattern of Fos expression in the olivo-cerebellar pathway. J Neurocytol 2004; 33(1):49–74.
39. Batini C, Buisseret-Delmas C, Conrath-Verrier M. Olivo-cerebellar activity during harmaline-induced tremor. A 2-[14C]deoxyglucose study. Neurosci Lett 1979; 12(2–3):241–246.

40. Batini C, Buisseret-Delmas C, Conrath-Verrier M. Harmaline-induced tremor. I. Regional metabolic activity as revealed by [14C]2-deoxyglucose in cat. Exp Brain Res 1981; 42(3–4):371–382.
41. Bernard JF, Buisseret-Delmas C, Compoint C, Laplante S. Harmaline-induced tremor. III. A combined simple units, horseradish peroxidase, and 2-deoxyglucose study of the olivocerebellar system in the rat. Exp Brain Res 1984; 57(1):128–137.
42. Batini C, Bernard JF, Buisseret-Delmas C, Conrath-Verrier M, Horcholle-Bossavit G. Harmaline-induced tremor. II. Unit activity correlation in the interposito-rubral and oculomotor systems of cat. Exp Brain Res 1981; 42(3–4):383–391.
43. Sjolund B, Bjorklund A, Wiklund L. The indolaminergic innervation of the inferior olive. 2. Relation to harmaline-induced tremor. Brain Res 1977; 131(1):23–37.
44. Compoint C, Buisseret-Delmas C. Origin, distribution and organization of the serotoninergic innervation in the inferior olivary complex of the rat. Arch Ital Biol 1988; 126(2):99–110.
45. Veasey SC, Fornal CA, Metzler CW, Jacobs BL. Single-unit responses of serotonergic dorsal raphe neurons to specific motor challenges in freely moving cats. Neuroscience 1997; 79(1):161–169.
46. Veasey SC, Fornal CA, Metzler CW, Jacobs BL. Response of serotonergic caudal raphe neurons in relation to specific motor activities in freely moving cats. J Neurosci 1995; 15(7 Pt 2):5346–5359.
47. Bishop GA, Ho RH. Cell bodies of origin of serotonin-immunoreactive afferents to the inferior olivary complex of the rat. Brain Res 1986; 399(2):369–373.
48. Sugihara I, Lang EJ, Llinas R. Serotonin modulation of inferior olivary oscillations and synchronicity: a multiple-electrode study in the rat cerebellum. Eur J Neurosci 1995; 7(4):521–534.
49. Mehta H, Saravanan KS, Mohanakumar KP. Serotonin synthesis inhibition in olivocerebellar system attenuates harmaline-induced tremor in Swiss albino mice. Behav Brain Res 2003; 145(1–2):31–36.
50. Arshaduddin M, Al Kadasah S, Biary N, Al Deeb S, Al Moutaery K, Tariq M. Citalopram, a selective serotonin reuptake inhibitor augments harmaline-induced tremor in rats. Behav Brain Res 2004; 153(1):15–20.
51. Wiklund L, Sjolund B, Bjorklund A. Morphological and functional studies on the serotoninergic innervation of the inferior olive. J Physiol (Paris) 1981; 77(2–3):183–186.
52. Costall B, Kelly DM, Naylor RJ. The importance of 5-hydroxytryptamine for the induction of harmine tremor and its antagonism by dopaminergic agonists assessed by lesions of the midbrain raphe nuclei. Eur J Pharmacol 1976; 35(1):109–119.
53. Kelly DM, Naylor RJ. Mechanisms of tremor induction by harmine. Europ J Pharmacol 1974; 27:14–24.
54. Headley PM, Lodge D, Duggan AW. Drug-induced rhythmical activity in the inferior olivary complex of the rat. Brain Res 1976; 101(3):461–478.
55. Welsh JP, Chang B, Menaker ME, Aicher SA. Removal of the inferior olive abolishes myoclonic seizures associated with a loss of olivary serotonin. Neuroscience 1998; 82(3):879–897.
56. Llinas R, Yarom Y. Oscillatory properties of guinea-pig inferior olivary neurones and their pharmacological modulation: an *in vitro* study. J Physiol 1986; 376:163–182.
57. Placantonakis DG, Schwarz C, Welsh JP. Serotonin suppresses subthreshold and suprathreshold oscillatory activity of rat inferior olivary neurones *in vitro*. J Physiol 2000; 524(Pt 3):833–851.

58. Groenewegen HJ, Boesten AJ, Voogd J. The dorsal column nuclear projections to the nucleus ventralis posterior lateralis thalami and the inferior olive in the cat: an autoradiographic study. J Comp Neurol 1975; 162(4):505–517.

59. Ho BT, Fritchie GE, Idanpaan-Heikkila JE, Tansey LW, McIsaac WM. 3H Harmaline distribution in monkey brain; pharmacological and autoradiographic study. Br Res 1970; 22(3):397–401.

60. Helmchen C, Hagenow A, Miesner J et al. Eye movement abnormalities in essential tremor may indicate cerebellar dysfunction. Brain 2003; 126(Pt 6):1319–1332.

61. Phillips MI, Knowles WD, January CT. Different times of development of tremor to harmaline and oxotremorine in neonatal rats. Neurosci Lett 1978; 9(3):255–259.

62. Singer C, Sanchez-Ramos J, Weiner WJ. Gait abnormality in essential tremor. Mov Disord 1994; 9(2):193–196.

63. Hubble JP, Busenbark KL, Pahwa R, Lyons K, Koller WC. Clinical expression of essential tremor: effects of gender and age. Mov Disord 1997; 12(6):969–972.

64. Hallett M, Dubinsky RM. Glucose metabolism in the brain of patients with essential tremor. J Neurol Sci 1993; 114(1):45–48.

65. Wills AJ, Jenkins IH, Thompson PD, Findley LJ, Brooks DJ. Red nuclear and cerebellar but no olivary activation associated with essential tremor: a positron emission tomographic study. Ann Neurol 1994; 36(4):636–642.

66. Boecker H, Wills AJ, Ceballos-Baumann A et al. The effect of ethanol on alcohol-responsive essential tremor: a positron emission tomography study. Ann Neurol 1996; 39(5):650–658.

67. Sinton CM, Krosser BI, Walton KD, Llinas RR. The effectiveness of different isomers of octanol as blockers of harmaline-induced tremor. Pflugers Arch 1989; 414(1):31–36.

68. Bushara KO, Goldstein SR, Grimes GJ Jr, Burstein AH, Hallett M. Pilot trial of 1-octanol in essential tremor. Neurology 2004; 62(1):122–124.

69. Shill HA, Bushara KO, Mari Z, Reich M, Hallett M. Open-label dose-escalation study of oral 1-octanol in patients with essential tremor. Neurology 2004; 62(12):2320–2322.

5

Neuropathology and Neurochemistry of Essential Tremor

Ali Rajput and Alex Rajput

*Royal University Hospital and University of Saskatchewan,
Saskatoon, Saskatchewan, Canada*

I. NEUROPATHOLOGY

Essential tremor is the most common pathological tremor in humans (1) and is estimated to be 10–20 times as common as Parkinson's disease (2). Yet, the scientific information on essential tremor is only a small fraction of the Parkinson's disease literature. Essential tremor is regarded as a dysfunction within the central nervous system (CNS), but the site and nature of the pathological process remain unknown. Pathological studies of essential tremor are scarce.

To date, there are <50 essential tremor patients who have had detailed neuro-pathological studies (3). Routine neuropathological studies have thus far failed to identify specific anatomical sites or pathological processes characteristic of essential tremor.

The literature to date indicates that the pathology in essential tremor is in the cerebellum or its brain stem connections. Nearly 50% of the essential tremor patients have been reported to have difficulty with tandem gait (4) and clinical evidence of cerebellar ataxia and dysmetria is reported in some patients (3,5,6). Electrophysiological studies indicate that 58% of essential tremor cases have intention tremor resembling that seen in cerebellar disorders and some degree of hypermetria (7); however, most essential tremor patients do not manifest clinical ataxia or dysmetria (8). One well documented essential tremor patient had resolution of ipsilateral tremor following cerebellar stroke (9). The magnetic resonance imaging (MRI) studies in this case indicated an ischemic lesion of the deep cerebellar nuclei and their efferent fibers into the superior cerebellar peduncle with involvement of the superior cerebellar cortex (9). This patient did not have an autopsy study; therefore, the precise anatomical site of the lesion was not fully identified.

Positron emission tomography (PET) studies show an increase in the cerebellar blood flow coinciding with the emergence of postural tremor in essential tremor patients (10). Alcohol ingestion, which decreases the amplitude of essential tremor in most patients, has been noted to produce an increase of blood flow in the inferior olivary nucleus in essential tremor patients but not in control subjects (11). These diverse observations have been interpreted as evidence that the cerebellum and its afferent and efferent pathways are critical in the production of essential tremor.

In the overwhelming majority of patients, essential tremor is a monosymptomatic disorder characterized by postural and/or kinetic tremor. The tremor is restricted in most patients to the upper limbs and/or head (3). We will classify such patients as pure essential tremor for the purpose of this chapter. Pathological observations of pure essential tremor were first reported by Hassler in 1939 (12). He studied one patient and noted that the number of small neurons in the striatum was reduced. Mylle and van Bogaert (13) also reported two such patients. Both had a history of psychiatric disorders and one also suffered from a stroke. Both of these patients were noted to have neuronal loss of cerebellar Purkinje cells and cells in the globus pallidus. One patient had neuronal loss in the inferior olivary nucleus and one had neuronal loss in the cerebellar dentate nucleus. One of these patients also had status cribrosus involving the caudate and the putamen. Lapresle et al. (14) reported one pure essential tremor patient with no histological abnormalities in the brain. Rajput et al. (15) reported five pure essential tremor cases. One 83-year-old patient had bilateral status lacunaris while the other four had no histological abnormalities in the brain. A more recent study added three pure essential tremor cases to this series (3). One of these three, an 80-year-old female with diabetes mellitus and coronary artery disease, had loss of cerebellar Purkinje cells. These studies indicate that pure essential tremor patients have no consistent brain pathology on routine histopathological examination (3,12–15).

Although clinically mild cerebellar dysfunction has been reported in some essential tremor patients, autopsy studies in such patients are very rare. Rajput et al. (3) reported two such patients, a mother and child. No cerebellar pathology was identified on routine histological studies in either of these two cases. There are no other pathological studies reported in essential tremor patients with clinical features suggestive of cerebellar dysfunction.

In the third clinical profile in essential tremor, patients have classical essential tremor but also manifest resting tremor but no other motor features of parkinsonism (3,15). We will classify these patients as essential tremor plus resting tremor. Herskovits and Black (16) reported one essential tremor plus resting tremor autopsy. This patient had multiple cerebral infarcts but no other pathological changes. Rajput et al. (3) longitudinally followed 20 essential tremor patients. Six (30%) of those developed resting tremor later in the course of illness. At autopsy, one patient had a cerebral hemisphere infarct and one patient suffered from neuroleptic malignant syndrome with multiple perivascular hemorrhages in the brain. The remaining four essential tremor plus resting tremor patients had no histological abnormalities in the brain (3).

The literature on the association between essential tremor and parkinsonism is controversial. Since resting tremor is a well known feature in some essential tremor cases, only those patients who have all three major motor manifestations of parkinsonism-resting tremor, bradykinesia and rigidity—can be included in this group (15). We will classify patients having clinical features of essential tremor and of parkinsonism as essential tremor plus parkinsonism. The literature is somewhat confusing as the terms Parkinson syndrome and Parkinson's disease have been used interchangeably in most clinical studies. For the purpose of determining the cause of parkinsonism in essential tremor patients, autopsy studies are essential. Parkinson's disease is pathologically characterized by marked loss of substantia nigra pigmented neurons and presence of Lewy body inclusions (21–24).

Pathological studies of essential tremor plus parkinsonism cases are scarce. Quinn et al. (25) reported one such patient. This patient had normal histological examination; notably, the substantia nigra was normal. The cause of parkinsonism in this patient was not identified, and there was no other pathological process which could be considered as the basis of essential tremor. Yahr et al. (26) studied one large essential tremor family. In five generations, they evaluated 36 patients—13 of whom had essential tremor. In one generation, three brothers had essential tremor plus parkinsonism, including a pair of twins. The twin brothers died of intestinal neoplasms and autopsy was done on one case, revealing Lewy body inclusions in the substantia nigra and the locus caeruleus and marked loss of substantia nigra pigmented neurons. There were no other pathological findings. Although the history of essential tremor in this family was documented over five generations, the Parkinson's disease was restricted to only the members of one generation—three brothers. Thus, a genetic link with Parkinson's disease was not evident in this family.

Rajput et al. (3) longitudinally followed 20 essential tremor patients who came to autopsy. Six (30%) of those had essential tremor plus parkinsonism. The cause of parkinsonism was diverse in this group. One patient had Lewy body disease (21,23) and no other histological abnormality. One patient had basal ganglia status cribrosus. Two of the essential tremor plus parkinsonism patients had pathological findings characteristic of progressive supranuclear palsy. In two patients, the parkinsonism was attributed to neuroleptic use and there was no brain pathology (3).

In summary, in the essential tremor plus parkinsonism patients, the only pathological process was that which accounted for the parkinsonism. There were no consistent pathological changes that can be attributed as the basis of essential tremor.

Essential tremor patients are reported to have a higher frequency of dystonia and dystonia patients have been reported to have more frequent essential tremor than expected in the general population (20). There are no pathological reports on patients who have essential tremor and dystonia.

II. NEUROCHEMISTRY

In contrast to the well-defined biochemical defect in Parkinson's disease (27), there are no characteristic findings in essential tremor. Clues for biochemical abnormalities may be gleaned by what medications are effective for essential tremor. Treatment and pathophysiology of tremor are discussed in more detail elsewhere in this book.

Essential tremor is strictly a human disorder. As yet, there is no good animal model which could be used for biochemical studies of essential tremor (28).

A. Proteins

Stibler and Kjellin reported on cerebrospinal fluid (CSF) proteins in patients with tremor of different causes (chronic alcoholism, Parkinson's disease, and essential tremor) (29). Abnormal CSF proteins were found in 94% (15/16) of the essential tremor patients. Protein electrophoresis of CSF was inconclusive.

Somatostatin is believed to have neurotransmitter or synapse modulating functions. While somatostatin levels in CSF are low in Parkinson's disease, essential tremor patients have levels similar to controls (30). CSF somatostatin levels of 14 essential tremor patients before and after 2 weeks treatment with a GABA-agonist, (Progabide, SL76002) were virtually unchanged (30).

Secretogranin II and Chromogranins A and B are precursor peptides found in neuronal large dense core vesicles. CSF levels of peptides derived from these three precursors are higher than other peptides. Eder et al., found no differences in proteolytic processing of chromogranins/secretogranin in essential tremor ($n = 2$), Parkinson's disease, Alzheimer's disease, and multiple sclerosis compared with controls (31).

B. Amino Acids

Mally and Baranyi in 1994 (32) reported on CSF in 19 essential tremor cases and 10 controls. They noted elevation of the excitatory amino acids aspartate (significant) and glutamate (nonsignificant) compared with controls. The amino acids threonine, serine, and glycine were reduced in essential tremor cases. Two years later, Mally and colleagues (33) compared amino acid composition in both CSF and serum of essential tremor patients with controls. They reported reduced concentrations of some amino acids (glutamine, glycine, isoleucine, leucine, threonine, and asparagine) in the serum of essential tremor cases ($n = 20$) compared to controls ($n = 10$). Serum glutamate and aspartate were found at significantly higher concentrations in essential tremor than controls. Glutamate and aspartate changes in CSF were similar but not identical. Some amino acids had an opposite shift and CSF concentrations did not always correlate with serum concentrations. While glutamate concentration was higher in the CSF of essential tremor patients, aspartate concentration was lower in the essential tremor cases compared with controls. The inhibitory amino acid glycine was in lower concentration in both serum and CSF of essential tremor, while gamma amino butyric acid (GABA) concentration was lower in CSF of essential tremor and not detected in serum of either essential tremor or controls. This suggests a role for overactivity via the excitatory amino acids with a possible role of decreased central inhibition as reflected by diminished GABA levels (33).

A recent study reported no difference in ventricular CSF glutamate levels between essential tremor ($n = 6$) and Parkinson's disease ($n = 22$) cases (34).

C. Adrenergic System and Catecholamines

Beta-blockers are a mainstay of essential tremor therapy. Selective beta-1 antagonists are reported to be less beneficial than propranolol—a nonselective beta antagonist (35–37).The mechanism of action is believed to involve both peripheral and central adrenergic effects of drugs. The peripheral effects are thought to be due to a blockade of beta-2 receptors in muscle spindle. The central effects are less certain. Abila et al., proposed that the improvement in essential tremor, physiological, and isoprenaline-induced tremors by beta-adrenergic agents is due to blockade of beta-2 receptors in muscle spindles (35). Because selective beta-1 antagonists still provide benefit, there is likely central adrenergic overactivity in essential tremor.

Serum levels of catecholamines may not correlate with CSF or intracranial concentrations. Indeed, given the functional neuroimaging studies in essential tremor, one would expect regional as opposed to global biochemical differences in essential tremor. Rajput et al. (38) reported regional differences in a small sample of autopsy verified essential tremor frozen brain samples. Mean noradrenaline levels in three essential tremor brains was higher than those of three control brains in cerebellar cortex, dentate nucleus, inferior olive, and locus caeruleus, but was not elevated in the red nucleus. The noradrenaline increase was the greatest in the locus caeruleus, dentate, and inferior olive and the least marked in the cerebellar cortex (38). Dopamine levels in those regions were not different between essential tremor and control brains. Aspartate, glutamate, glutamine, glycine, taurine, serine alanine, and GABA levels in these brain areas were similar in essential tremor and control brains (Rajput et al., unpublished data).

Barkhatova and Ivanova-Smolenskaia (39) reported on catecholamine metabolism in 40 essential tremor patients. They observed decreased catecholamine urinary excretion, particularly norepinephrine, but the catecholamine precursor DOPA was not altered. The urinary excretion of vanillylmandelic acid, a catecholamine metabolite, was reduced. In contrast to the altered urinary levels, blood levels in essential tremor were not appreciably different from controls. These results have not been replicated (39). Lenman et al. (40) found no change in urinary monoamine metabolites in essential tremor patients compared with controls.

Beta-carboline alkaloids induce tremor when given to lab animals (41) and to humans (42,43). These are naturally occurring compounds, with both endogenous and exogenous sources including plant-derived food items. Louis and colleagues reported elevated blood harmane concentration in essential tremor cases compared with controls ($p = 0.01$) (44). Values were similar in essential tremor cases with and without affected family members. Harmine concentrations were also elevated in essential tremor cases compared with controls but the difference was not statistically significant. They point out that the normal physiological levels of harmane in humans have not been established. As many beta-carboline alkaloids are lipophilic, the brain and CSF concentrations may well be significantly higher than that detected in serum.

Rate limiting steps for synthesis of dopamine, norepinephrine and serotonin are the hydroxylation of tyrosine (dopamine, norepinephrine) and tryptophan (serotonin). Tetrahydrobiopterin (BH4) cofactor is essential for this hydroxylation. CSF levels of BH4 were low in essential tremor ($n = 10$) compared with controls (45). These results were not specific, as patients with Parkinson's disease, Shy-Drager syndrome, progressive supranuclear palsy, Huntington's disease, and presenile dementia also had reduced levels (45).

D. GABA

GABA is an inhibitory neurotransmitter, which causes cellular hyperpolarization via its action on the chloride channel (46). Medications which potentiate GABA activity, including barbiturates and benzodiazepines, may be effective for essential tremor. Ethanol also enhances activity of GABA receptors (46). Response to ethanol, however, is not specific for essential tremor (47).

Other medications related to GABA have been used to treat tremor. Tariq et al. (48) reported on the beneficial effect of baclofen, a GABA$_B$ agonist, on harmaline induced tremors in rats. Gabapentin, an anticonvulsant structurally similar to GABA, has been reported as effective as monotherapy for essential tremor (49) but this has not been confirmed by others (50,51). Progabide, a GABA-agonist, was found to be ineffective in essential tremor (52).

Theophylline and propranolol both improve tremor in essential tremor (53). In mice neocortical slices, theophylline but not propranolol stopped adenosine potentiated N-methyl-D-aspartate (NMDA) depolarization. GABA alone did not alter NMDA depolarization. However, after chronic treatment with propranolol or theophylline, GABA significantly enhanced NMDA depolarization. The authors postulate upregulation of GABA receptor function, and increased GABA sensitivity may be involved in the chronic benefit of propranolol as opposed to the early effects of non-selective peripheral beta-receptor blockade (53).

E. Adenosine

Adenosine receptors are widely distributed in the CNS. Caffeine blocks adenosine's modulation of dopamine receptors and/or dopamine release and adenosine antagonists may have a role in the treatment of tremor and Parkinson's disease (54). An adenosine antagonist, theophylline, was reported to have similar efficacy to propranolol and was superior to placebo in a small blinded, cross-over, controlled study. Acutely, theophylline should increase neurotransmitter release (including norepinephrine, glutamate, and aspartate) but chronic use causes reduced neurotransmitter release, and hence its therapeutic action on tremor (55).

Despite the potential role of adenosine receptors in essential tremor, there are no reports of altered adenosine levels in essential tremor patients. Adenosine is a short-lived molecule and would be difficult to study. Adenosine is also not considered a classic neurotransmitter, but rather is produced from metabolism of adenosine nucleotides [e.g., adenosine triphosphate (ATP)] (46).

III. CONCLUSIONS

Routine histological studies of essential tremor brains have revealed no abnormalities. A handful of cases are reported to have cerebellar Purkinje cell loss but there are no inclusions or other findings typical or pathognomonic of essential tremor. As the remainder of the neurological examination is typically normal, it is more likely that one would find a functional (neurotransmitter or neurochemical) abnormality. There are no diagnostic tests or investigations to confirm the diagnosis of essential tremor. Reports of catecholamine metabolism are conflicting. Functional neuroimaging, human biochemical studies and possibly animal model(s) of essential tremor will help us gain a better understanding of the disorder. More detailed morphometric studies including special staining techniques could help us to identify the structural pathology of essential tremor which as yet has not been reported.

REFERENCES

1. Louis ED, Marder K, Cote L, Pullman S, Ford B, Wilder D, Tang MX, Lantigua R, Gurland B, Mayeux R. Differences in the prevalence of essential tremor among elderly African Americans, whites, and Hispanics in northern Manhattan, NY. Arch Neurol 1995; 52:1201–1205.
2. Rautakorpi I, Takala J, Marttila RJ, Sievers K, Rinne UK. Essential tremor in a Finnish Population. Acta Neurol Scandinav 1982; 66:58–67.
3. Rajput A, Robinson C, Rajput AH. Essential tremor course and disability: A clinico-pathological study of 20 cases. Neurology 2004; 62:932–936.
4. Singer C, Sanchez-Ramos J, Weiner WJ. Gait abnormality in essential tremor. Mov Disord 1994; 9(2):193–196.
5. Critchley E. Clinical manifestations of essential tremor. J Neurol Neurosurg Psychiatry 1972; 35:365–372.
6. Deuschl G, Elble RJ. The pathophysiology of essential tremor. Neurology 2000; 54(suppl 4):S14–S20.
7. Deuschl G, Wenzelburger R, Loffler K, Raethjen J, Stolze H. Essential tremor and cerebellar dysfunction—Clinical and kinematic analysis of intentional tremor. Brain 2000; 123:1568–1580.
8. Elble RJ. Diagnostic criteria for essential tremor and differential diagnosis. Neurology 2000; 54(suppl 4):S2–S6.
9. Dupuis MJM, Delwaide PJ, Boucquey D, Gonsette RE. Homolateral disappearance of essential tremor after cerebellar stroke. Mov Disord 1989; 4(2):183–187.
10. Colebatch JG, Findley LJ, Frackowiak RSJ, Marsden CD, Brooks DJ. Preliminary report: activation of the cerebellum in essential tremor. Lancet 1990; 336:1028–1030.
11. Boecker H, Wills AJ, Ceballos-Baumann, Samuel M, Thomas DG, Marsden CD. The effect of ethanol on alcohol-responsive essential tremor: a positron emission tomography study. Ann Neurol 1996; 39:650–658.
12. Hassler R. Zur pathologischen Anatomie des senilen und des parkinsonistischen Tremor. J Psychol Neurol (Lpz) 1939; 49:193–230.
13. Mylle G, van Bogaert L. Du tremblement essential non familial. Mschr Psychiat Neurol 1948; 115:80–90.
14. Lapresle J, Rondot P, Said G. Tremblement idiopathique de repos, d' attitude et d'action: Etude anatomo-clinique d'une observation. Revue Neurologique, Paris 1974; 130:343–348.
15. Rajput AH, Rozdilsky B, Ang L, Rajput A. Significance of parkinsonian manifestations in essential tremor. Can J Neurol Sci 1993; 20:114–117.
16. Herskovits E, Blackwood W. Essential (familial, hereditary) tremor: a case report. J Neurol Neurosurg Psychiatry 1969; 32:509–511.
17. Geraghty JJ, Jankovic J, Zetusky WJ. Association between essential tremor and Parkinson's disease. Ann Neurol 1985; 17:329–333.
18. Hornabrook RW, Nagurney JT. Essential tremor in Papua, New Guinea. Brain 1976; 99:659–672.

19. Lang AE, Kierans C, Blair RDG. Association between familial tremor and Parkinson's disease. Ann Neurol 1986; 19:306–307.
20. Koller WC, Busenbark K, Miner K. The relationship of essential tremor to other movement disorders: report on 678 patients. essential tremor study group. Ann Neurol 1994; 35(6):717–723.
21. Gibb WRG, Lees AJ. The Relevance of the Lewy body to the pathogenesis of idiopathic Parkinson's disease. J Neurol Neurosurg Psychiatry 1988; 51:745–752.
22. Rajput AH, Rozdilsky B, Rajput A. Accuracy of clinical diagnosis in parkinsonism–a prospective study. Can J Neurol Sci 1991; 18:275–278.
23. Duvoisin R, Golbe LI. Toward a definition of Parkinson's disease. Neurology 1989; 39:746.
24. Jellinger K. The pathology of Parkinsonism. In: Marsden CD, Fahn S, eds. Movement Disorders 2. London: Butterworths and Co., 1987:124–165.
25. Quinn N, Parkes D, Janota I, Marsden CD. Preservation of the substantia nigra and locus coeruleus in a patient receiving levodopa (2 kg) plus decarboxylase inhibitor over a four-year period. Mov Disord 1986; 1(1):65–68.
26. Yahr MD, Orosz D, Purohit DP. Co-occurrence of essential tremor and Parkinson's disease: clinical study of a large kindred and autopsy findings. Parkinsonism & Related Disorders 2003; 9:225–231.
27. Ehringer H, Hornykiewicz O. Distribution of noradrenaline and dopamine (3-hydroxytyramine) in human brain: their behaviour in extrapyramidal system diseases. Klin Wochenschr 1960; 38:1236–1239.
28. Rajput AH. Contributions of human brain biochemical studies to movement disorders. Parkinsonism & Related Disorders 2002; 8:425–431.
29. Stibler H, Kjellin KG. Isoelectric focusing and electrophoresis of the CSF proteins in tremor of different origins. J Neurol Sci 1976; 30:269–285.
30. Christensen SE, Dupont E, Mondrup K, de Fine Olivarius B, Orskov H. Parkinson's disease and benign essential tremor: somatostatin-like immunoreactivity in the cerebrospinal fluid. Adv Neurol 1984; 40:325–331.
31. Eder U, Leitner B, Kirchmair R, Pohl P, Jobst KA, Smith AD, Mally J, Benzer A, Riederer P, Reichmann H, Saria A, Winkler H. Levels and proteolytic processing of chromogranin A and B and secretogranin II in cerebrospinal fluid in neurological diseases. J Neural Transm 1998; 105:39–51.
32. Mally J, Baranyi M. Change in the concentrations of amino acids in cisternal CSF of patients with essential tremor. J Neurol Neurosurg Psychiatry 1994; 57(8):1012–1013.
33. Mally J, Baranyi M, Vizi ES. Change in the concentrations of amino acids in CSF and serum of patients with essential tremor. J Neural Transm 1996; 103:555–560.
34. Mandybur GT, Miyagi Y, Yin W, Perkins E, Zhang JH. Cytotoxicity of ventricular cerebrospinal fluid from Parkinson patients: correlation with clinical profiles and neurochemistry. Neurol Res 2003; 25:104–111.
35. Abila B, Wilson JF, Marshall RW, Richens A. The tremorolytic action of β-adrenoceptor blockers in essential, physiological and isoprenaline-induced tremor is mediated by β-adrenoceptors located in a deep peripheral compartment. Br J Clin Pharmacol 1985; 20:369–376.
36. Ljung O. Treatment of essential tremor with metoprolol. New Engl J Med 1979; 301:1005.
37. Larsen TA, Teravainen H, Calne DB. Atenolol vs propranolol in essential tremor: a controlled quantitative study. Acta Neurol Scand 1982; 66:547–554.

38. Rajput AH, Hornykiewicz O, Deng Y, Birdi S, Miyashita H, Macaulay R. Increased noradrenaline levels in essential tremor brain. Neurology 2001; 56 (suppl 3):A302.
39. Barhkatova VP, Ivanova-Smolenskaia IA. Catecholamine metabolism in essential tremor. Zh Nevropatol Psikhiatr IM S S Korsakova 1990; 90:10–14.
40. Lenman JAR, Turnbull MJ, Reid A, Fleming AM. Urinary monoamine metabolites excretion in disorders of movement. J Neurol Sci 1977; 32:219–225.
41. Fuentes LA, Longo VG. An investigation on the central effects of harmine, harmaline and related ß-carbolines. Neuropharmacology 1991; 10:15–23.
42. Lewin L. Utersuchungen uber Banisteria caapi Sp. Arch Exp Pathol Pharmacol 1928; 129:133–149.
43. Pennes HH, Hoch PH. Psychotomimetics, clinical and theoretical considerations: harmine, Win-2299 and Nalline. Am J Psychiatry 1957; 13:885–892.
44. Louis ED, Zheng W, Jurewicz EC, Watner D, Chen J, Factor-Litvak P, Parides M. Elevation of blood beta-carboline alkaloids in essential tremor. Neurology 2002; 59:1940–1944.
45. Williams AC, Levine RA, Chase TN, Lovenberg W, Calne DB. CSF hydroxylase cofactor levels in some neurological diseases. J Neurol Neurosurg Psychiatry 1980; 43:735–738.
46. Siegel GJ, Agranoff B, Albers RW, Fisher SK, Uhler MD, eds. Basic Neurochemistry: Molecular Cellular and Medical Aspects. 6th ed. New York: Lippincott-Raven, 1999.
47. Rajput AH, Jamieson H, Hirsch S, Quraishi A. Relative efficacy of alcohol and propranolol in action tremor. Can J Neurol Sci 1975; 2:31–35.
48. Tariq M, Arshaduddin M, Biary N, Al Moutaery K, Al Deeb S. Baclofen attenuates harmaline induced tremors in rats. Neurosci Lett 2001; 312:79–82.
49. Gironelli A, Kulisevsky J, Barbanoj M, Lopez-Villegas D, Hernandez G, Pascual-Sedano B. A randomized placebo-controlled comparative trial of gabapentin and propranolol in essential tremor. Arch Neurol 1999; 56(4):475–480.
50. Pahwa R, Lyons K, Hubble JP, Busenbark K, Rienerth JD, Pahwa AK. Double-blind controlled trial of gabapentin in essential tremor. Mov Disord 1998; 13(3):465–467.
51. Louis ED. A new twist for stopping the shakes? Revisiting GABAergic therapy for essential tremor. Arch Neurol 1999; 56(7):807–808.
52. Mondrup K, Dupont E, Pedersen E. The effect of the GABA-agonist, progabide, on benign essential tremor. Acta Neurol Scand 1983; 68:248–252.
53. Mally J, Stone TW. The effect of theophylline on essential tremor: the possible role of GABA. Pharmacol Biochem Behav 1991; 39:345–349.
54. Mally J, Stone TW. Potential role of adenosine antagonist therapy in pathological tremor disorders. Pharmacol Ther 1996; 72:243–250.
55. Mally J, Stone TW. Efficacy of an adenosine antagonist, theophylline, in essential tremor: comparison with placebo and propranolol. J Neurol Sci 1995; 132:129–132.

6

Differential Diagnosis and Clinical Characteristics of Essential Tremor

Rodger J. Elble

Southern Illinois University School of Medicine, Springfield, Illinois, USA

I. CLINICAL CLASSIFICATION OF TREMOR

Tremor is an involuntary oscillation of a body part and is commonly classified according to the behavioral circumstances in which it occurs (Table 6.1) (1). Tremor may occur during attempted relaxation (rest tremor), during a voluntarily held posture (postural tremor), or during a voluntary movement (kinetic tremor).

The classification schema in Table 6.1 has been expanded to include subtypes of tremor with unique characteristics. For example, pill-rolling rest tremor

Table 6.1   Behavioral Classification of Tremor [with Permission from Elble (61)]

Type of tremor	Definition	Example circumstances
Rest tremor	Occurs in a body part that is supported in such a way that skeletal muscle activation is neither necessary nor intended	The patient is recumbent on a bed or seated on a couch, with the body part supported. Tremor is often enhanced by the performance of cognitive tasks or motor tasks with other body parts, and it is often suppressed, at least temporarily, by voluntary muscle contraction.
Postural tremor	Occurs in an attempt to hold a body part motionless against the force of gravity	Extending the upper limbs horizontally; pointing at objects; sitting erectly without support for the upper body; protruding the tongue
Kinetic tremor	Occurs during a voluntary movement	Nose-finger-nose testing; heel-knee-shin testing; reaching; writing; drawing; pouring water into a cup; drinking from a cup; eating with utensils; speaking
Isometric tremor	Occurs during a muscle contraction against a rigid stationary object	Pushing against a wall; flexing the wrist against a table; making a fist
Action tremor	Occurs during any voluntary contraction of skeletal muscle	May be any combination of postural, kinetic, and isometric tremor

is a rest tremor in which the fingers and wrist move in a manner reminiscent of a voluntary rhythmic manipulation of small objects in the hand. Degeneration or pharmacologic blockade (as with neuroleptics) of the nigrostriatal dopaminergic pathway produces this unique tremor, and idiopathic Parkinson's disease is the most common etiology.

Kinetic tremor may increase dramatically in the pursuit of a visual target, particularly as the target is approached by the hand or foot, and this form of kinetic tremor is called intention tremor. True intention tremor has crescendo and somewhat paroxysmal accentuation as the target is approached, resulting in considerable disability. Little or no tremor may be present during posture or during the initial movement toward the target. Intention tremor is usually caused by damage to the deep cerebellar nuclei (dentate and globose-emboliform) or their efferent pathway to the contralateral ventrolateral thalamus.

Some kinetic tremors are called task-specific tremor because they are largely or solely limited to a specific task or movement, such as writing, speaking, smiling, or standing (2,3). Focal action tremors are limited to one anatomical site such as the head, voice, tongue, or hand, and such tremors may be task-specific. Position-specific and position-sensitive action tremors are produced or greatly exacerbated by specific postures (2,3).

II. CLINICAL CHARACTERISTICS OF ESSENTIAL TREMOR

Essential tremor is typically a mixture of postural and kinetic tremors, although either form of tremor may occur in isolation. Essential tremor nearly always affects the hands (~95% of patients) but also affects the head (~34%), face (~5%), voice (~12%), trunk (~5%), and lower extremities (~20%) (4–6). Thus, most patients have tremor in the upper limbs, frequently in isolation. Tremor in the lower limbs is usually asymptomatic.

Isolated head tremor may occur, but in cases of isolated head tremor, one must always consider the diagnosis of tremor-predominant torticollis in which cervical dystonia may be very subtle (3). For this reason, many investigators regard cases of pure head tremor as probable essential tremor rather than definite essential tremor (7). Position sensitivity, task specificity, and focality increase the likelihood of an underlying dystonia or some other disorder unrelated to essential tremor (2,3). Tremor may exist for several years before any sign of dystonia (8–10). Nevertheless, the possibility that focal, position-specific, and task-specific tremors are at times a variant of essential tremor cannot be dismissed with certainty (3,7).

Rest tremor occurs rarely in elderly patients with advanced essential tremor (11). Therefore, coexistent Parkinson's disease or some other cause of parkinsonism should be suspected in patients with rest tremor. In most instances, the "rest tremor" in essential tremor is actually a postural tremor that is caused by incomplete muscle relaxation. Patients are often examined while seated on a table that does not provide complete support for the head, neck, torso, and proximal limb muscles. Consequently, the muscles of these body parts may be active against gravity, producing a tremor that is mistakenly classified as rest tremor. This common error can be avoided by examining patients in recumbent and seated positions with complete body support. Essential tremor does not cause pill-rolling rest tremor in the hands or rest tremor in the feet (12).

Classic essential tremor is a monosymptomatic disorder with no neurologic signs or symptoms other than tremor (3,13). Muscle tone is normal, and there is no weakness or problem with coordination other than that which is attributable to tremor. Cogwheeling may be palpable during the manual testing of muscle tone, particularly when muscle tone is enhanced by voluntary action of another body part (Froment's sign) (1).

Essential tremor develops insidiously and progresses gradually at a variable rate, as determined by factors that are as yet unknown (14–16). Essential tremor affects people of all ages, but its prevalence increases with age, affecting at least 5% of people age ≥65 years (17–21). The uncertainty in prevalence estimates is largely due to the lack of reliable methods for distinguishing very mild essential tremor from physiologic tremor. This distinction is particularly difficult in older people (18,19).

The extent to which other neurologic signs may occur in essential tremor is a topic of continuing controversy (7,13). Some patients with advanced essential tremor have impaired tandem walking (22). These patients tend to be elderly, but the confounding influence of age-associated neurologic impairment is probably not the only explanation (22). Subclinical deficits in cognitive function have been found in two small studies of elderly patients with advanced essential tremor, but larger studies with better controls and less recruitment bias are needed to confirm these deficits (23,24). Impaired hearing may be more common in patients with essential tremor (25). Regardless, additional neurologic signs or symptoms should alert the clinician to the presence of some other neurologic disorder, either in isolation or in combination with essential tremor.

The characteristics of essential tremor in the upper limbs are nonspecific, and identical action tremor can be the sole presenting symptom in patients with Parkinson's disease and dystonia (8–10,26,27). Furthermore, essential tremor is common in the general population (at least 5% of people ≥65 years), and it must be just as common among patients with Parkinson's disease, dystonia, and other neurologic conditions. Therefore, it is not surprising that action tremor resembling essential tremor has been observed in patients and families with many other common neurologic disorders, including Parkinson's disease, dystonia, migraine, and peripheral neuropathy (7). Whether these patients had essential tremor or another disease resembling essential tremor is unknown because there is no sensitive and specific neurophysiologic test or biological marker for essential tremor. At present, there is no conclusive evidence for a pathophysiologic relationship between essential tremor and other neurologic diseases (13).

III. DIAGNOSTIC CRITERIA FOR ESSENTIAL TREMOR

A. Clinical Diagnostic Criteria

The Movement Disorder Society sponsored an international meeting of specialists in Kiel Germany in July 1997, with the specific aim of producing a consensus statement on the terminology and diagnostic criteria for tremor disorders (3). The consensus diagnostic criteria for classic essential tremor are summarized in Table 6.2. The views contained in Table 6.2 are still widely held.

The Movement Disorder Society did not address the problem of distinguishing mild essential tremor from physiologic tremor. This distinction is critically important in genetic studies of familial essential tremor. Consequently, many researchers supplement the diagnostic criteria in Table 6.2 with amplitude criteria based on a clinical rating scale such as the tremor rating scale of Fahn and coworkers (28). For example, Louis and coworkers defined definite essential tremor as grade 2 (1–2 cm amplitude) postural tremor in at least one upper limb and either grade 2 kinetic tremor in 4 of 5 tasks or grade 2 kinetic tremor in one task and grade 3 (>3 cm amplitude) kinetic tremor in a second task (29). The five tasks were pouring water between two cups, drinking water from a cup, using a spoon to drink water, finger-nose-finger test and drawing

Table 6.2 Diagnostic Criteria for Essential Tremor, from the Consensus Statement of the Movement Disorder Society (3)

Diagnosis	Inclusion criteria	Exclusion criteria
Classic essential tremor	Either of the following is true: 1. Bilateral, largely symmetric postural or kinetic tremor of the hands and forearms that is visible and persistent. 2. Additional or isolated head tremor without evidence of dystonia (e.g., abnormal posturing)	1. Other abnormal neurologic signs, especially dystonia 2. Presence of known causes of enhanced physiologic tremor (e.g., drugs, anxiety, depression, hyperthyroidism), including current or recent exposure to tremorogenic drugs or the presence of a drug withdrawal state 3. Historic or clinical evidence of psychogenic tremor 4. Convincing evidence of sudden onset or stepwise progression (e.g., following a neurologic trauma) 5. Primary orthostatic tremor 6. Isolated voice tremor 7. Isolated position-specific or task-specific tremors, including occupational tremors and primary writing tremor 8. Isolated tongue or chin tremor 9. Isolated leg tremor
Indeterminate tremor syndrome	Satisfies the inclusion criteria for classic essential tremor, but the patient has equivocal neurologic signs or concomitant neurologic signs of doubtful significance (e.g., a mildly unsteady gait, mild dementia in an elderly patient, or mild extrapyramidal signs such as hypomimia, reduced arm swing, and mild bradykinesia)	Same as for classic essential tremor

Archimedes spirals. Such amplitude criteria are obviously very conservative and will exclude all patients with very mild essential tremor. Consequently, some investigators supplement the clinical criteria in Table 6.2 with the results of electrophysiologic testing.

B.   Electrophysiologic Criteria

The *sine qua non* of essential tremor is a rhythmic 4–12 Hz entrainment of motor
unit activity that forces the upper limbs into oscillation (30). Head tremor has a
frequency of 3–9 Hz (31). Older patients usually exhibit tremor frequencies
in the lower range of 4–12 Hz, overlapping with the frequency ranges of
Parkinson's disease action tremor and dystonic tremors (3,32). Younger patients
exhibit higher tremor frequencies that often extend into the frequency range of
physiologic hand tremor (8–12 Hz) (33). Tremor frequency tends to decrease
slowly at an average rate of 0.07 Hz per year (34).

The frequency of oscillation is independent of reflex arc length and mechanical properties (inertia and stiffness) of the body part. Consequently, the frequency of moderate-severe (>1 cm) hand tremor changes <1 Hz when large
inertial loads are attached to the hand (35–37). This diagnostic maneuver, combined with electromyography (EMG), accelerometry and spectral analysis, has
been used in the diagnosis of essential tremor and other action tremors of
central origin. In general, any of the following four electrophysiologic outcomes
may occur when inertial (mass) loads are used to study hand tremor and forearm
EMG (36):

1.   There is no rhythmic entrainment of EMG despite rhythmic oscillation
     of the limb, measured with accelerometry. The tremor frequency
     decreases when an inertial load is attached to the limb, in proportion
     to the square root of 1/inertia. This ultra-normal behavior is character-
     istic of tremor that emerges from the mechanical properties of the
     trembling hand, without a substantial contribution from the stretch
     reflex or central oscillation.
2.   Evidence of motor-unit entrainment is found in the EMG, and the fre-
     quency of the hand oscillation and EMG entrainment both decrease
     with inertial loading and are equal. Hence, the mechanical resonance
     frequency of the wrist is imposed on the EMG pattern or, in other
     words, the oscillating musculoskeletal system dictates the frequency
     of motor-unit entrainment through somatosensory feedback. Thus,
     one may conclude that the tremor is due to a stretch-reflex response
     to mechanical oscillation. Most patients with enhanced physiologic
     tremor have this pattern.
3.   The wrist oscillation and EMG entrainment have the same frequencies
     in the unloaded condition. In the loaded condition, two frequencies
     may be seen in the accelerometry: a lower-frequency oscillation
     corresponding to the mechanical-reflex resonance frequency and a
     higher-frequency oscillation with associated EMG entrainment. This
     high-frequency oscillation is interpreted as a central neurogenic oscil-
     lation because its frequency does not decrease with inertial loading and
     bears no relationship to reflex arc length (i.e., loop conduction time).

4. The wrist oscillation and EMG entrainment have the same frequency in the loaded and unloaded condition (frequency decreases <1 Hz). This result is interpreted as a sign of strong central neurogenic oscillation, with stretch-reflex and limb mechanics playing no major mechanistic role in tremor rhythmogenesis.

Most patients with moderate to severe essential tremor have pattern #4 above (30,32,38). Patients with mild to moderate tremor commonly exhibit pattern #3, but pattern #4 may occur when the neurogenic oscillation frequency is nearly the same as the mechanical resonant frequency of the wrist ($\sim$6–9 Hz) (36,37). Pattern #2 occurs when the motor-unit entrainment is so irregular and intermittent that it produces only a series of perturbations to the mechanical-reflex system, resulting in an enhanced mechanical-reflex oscillation (36,39). Pattern #1 is unequivocally normal (36). Progression from pattern #2 to pattern #4 is believed to reflect an increasing strength of central neurogenic oscillation as essential tremor progresses or is enhanced by drugs, fatigue, or other provocative maneuvers.

Pattern #3 or #4 is found in about 8% of ostensibly normal adults (37). Thus, the specificity of these patterns is 0.92. We have studied 83 people who were initially questionably abnormal (grade 1 postural and kinetic hand tremor: <1 cm amplitude) but were ultimately judged years later to have probable essential tremor. Forty-two of these patients had pattern #3 or #4 at the time of their initial exam. Thus, the sensitivity of this test for diagnosing mild essential tremor in people with questionably abnormal clinical exams is only 0.51. By contrast, all patients with clinically definite essential hand tremor (grade 2 or greater) exhibit pattern #3 or #4 (30,32,38).

Thus, the presence of pattern #3 or #4 in a person with questionably abnormal tremor is support for the diagnosis of essential tremor or some other central neurogenic action tremor. However, the absence of this pattern in questionably abnormal people cannot be interpreted as an indication of normalcy. Furthermore, it must be emphasized that patterns #3 and #4 are not specific for essential tremor and may be produced by any etiology of central neurogenic tremor, including Parkinson's disease and dystonia (40).

C. Genetic Criteria

The common view is that 50% of patients inherit essential tremor through an autosomal dominant gene, but the true prevalence of hereditary versus sporadic essential tremor is uncertain (41). Studies of autosomal dominant pedigrees have identified disease loci on chromosome 3q13 (hereditary essential tremor, type 1) and on chromosome 2p22-p25 (42,43). Additional genetic loci are likely, and no genes have been identified with certainty (44). Sporadic cases are common, and clinical subtypes probably exist, particularly in older patients (45). Thus, a family history of tremor is not used as a diagnostic criterion, and no genetic test is available.

D. Pharmacologic Criteria

Many patients report a dramatic improvement in their tremor after the consumption of ethanol, and beta-adrenergic blockers are known to be beneficial in the treatment of essential tremor. However, these effects are too unpredictable and nonspecific to be used diagnostically (1,46).

IV. DIFFERENTIAL DIAGNOSIS OF ESSENTIAL TREMOR

Other conditions are frequently mistaken for essential tremor (Table 6.3) (47). These conditions include drug- and toxin-induced tremor, cortical tremor (rhythmic cortical myoclonus), cerebellar outflow tremor (intention tremor with terminal dysmetria and other signs of ataxia), tardive tremor, focal dystonia, neuropathic tremor, posttraumatic tremor, Parkinson's disease, and psychogenic tremor. Thyrotoxicosis and hyperadrenergic states produced by systemic disease, psychiatric conditions, or drugs can cause an enhanced physiologic tremor that is clinically indistinguishable from mild essential tremor. However, the frequency of this enhanced physiologic tremor usually decreases >1 Hz when large inertial loads are applied to the limb (32,36).

Essential tremor affects both upper limbs in $>90\%$ of cases and is usually symmetric or nearly symmetric (48). The presence of unilateral or highly asymmetric tremor increases the likelihood of other diagnoses such as early Parkinson's disease or focal dystonia. Isolated head tremor should raise the suspicion of focal cervical dystonia. Tremulous cervical dystonia is often suppressed by sensory tricks (geste antagoniste), whereas essential tremor is not (49,50).

Action tremor is seen in all forms of dystonia, and the dystonia can be very difficult to appreciate when tremor is severe (2,3,8–10,51–54). Some patients with head tremor and upper extremity tremor may exhibit abnormal postures, such as head tilt, wrist extension, wrist flexion, and excessive finger flexion (e.g., during writing). In some instances, these postures are merely compensatory measures that patients use to reduce tremor, but frequently these abnormal postures are signs of underlying dystonia, as in torticollis and writer's cramp. Electrophysiologic studies are helpful in some cases (10,31,50,55,56).

Orthostatic tremor is a lower extremity tremor that occurs on standing and is produced by uniquely high-frequency 14–18 Hz bursts of motor unit activity. The upper limbs become involved if they are used for support, and the tremor rhythm is uniquely and characteristically synchronous among all four extremities (57,58).

Psychogenic tremors exhibit erratic frequency and amplitude fluctuations, and they frequently resolve and recur spontaneously. Tremor is usually reduced or abolished when the patient is distracted with motor or cognitive tasks, and the frequency of tremor changes to the frequency of voluntary repetitive movements of the ipsilateral or contralateral limb (36,59,60). These characteristics are easily captured with electrophysiologic studies (36,59,60).

Table 6.3   Differential Diagnosis of Essential Tremor (3,61)

Etiology	Tremor type and distribution	Features that are uncharacteristic of essential tremor
Thyrotoxicosis and hyperadrenergic conditions (e.g., anxiety)	Enhanced physiologic tremor, producing a mixture of mild postural and kinetic tremor, mainly in the hands but can have a more-or-less diffuse distribution	May be difficult or impossible to distinguish from mild essential tremor. The frequency of tremor and associated motor unit entrainment usually decrease more than 1 Hz when large inertial loads are applied to the limb.
Focal and task-specific tremors	Action tremor in the affected body part (e.g., in the hand or voice)	Tremor is limited to the affected body part and is specific for a particular motor act (e.g., writing, speaking)
Focal, generalized, and task-specific dystonias	Action tremor and dystonia in the affected body part(s). Action tremor also may occur in other body parts with little or no dystonia and may precede the onset of dystonia by several years.	Dystonia, which may be subtle (e.g., abnormal head tilt or hand posture)
Parkinson's disease	Mixture of rest and action tremors; occasionally, action tremor alone. Action tremor may be the sole presenting symptom and may precede other signs by several years.	Bradykinesia, rigidity, shuffling gait, hypophonia, hypomimia, pill-rolling rest tremor in the hands, rest tremor in the feet
Orthostatic tremor	Postural tremor in the torso and lower limbs while standing; may also occur in the upper limbs when leaning against a support. Produces a sense of poor balance that is relieved by walking.	High-frequency 14–18 Hz entrainment of motor unit activity that is very rhythmic and synchronous among ipsilateral and contralateral muscles
Cerebellar nuclear outflow tract lesions (deep cerebellar nuclei and brachium conjunctivum)	Intention tremor in the upper or lower limbs. There is often little postural tremor except when limb position is guided by a visual target (e.g., pointing or reaching).	Other signs of cerebellar ataxia except when the lesion is in the vicinity of the ventrolateral thalamus (e.g., a ventrolateral thalamic infarct)

(continued)

Table 6.3 *Continued*

Etiology	Tremor type and distribution	Features that are uncharacteristic of essential tremor
Fragile X premutation carrier syndrome in men	Action tremor in the upper limbs that resembles essential tremor	Ataxia, parkinsonism, peripheral neuropathy and cognitive decline beginning after age 50. T2 signal magnetic resonance imaging scan abnormalities in the middle cerebellar peduncles.
Neuropathic tremor	Postural and kinetic tremor in the involved extremities but not always in proportion to the severity of the neuropathy	Other signs of peripheral neuropathy. Visible involvement of the lower limbs and lack of involvement of the head and voice.
Toxic or drug-induced tremor	Usually a mixture of postural and kinetic tremor, but rest tremor and intention tremor may occur, depending upon the offending drug and severity of intoxication.	Irregular rhythm with asterixis and myoclonus. Diffuse and fairly uniform bodily distribution in many patients. Other systemic signs and symptoms.
Cortical tremor (a.k.a. rhythmic cortical myoclonus)	Irregular high-frequency (>7 Hz) postural and kinetic tremor associated with action myoclonus	Action myoclonus, giant somatosensory cortical-evoked potentials, and enhanced long-loop somatosensory reflexes (C-reflex)
Rubral or midbrain tremor (a.k.a. Holmes tremor)	A mixture of rest, postural, and intention tremor, usually caused by lesions in the vicinity of the red nucleus, causing an interruption of nigrostriatal and brachium conjunctival pathways	Usually associated with other signs of brainstem or cerebellar damage, most commonly produced by stroke or trauma. Typically unilateral. Frequency is 2–5 Hz.

A careful drug history is mandatory in all patients with tremor. Many drugs produce parkinsonian rest tremor (neuroleptics, metoclopramide), action tremor (beta-adrenergic agonists, valproic acid, thyroxin, tricyclic antidepressants, selective serotonin reuptake inhibitors, tocainamide, methylxanthines, and lithium), and mixed rest and action tremors (lithium, amiodarone, valproic acid, and neuroleptics) (61).

The problem of distinguishing essential tremor from other neurologic conditions is illustrated by the recent discovery that male carriers of premutations (50–200 CGG repeats) in the fragile X mental retardation 1 gene (FMR1) frequently develop an action tremor resembling essential tremor (62,63). These male carriers are typically age ≥50 years, and they commonly develop disabling action tremor, ataxia, parkinsonism, peripheral neuropathy and cognitive decline as their condition progresses. Magnetic resonance imaging scan of the head usually reveals generalized brain atrophy and T2 signal abnormalities in the middle cerebellar peduncles (64). The population frequency of the premutation carrier state in males is ∼1 in 800, so this hereditary neurodegenerative syndrome is probably underrecognized and may be incorrectly diagnosed as essential tremor. The premutation predisposes the carrier to having a child with fragile X mental retardation.

V. CONCLUSIONS

The discovery of the fragile X premutation carrier syndrome should deter those clinicians who are tempted to lump various tremor disorders under the rubric of essential tremor. Any deviation from the definition of classic essential tremor in Table 6.2 can lead to a possible misdiagnosis. The clinical characteristics of essential tremor in the upper limbs are nonspecific, and identical action tremor can be the sole presenting symptom in patients with Parkinson's disease and dystonia (8–10,26,27). Furthermore, essential tremor is common in the general population, and it will therefore occur commonly in patients with other neurologic disorders, such as Parkinson's disease, dystonia and ataxia. Classic essential tremor, as defined in Table 6.2, is a distinct clinical entity that is faithfully reproduced in families with hereditary essential tremor (42–44,65). The existence of putative subtypes, variants and related illnesses will not be resolved until we have specific genetic tests or other biologic markers for essential tremor.

ACKNOWLEDGMENTS

Supported by NS20973 from the National Institute of Neurological Disorders and Stroke and by the Spastic Research Foundation of Kiwanis International, Illinois-Eastern Iowa District.

REFERENCES

1. Findley LJ. Classification of tremors. J Clin Neurophysiol 1996; 13(2):122–132.
2. Soland VL, Bhatia KP, Volonte MA, Marsden CD. Focal task-specific tremors. Mov Disord 1996; 11(6):665–670.
3. Deuschl G, Bain P, Brin M. Consensus statement of the Movement Disorder Society on tremor. Ad Hoc Scientific Committee. Mov Disord 1998; 13(suppl 3):2–23.

4. Gerstenbrand F, Klingler D, Pfeiffer B. Der essentialle tremor, phanomenologie und epidemiologie. Nervenarzt 1983; 43:46–53.
5. Findley LJ, Gresty MA. Head, facial, and voice tremor. Adv Neurol 1988; 49:239–253.
6. Hsu YD, Chang MK, Sung SC, Hsein HH, Deng JC. Essential tremor: clinical, electromyographical and pharmacological studies in 146 Chinese patients. Chung Hua I Hsueh Tsa Chih (Taipei) 1990; 45(2):93–99.
7. Jankovic J. Essential tremor: a heterogenous disorder. Mov Disord 2002; 17(4):638–644.
8. Yanagisawa N, Goto A, Narabayashi H. Familial dystonia musculorum deformans and tremor. J Neurol Sci 1972; 16(2):125–136.
9. Rivest J, Marsden CD. Trunk and head tremor as isolated manifestations of dystonia. Mov Disord 1990; 5(1):60–65.
10. Münchau A, Schrag A, Chuang C, MacKinnon CD, Bhatia KP, Quinn NP, Rothwell JC. Arm tremor in cervical dystonia differs from essential tremor and can be classified by onset age and spread of symptoms. Brain 2001; 124(Pt 9):1765–1776.
11. Rajput AH, Rozdilsky B, Ang L, Rajput A. Significance of parkinsonian manifestations in essential tremor. Can J Neurol Sci 1993; 20(2):114–117.
12. Brooks DJ, Playford ED, Ibanez V, Sawle GV, Thompson PD, Findley LJ, Marsden CD. Isolated tremor and disruption of the nigrostriatal dopaminergic system: an 18F-dopa PET study. Neurology 1992; 42(8):1554–1560.
13. Elble RJ. Essential tremor is a monosymptomatic disorder. Mov Disord 2002; 17(4):633–637.
14. Elble RJ. The role of aging in the clinical expression of essential tremor. Experimental Gerontology 1995; 30:337–347.
15. Louis ED, Jurewicz EC, Watner D. Community-based data on associations of disease duration and age with severity of essential tremor: implications for disease pathophysiology. Mov Disord 2003; 18(1):90–93.
16. Louis ED, Barnes L, Albert SM, Cote L, Schneier FR, Pullman SL, Yu Q. Correlates of functional disability in essential tremor. Mov Disord 2001; 16(5):914–920.
17. Paulson GW. Benign essential tremor in childhood: Symptoms, pathogenesis, treatment. Clin Pediatr (Phila) 1976; 15(1):67–70.
18. Elble RJ. Tremor in ostensibly normal elderly people. Mov Disord 1998; 13(3):457–464.
19. Louis ED, Wendt KJ, Ford B. Senile tremor: what is the prevalence and severity of tremor in older adults? Gerontology 2000; 46:12–16.
20. Louis ED, Dure LSt, Pullman S. Essential tremor in childhood: a series of nineteen cases. Mov Disord 2001; 16(5):921–923.
21. Bergareche A, De La Puente E, Lopez De Munain A, Sarasqueta C, De Arce A, Poza JJ, Marti-Masso JF. Prevalence of essential tremor: a door-to-door survey in Bidasoa, Spain. Neuroepidemiology 2001; 20(2):125–128.
22. Stolze H, Petersen G, Raethjen J, Wenzelburger R, Deuschl G. The gait disorder of advanced essential tremor. Brain 2001; 124(Pt 11):2278–2286.
23. Gasparini M, Bonifati V, Fabrizio E, Fabbrini G, Brusa L, Lenzi GL, Meco G. Frontal lobe dysfunction in essential tremor: a preliminary study. J Neurol 2001; 248(5):399–402.
24. Lombardi WJ, Woolston DJ, Roberts JW, Gross RE. Cognitive deficits in patients with essential tremor. Neurology 2001; 57(5):785–790.

25. Ondo WG, Sutton L, Dat Vuong K, Lai D, Jankovic J. Hearing impairment in essential tremor. Neurology 2003; 61(8):1093–1097.
26. Farrer M, Gwinn-Hardy K, Muenter M, DeVrieze FW, Crook R, Perez-Tur J, Lincoln S, Maraganore D, Adler C, Newman S, MacElwee K, McCarthy P, Miller C, Waters C, Hardy J. A chromosome 4p haplotype segregating with Parkinson's disease and postural tremor. Hum Mol Genet 1999; 8(1):81–85.
27. Lee MS, Kim YD, Im JH, Kim HJ, Rinne JO, Bhatia KP. 123I-IPT brain SPECT study in essential tremor and Parkinson's disease. Neurology 1999; 52(7):1422–1426.
28. Fahn S, Tolosa E, Marín C. Clinical rating scale for tremor. In: Jankovic J, Tolosa E, eds. Parkinson's Disease and Movement Disorders, 2nd ed. Baltimore: Williams & Wilkins, 1993:225–234.
29. Louis ED, Ford B, Bismuth B. Reliability between two observers using a protocol for diagnosing essential tremor. Mov Disord 1998; 13(2):287–293.
30. Elble RJ. Physiologic and essential tremor. Neurology 1986; 36:225–231.
31. Valls-Sole J, Tolosa ES, Nobbe F, Dieguez E, Munoz E, Sanz P, Valldeoriola F. Neurophysiological investigations in patients with head tremor. Mov Disord 1997; 12(4):576–584.
32. Deuschl G, Krack P, Lauk M, Timmer J. Clinical neurophysiology of tremor. J Clin Neurophysiol 1996; 13(2):110–121.
33. Elble RJ, Higgins C, Leffler K, Hughes L. Factors influencing the amplitude and frequency of essential tremor [published erratum appears in Mov Disord 1995; 10(3):411]. Mov Disord 1994; 9(6):589–596.
34. Elble RJ. Essential tremor frequency decreases with time. Neurology 2000; 55(10):1547–1551.
35. Deuschl G, Elble RJ. The pathophysiology of essential tremor. Neurology 2000; 54(11):S14–S20.
36. Elble RJ, Deuschl G. Tremor. In: Brown WF, Bolton CF, Aminoff M, eds. Neuromuscular Function and Disease: Basic, Clinical, and Electrodiagnostic Aspects. Philadelphia: W. B. Saunders Co., 2002:1759–1779.
37. Elble RJ. Characteristics of physiologic tremor in young and elderly adults. Clin Neurophysiol 2003; 114(4):624–635.
38. Louis ED, Pullman SL. Comparison of clinical vs. electrophysiological methods of diagnosing of essential tremor. Mov Disord 2001; 16(4):668–673.
39. Elble RJ. Inhibition of forearm EMG by palatal myoclonus. Movement Disorders 1991; 6:324–329.
40. Hömberg V, Hefter H, Reiners K, Freund H-J. Differential effects of changes in mechanical limb properties on physiological and pathological tremor. J Neurology, Neurosurgery and Psychiatry 1987; 50:568–579.
41. Louis ED, Ottman R. How familial is familial tremor? The genetic epidemiology of essential tremor. Neurology 1996; 46(5):1200–1205.
42. Gulcher JR, Jonsson P, Kong A, Kristjansson K, Frigge ML, Karason A, Einarsdottir IE, Stefansson H, Einarsdottir AS, Sigurthoardottir S, Baldursson S, Bjornsdottir S, Hrafnkelsdottir SM, Jakobsson F, Benedickz J, Stefansson K. Mapping of a familial essential tremor gene, FET1, to chromosome 3q13. Nature Genetics 1997; 17(1):84–87.
43. Higgins JJ, Pho LT, Nee LE. A gene (ETM) for essential tremor maps to chromosome 2p22–p25. Mov Disord 1997; 12(6):859–864.

44. Kovach MJ, Ruiz J, Kimonis K, Mueed S, Sinha S, Higgins C, Elble S, Elble R, Kimonis VE. Genetic heterogeneity in autosomal dominant essential tremor. Genet Med 2001; 3(3):197–199.

45. Louis ED, Ford B, Barnes LF. Clinical subtypes of essential tremor. Arch Neurol 2000; 57(8):1194–1198.

46. Rajput AH, Jamieson H, Hirsh S, Quraishi A. Relative efficacy of alcohol and propranolol in action tremor. Can J Neurol Sci 1975; 2(1):31–35.

47. Schrag A, Münchau A, Bhatia KP, Quinn NP, Marsden CD. Essential tremor: an over-diagnosed condition? J Neurol 2000; 247(12):955–959.

48. Louis ED, Wendt KJ, Pullman SL, Ford B. Is essential tremor symmetric? Observational data from a community-based study of essential tremor. Arch Neurol 1998; 55(12):1553–1559.

49. Deuschl G, Heinen F, Kleedorfer B, Wagner M, Lucking CH, Poewe W. Clinical and polymyographic investigation of spasmodic torticollis. J Neurol 1992; 239(1):9–15.

50. Masuhr F, Wissel J, Muller J, Scholz U, Poewe W. Quantification of sensory trick impact on tremor amplitude and frequency in 60 patients with head tremor. Mov Disord 2000; 15(5):960–964.

51. Sheehy MP, Marsden CD. Writers' cramp-a focal dystonia. Brain 1982; 105(Pt 3):461–480.

52. Jedynak CP, Bonnet AM, Agid Y. Tremor and idiopathic dystonia. Mov Disord 1991; 6(3):230–236.

53. Pal PK, Samii A, Schulzer M, Mak E, Tsui JK. Head tremor in cervical dystonia. Can J Neurol Sci 2000; 27(2):137–142.

54. Hillel AD. The study of laryngeal muscle activity in normal human subjects and in patients with laryngeal dystonia using multiple fine-wire electromyography. Laryngoscope 2001; 111(4 Pt 2 suppl 97):1–47.

55. Elble RJ, Moody C, Higgins C. Primary writing tremor. A form of focal dystonia? Mov Disord 1990; 5(2):118–126.

56. Deuschl G, Heinen F, Guschlbauer B, Schneider S, Glocker FX, Lucking CH. Hand tremor in patients with spasmodic torticollis. Mov Disord 1997; 12(4):547–552.

57. Sander HW, Masdeu JC, Tavoulareas G, Walters A, Zimmerman T, Chokroverty S. Orthostatic tremor: an electrophysiological analysis. Mov Disord 1998; 13(4):735–738.

58. Köster B, Lauk M, Timmer J, Poersch M, Guschlbauer B, Deuschl G, Lucking CH. Involvement of cranial muscles and high intermuscular coherence in orthostatic tremor. Ann Neurol 1999; 45(3):384–388.

59. Kim YJ, Pakiam AS-I, Lang AE. Historical and clinical features of psychogenic tremor: a review of 70 cases. Can J Neurol Sci 1999; 26:190–195.

60. O'Suilleabhain PE, Matsumoto JY. Time-frequency analysis of tremors. Brain 1998; 121:2127–2134.

61. Elble RJ. Diagnostic criteria for essential tremor and differential diagnosis. Neurology 2000; 54(11):S2–S6.

62. Leehey MA, Munhoz RP, Lang AE, Brunberg JA, Grigsby J, Greco C, Jacquemont S, Tassone F, Lozano AM, Hagerman PJ, Hagerman RJ. The fragile X premutation presenting as essential tremor. Arch Neurol 2003; 60(1):117–121.

63. Berry-Kravis E, Lewin F, Wuu J, Leehey M, Hagerman R, Hagerman P, Goetz CG. Tremor and ataxia in fragile X premutation carriers: blinded videotape study. Ann Neurol 2003; 53(5):616–623.
64. Jacquemont S, Hagerman RJ, Leehey M, Grigsby J, Zhang L, Brunberg JA, Greco C, Des Portes V, Jardini T, Levine R, Berry-Kravis E, Brown WT, Schaeffer S, Kissel J, Tassone F, Hagerman PJ. Fragile X premutation tremor/ataxia syndrome: molecular, clinical, and neuroimaging correlates. Am J Hum Genet 2003; 72(4):869–878.
65. Bain PG, Findley LJ, Thompson PD, Gresty MA, Rothwell JC, Harding AE, Marsden CD. A study of hereditary essential tremor. Brain 1994; 117(Pt 4):805–824.

7

The Clinical Assessment of Essential Tremor

Peter G. Bain

Imperial College London, London, UK

I. INTRODUCTION

Assessment of essential tremor is fundamental to the process of developing an understanding of the condition, documenting its natural history and evaluating the effects of therapy. Although tremor is simply defined as "an involuntary rhythmical, oscillatory movement of a body part" the process of assessing essential tremor is complicated by several factors (1). These include natural predominantly amplitude variations in the tremor and the fact that essential tremor may spread from the arms to other parts of the body. There are also complex interactions between essential tremor, the sufferer, society, and the observer.

II. ESSENTIAL TREMOR—BEHAVIORAL CHARACTERISTICS

It is important to appreciate that essential tremor has natural amplitude and, to a lesser extent, frequency variability. Beat to beat amplitude fluctuations in essential tremor are apparent in drawings of Archimedes spirals (Fig. 7.1) and amplitude fluctuations of up to 50% were recorded, in spite of careful standardization of the recording conditions, in accelerometer based test-retest studies of untreated essential tremor (2).

The frequency and amplitude characteristics of essential tremor also change with different tasks, for example holding a cup, drawing a spiral or using a joystick to track a projectile (3,4). In addition, the characteristics of essential tremor are influenced by a variety of complex factors that include the experimental environment, the patient's physical, emotional, and mental state as well as the tremor's natural perturbations (5–7). This behavioral variability of essential tremor causes a problem for accurate measurements; a difficulty that becomes acute when it is necessary to know whether or not a change in tremor magnitude is the result of a specific intervention. However, the problem

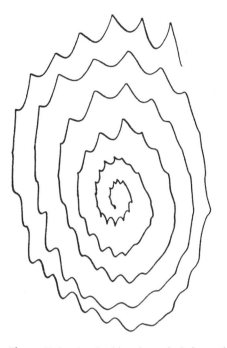

Figure 7.1 An Archimedes spiral drawn by a patient suffering from essential tremor showing natural fluctuations in tremor magnitude.

for tremor experts is that the natural behavioral fluctuations of essential tremor have not been studied in detail. This raises the practical issue of how best to obtain a representative tremor sample. There is no rigorous answer to this sampling problem. In practice clinicians compare a patient's tremor magnitude with that documented in the past. In addition the patient and their family may provide evidence from everyday activities to suggest that a significant change in tremor behavior has occurred, although this information can be clouded by poor quality observation or recall.

III. MEASURING ESSENTIAL TREMOR IN THERAPEUTIC TRIALS

It is now accepted that in order to reduce the chances of producing misleading results randomized double-blind studies are necessary for accurately assessing new and many old putative symptomatic treatments. This is particularly important in essential tremor, because problems caused by fluctuations in tremor magnitude make random allocation of patients within a therapeutic trial a virtual necessity, if bias is to be avoided. There is also a strong case for including a placebo. Even though effective treatments presently exist, it has been demonstrated that the magnitude of untreated essential tremor decreases with serial assessments, perhaps because patients become more familiar and thus more relaxed as the test situation is repeated (2). This inevitably leads to an over-estimate of the beneficial effects of trial medications unless the size of this false positive effect can be determined from the placebo response and subtracted from the effect of each active treatment (8).

Interpreting data derived from trials involving essential tremor patients is a complex task. Firstly, it is useful to consider whether bias was excluded by an adequate trial design. Secondly, the results should be examined to determine whether they are significant both from a statistical and a clinical perspective. Clearly the degree of statistical significance does not simply correlate with the degree of clinical benefit. Thirdly, it is useful to divide trial data into five categorical domains: (i) electronic-physiological indices of tremor magnitude [e.g., accelerometer or electromyographic (EMG) derived data]; (ii) impairment (i.e., tremor severity as measured by clinical rating scales or rating tremor visible in spiral drawings or handwriting); (iii) objective functional performance-test measurements (e.g., 9-hole pegboard test or the amount of water spilt from a cup); (iv) disability; and (v) social handicap or quality of life.

It is also necessary to be aware of other methodological issues that may influence the results of a tremor study, such as the timing of the tremor measurements and the precise dosage and method of drug administration. In addition, the outcome measures deployed in a study should have been assessed for reliability, validity, and responsiveness (9). Reliability estimates the capacity of an instrument (e.g., accelerometer or rating scale) to measure tremor in an accurate, reproducible and consistent way. Validity, in this context, considers whether that instrument actually reflects tremor, whilst responsiveness determines whether the instrument is sensitive to clinically important changes in essential tremor severity.

IV. CLINICAL MEASUREMENT OF IMPAIRMENT, DISABILITY, AND SOCIAL HANDICAP CAUSED BY ESSENTIAL TREMOR

Clinical methods for quantifying tremor severity are cheap, quick, and easy to perform, which allows them to be widely deployed. Furthermore, these simple methods provide readily comprehensible indices of tremor severity, which is perhaps their most significant advantage over physiological techniques. Disease specific clinical instruments presently exist for documenting impairments caused by essential tremor as well as its impact on patients in terms of disability and to a lesser extent social handicap. There are also generic instruments for measuring quality of life, which can also be applied to patients with essential tremor.

A. Subjective Clinical Measures of Tremor

1. Clinical Rating Scales for Essential Tremor

A variety of tremor rating scale designs have been used in therapeutic trials for measuring changes in the magnitude of essential tremor. There has been little discussion about their relative merits and the composition of these scales has differed considerably. Nevertheless, certain points should be considered:

First, the severity of tremor should obviously be related to the parts of the body that are affected;

Second, information is lost if tremors from different anatomical sites are averaged;

Third, scoring tremor magnitude separately for different tremor components (e.g., postural or kinetic tremor) makes sense, as these components have different influences on resultant disability and social handicap;

Fourth, an analogue scale has mathematical advantages over one that is based on discrete steps and finally, the number of steps within a discrete-step scale should be optimized, because the number of gradations on the scale influences reliability.

Scales with few gradations (e.g., a 0–3 scale) are easier to score than those with a greater number of increments (e.g., a 0–10 scale). However, increasing the number of steps also decreases the significance of a "unit" error, so that true score variance is altered advantageously for reliability (10–12).

Presently there is only one tremor-specific rating scale that incorporates these design features (Appendix 1) (12). This scale was designed by Bain and colleagues and was chosen after experimenting with various alternative designs because raters found it easy to use. It is an analog (0–10) tremor impairment scale in which the magnitudes of the various tremor components are scored separately for each limb and, if appropriate, other body parts. The scale includes a supplementary mild-moderate-severe framework to facilitate scoring. It has been tested for validity and inter- and intra-rater reliability, using Cohen's kappa coefficients (3,12,13). The results of these evaluations showed that the tremor scores assigned by raters employing this scale correlated well with patient self-assessments of their own tremor-related disability, and that the reliability of the scoring was good (12). The degree of agreement between raters' scores was found to be in the moderate to almost perfect range for postural tremor of the upper limbs and head tremor (12).

One other tremor-specific rating scale, produced by Fahn, Tolosa, and Marin, is widely deployed and has been evaluated for reliability (Appendix 2) (14). It is a complex multi-modal scale that includes ratings of tremor impairment (on a discrete 5-point scale) as well as tremor-induced disability and social handicap (14). It is divided into three sub-sections that reflect (a) tremor impairment (intrinsically weighted for upper limb tremor), (b) functional tasks (writing, drawing and pouring water), and (c) disability and social handicap (Appendix 2). However, this scale saturates at tremor amplitudes of >2 cm and consequently is unsuitable for studies involving patients with severe essential tremor. This ceiling effect is much less of a problem for rating essential tremor with the scale designed by Bain and colleagues (12,14).

2.   Spirographic and Handwriting Analysis

It is a simple matter to obtain specimens of handwriting and spirals from tremulous patients. Therefore it would be convenient if the tremor apparent in a spiral or piece of handwriting could be scored reliably, particularly if the score correlated with tremor invoked disability. Fortunately, this is the case for essential tremor (3,12). Typically patients are instructed to draw a spiral (from inside to out) with each hand in turn, whilst holding the pen held in a normal way (rather than at the top), as spirography is rather over-sensitive to fine tremors even when the pen is held normally (12,13). The tremor visible in a spiral can then be scored independently by "blinded" raters, using a 0–10 subjective scoring system (3,12,13). The inter-rater and intra-rater reliability of this method of scoring essential tremor with spirals is good (12). Furthermore, the spiral scores correlate with those obtained with a tremor rating scale, patient self-assessments of tremor induced disability and the magnitude of upper limb tremor measured by uni-axial accelerometry (12). The process of scoring essential tremor with spirals can be facilitated by cross-referencing a published collection of previously rated spirals (13).

There is no particular advantage in rating tremor in handwriting rather than spirals, as the latter are easier to score (12,13). However, handwriting specimens can often be obtained retrospectively from old work and thus can be particularly useful for following the natural history of essential tremor.

B.   Objective Functional Performance Tests

For patients with essential tremor functional performance tests provide objective measures of impaired upper limb function (focal disability). These techniques include the volumetric method, Gibson maze test and the nine-hole pegboard test.

1.   Volumetric Methods

There are two common variants of the volumetric method: (a) pouring water from one cup to another (a bimanual kinetic tremor test) (14) or (b) simply holding a cup of water for a specified time (which tests for unilateral postural tremor) (3,15). In the latter version of this test the patients are asked to hold a 100 mL plastic beaker full of water between the thumb and fingers with the elbow supported and flexed by $\sim 20°$, with the forearm in a semi-prone position and slightly elevated, as if about to raise the cup to drink. The volume of water remaining in the beaker after one minute is measured. This test is usually carried out three times for each hand and the mean for each hand is recorded (3). Furthermore, the method has been validated for patients with essential tremor as the data obtained by this method correlated with that obtained by spiral ratings and accelerometry (3). However, the volumetric method is insensitive to fine tremors and there is a ceiling effect when all the water is spilt (3,13–15). It can also be quite messy, particularly for patients with severe essential tremor. The volumetric method also allows "start-up time" (the time from the start of the test to first spilling water) to be measured, which provides insight into the patients' ability to suppress their tremor in the temporal domain (3,13).

A "hybrid" performance-based test of arm function was developed by Louis and colleagues for use in essential tremor and has been assessed for validity (16). This test involves 15 tasks, including pouring liquid, drinking from a glass, using a soup-spoon, carrying glasses on a tray, writing, putting different types of objects in various receptacles, using a touch-tone phone, using screwdrivers, threading a needle, and doing up eight buttons on a shirt. These functional tasks were separately scored with a 5-point scale (0: no difficulty; 1: mild difficulty; 2: moderate difficulty; 3: severe difficulty; 4: unable to perform task) by an observer (16). The test takes ~10 minutes to perform and the results correlate with those obtained with a tremor disability questionnaire, ratings of a videotaped examination, and quantitative computerized tremor analysis (16). However, the intricate nature of many of the tasks involved in this test would result in a low ceiling effect, making it more useful for assessing patients with mild essential tremor.

2.   The 9-Hole Pegboard Test

The 9-hole pegboard test is a reliable test of upper limb function (focal disability). The results can be recorded as the time taken to insert all 9 pegs or the average time taken to place each peg into a hole. Normal controls average ~2 seconds to place each peg (17). It is useful for documenting the impact of essential tremor on arm function. However, the results are influenced by factors other than tremor, for example co-existing arthritis or poor vision and the method is rather insensitive to fine tremors.

3.   The Gibson Maze Test

The Gibson maze test, which is a quantifiable form of spiral drawings, can be used to grade essential tremor severity (18,19). The patient is instructed to draw a line through a printed spiral maze, starting at the arrow in the center and aiming to get out via the maze's pathway without touching the spiral's printed boundaries or circular obstacles. The number of times the patient's drawn line touches one of these obstructions is scored, which gives the test objectivity. However, it is too subtle for some patients with severe essential tremor and it is affected by other co-morbidities.

C.   Assessing the Impact of Essential Tremor on Patients' Lives

The impact of essential tremor on patients' lives can be assessed in a variety of ways, including measures of disability, social handicap, and quality of life (Table 7.1). Although these entities do not measure tremor magnitude directly, they can illustrate the effect of essential tremor on patients' lives, which is important from a clinical perspective. An occupation involving fine manual work will be more disrupted by essential tremor than one requiring simple heavy labor.

Table 7.1 Simple Clinical Methods for Assessing Tremor Severity

---

Subjective clinical measures of tremor:
Clinical rating scales for essential tremor
Rating essential tremor with spirals
Rating essential tremor with handwriting

Objective functional performance tests:
Water spilt from a cup
9-hole pegboard test
Gibson maze

Impact of essential tremor on patients' lives:
Disability scales (essential tremor specific)
Handicap questionnaire (essential tremor specific)
Quality of life (generic instruments)

However, a patient with low amplitude essential tremor might be more embarrassed by it than someone with a tremor of greater amplitude; the response depending on personality and the society in which they mingle. Nevertheless a generic problem with this type of assessment is that they may be affected by concurrent symptoms or illness. In addition the distinction between measures of disability, social handicap, and quality of life are rather vague.

1. Disability Questionnaires

Disability is the difficulty that a patient encounters in performing their activities of daily living (ADL) (the loss of function caused by an impairment) and can be quantified using either generic or disease specific disability questionnaires, the latter tending to be more sensitive to the target condition. However, the reliability of this type of questionnaire depends on patients being able to give an accurate account of their own physical disability, which may not always be the case; particularly if there is co-existing cognitive impairment.

Examining ADL questionnaires designed specifically for essential tremor patients reveals that the main conundrum inherent in this method of assessment is the issue of what items should be incorporated within the questionnaire (12–14,20). In particular, what proportions of the questionnaire should reflect dominant hand function, bimanual function, toileting, mobility or other disabilities and how should these be relatively weighted? The main objective being to provide essential tremor patients with a questionnaire that is readily understood and which can be transcribed into numerical values for statistical analysis. There have been three major attempts to achieve this aim: the first comprises section C of the Fahn, Tolosa, Marin scale (14) (see Appendix 2); the second a tremor specific disability self-questionnaire shown in Appendix 3 (12) and the third another, rather similar, tremor specific disability questionnaire shown in

Appendix 4 (20). The Fahn, Tolosa, Marin scale uses both patients' and observers' scores, whilst the latter two instruments use patients' ratings only. Nevertheless data obtained from essential tremor patients with each of the latter two instruments correlated well with physicians' scores of tremor severity (12,20). However, correlations with the results of electronic-physiological tests, for example accelerometry, have been less robust probably because the relationship between tremor magnitude and tremor related disability is logarithmic and not linear (12,20,21).

2. Social Handicap

Social Handicap, which is the social and societal consequences of having a specific set of disabilities, can also be quantified and as far as the patient is concerned determines the real severity of essential tremor, as patients can have significant social handicap in spite of relatively minor disability; a not infrequent occurrence in clinical practice. For example, some patients find their head tremor more embarrassing than an upper limb tremor, even if the latter is of greater amplitude because it is more easily masked. Only one instrument has been specifically developed to study social handicap in essential tremor patients. It is largely qualitative and was used in a study of hereditary essential tremor to explore whether or not patients thought that they were handicapped by physical disability or the embarrassment caused by their tremors or both (see Appendix 5) (6,12,13).

3. Quality of Life Measures

Whether or not quality of life is a different entity to disability and/or social handicap is a matter of debate, as there does not appear to be a unifying concept underlying the most commonly deployed "quality of life" instruments, which may include measures of impairment, disability, and social handicap (17). Literally "quality of life" suggests a positive entity, whilst disability and social handicap imply a negative or disadvantaged state. It would be reasonable to propose that the term "quality of life" is used to represent the patients' overall subjective impressions of the state of their own lives, whilst handicap is a negative measure of the deficiencies in their quality of life. Thus if a patient scored 75% on a "quality of life" scale, in which normality was 100%, the resultant social handicap would be 25% (i.e., 100–75%). However, if this definition were to be generally accepted it would exclude most of the presently available "quality of life" instruments, which impose the designer's sense of values on patients and include items that address disability and impairment. However, the SEIQoL-DW allows patients to choose their own assessment domains and weight them according to their own perspective, but this scale has not been tested on patients with essential tremor (22).

V. PHYSIOLOGICAL OUTCOME MEASURES

The main physiological techniques used to measure essential tremor are shown in Table 7.2. There is no single ubiquitous solution as there are advantages and disadvantages to each of the techniques commonly employed.

A. Accelerometer Based Methods

Tremors can be quantified in terms of the frequency and magnitude of the oscillatory cycles. These parameters are usually measured using linear accelerometers, which are small piezo-resistive electronic devices that can be attached to the body. It requires at least six one-dimensional transducers to measure all the translational and rotational movement components of a limb (23,24). Nevertheless because essential tremor has higher frequency and lower amplitude characteristics than voluntary limb movements, linear accelerometers are the most widely used transducers for measuring essential tremor. Accelerometers are preferable to displacement and velocity transducers as they are more sensitive to higher frequency vibrations and introduce less noise (which is amplified by differentiation of velocity or displacement signals) (25). The accelerometers used in clinical practice are either uni-axial or tri-axial, the latter being preferable (26,27). Typically their sensitivity is of the order of $0.5-5 \text{ mV}/\text{ms}^{-2}$ with flat frequency responses from DC to $>100 \text{ Hz}$ (3,23–25). It is customary to process the signal to produce an average of several ($\sim 5-10$) overlapping spectra derived from overlapping samples of tremor within a one minute period which display the root mean square (RMS) magnitude of frequency components as a function of frequency (3,12). Typically the spectra range from DC—50 Hz with 500 lines of spectral resolution and about 100 dB dynamic range. For moderate to severe essential tremor the averaged spectrum has a single dominant peak and the dominant frequency of the tremor is taken as the frequency of the largest peak. Similarly the magnitude of RMS acceleration at the main peak is taken and can be converted into displacement

Table 7.2 Physiological Techniques for Measuring Essential Tremor

---

Physiological techniques:
Accelerometers
Electromyography (short- or long-term)
Mechanical systems
Kinematic measurement systems
Gyroscopic techniques
Computer tracking tasks
Graphic digitizing tablets

---

arithmetically, using the formula:

$$\text{Displacement} = \frac{\text{acceleration}}{4\pi^2 f^2}$$

where f is the tremor frequency. However, some judgement may be necessary in identifying the principal peak as in some cases there can be several harmonics of comparable size. For mild essential tremor the averaged spectrum typically has significant components at a broad spread of frequencies reflecting its multiple component origins, as is the case for normal physiological tremor (3,28,29). In this situation it is preferable to have an estimate of all the frequency components. The total power content of the spectrum should be measured by calculating the sum of the squares of all the frequency components (30). The spectrum can also be transformed to a velocity spectrum which has a total power content proportional to the kinetic energy dissipated by the tremor [$1/2 \times$ (mass of limb) $\times$ (velocity)^2].

However, there are several problems associated with accelerometer based measurements:

Firstly, the low frequency high displacement components of a tremor are the events most likely to disrupt a piece of work but produce little effect on the dominant peak of averaged auto-spectra.

Secondly, postural tremor magnitude measured by uni-axial accelerometers correlated poorly with patients' self-reported disability, possibly because the relationship is logarithmic (12,21).

Thirdly, performing a fast-Fourier transform (FFT) on a signal obtained from an essential tremor patient with an intention tremor is not ideal because the finger-nose-finger-test takes $\sim$2 seconds to perform (providing $\sim$10 tremor cycles) during which tremor amplitude escalates. This causes a nonstationary signal that in turn results in an inaccurate FFT.

B.   Electromyographic Recordings

1.   Short-Term Recordings

The EMG activity accompanying essential tremor may be recorded by pairs of silver/silver chloride electrodes arranged over the surface of tremulous muscles. Typically essential tremor is recorded for $\sim$1 minute and the EMG signal is amplified, filtered and if desired rectified before the bursts are measured from records stored on paper or computer. The amplitude of the EMG is inversely proportional to the distance between the motor unit and the electrode (31). The resultant rectified-filtered EMG is proportional to muscle force during static and dynamic muscular contractions and is proportional to the force fluctuations caused by tremor (32–35). However, the relationships between rectified-filtered EMG, muscle force and movement are significantly nonlinear (31,36). The extent of nonlinearity is a function of muscle type and measurement technique

(31,36). Thus the amplitude of the rectified-filtered (demodulated) EMG bursts is only a surrogate measure of essential tremor amplitude and is a reflection of the number of motor units producing tremor (37). The signal can also be processed in a similar way to that obtained from accelerometers to produce a spectrum of the magnitude of the frequency components of the EMG against frequency (38).

2.   Long-Term Electromyographic Recordings

A system using a portable cassette recorder coupled to surface EMG electrodes has been developed for obtaining 24 hour EMG samples of patients with essential tremor (37,39,40). This technique attempts to overcome the problem of obtaining representative tremor samples. It can be used to measure tremor occurrence rate, which is the proportion of time that rhythmic EMG activity occurs during a specified period, as well as the average EMG magnitude and tremor frequency over a given epoch. Tremor occurrence rate has been shown to correlate with clinical ratings of essential tremor severity (39,40). The technique has the considerable merit of assessing patients during their normal activities rather than in an artificial laboratory environment, where patients may (at least initially) be unduly tense and anxious. It also allows diurnal variations of tremor magnitude to be measured.

C.   Mechanical and Optically Based Systems

The earliest systems used for recording human tremor were mechanical and measured displacement with a tambour applied to the tremulous limb. Displacement of the tambour was transmitted through mechanical levers to produce a permanent record of the tremor on a rotating smoked drum (41). More recently a mechanical linkage device was devised to measure the three-dimensional position of the fingertip during postural tremor (21). The device accurately captured the three-dimensional movement associated with postural tremor in essential tremor. The measures derived from the device were: mean 3D-velocity, mean 3D-acceleration and mean 3D-dispersion. The logarithms of these measures strongly correlated with those obtained by clinical tremor ratings and self-reported tremor related disability and were shown to have good test-retest reliability (21). The performance of the device was superior to uni-axial accelerometry, probably because the former captured movement in three-dimensions. However, the device has limitations caused by nonlinear filtering effects that particularly effect high amplitude tremors and the authors concluded that the 0–10 clinical rating scale devised by Bain and colleagues performed as well or better than the device (13,21).

D.   Kinematic Measurement Systems

The limitations of these techniques to the measurement of rest or postural tremors led to the development of systems for studying kinetic tremor, for example that seen during the finger-nose-finger test. Subsequent developments have led to systems that have a minimum of two computer controlled cameras which can produce real time digital coordinates of the movement of several infra-red or light-emitting diodes on the patient (42,43). The best systems are portable and have sampling rates of 50 or 100 Hz, which is well above the required Nyquist folding frequencies for essential tremor and is thus sufficient to capture essential tremor without aliasing. However, data analysis is time consuming and presently there is scant experience with these systems in therapeutic studies. The continuing refinement of motion analysis systems may lead to more efficient ways of quantifying the kinetic/intention components of essential tremor that cannot be captured accurately with accelerometers.

E. Gyroscopic Techniques

Miniature solid state "gyroscopes" that sense rate of limb and trunk rotation have been adapted for measuring tremor (44). One device (Systron model QRS-11) weighs 26 g and measures 40 mm in diameter and 13 mm in height. It utilizes a vibrating quartz tuning fork that generates a torque when rotated around a predetermined axis (axis of symmetry). A second quartz fork is rigidly attached to the first and acts as a piezoelectric transducer that senses the torque, converting it into a voltage proportional to the rate of angular rotation and thereby acting as a gyroscope. The advantage of this method over standard accelerometer based systems is that the latter are affected by gravity (9.81 ms^{-2}), because as the axes of a linear accelerometer oscillate around the gravitational vector a component of gravity is recorded at tremor frequency. This causes a measurement error, which varies according to the angle between the gravitational vector and the accelerometer's axis. However, the bulk of the Systron device makes it unsuitable for recording digital tremor. It is also quite delicate and costly.

F. Computerized Tracking Tasks

Computerized tracking tasks have been used to quantify the severity of essential tremor (3). The tracking task was designed to provide a two-dimensional eye-hand coordination test, which involves patients tracking a target across an oscilloscope screen using a joystick control. The objective is to maintain superimposition of the tracking projectile on the target for the 1 minute duration of the sweep. The joystick is mounted on the arm of a chair and is held between the thumb and fingers of the hand with the forearm supported. It is thus predominantly sensitive to a visually dependent feedback form of kinetic tremor (as there is some hand movement), which causes vertical disparity between the target and tracking projectile. The tracking error being characterized by the integral of the modulus of the distance of the tracking projectile trace from a 1 mm deep neutral zone about the target trace (3). The technique is elegant because it measures the error produced by a tremor during a useful manual task.

G. Digitizing Tablets

The use of commercially available digitizing tablets for the measurement of the frequency and severity of essential tremor present during writing and drawing is receiving increasing attention (4,45). Digitizing tablets are much less expensive than EMG or accelerometer based techniques (<10% of the cost) and the signal does not require amplification. They can be used to measure tremor during writing and drawing. Furthermore, the results of inter-trial variability studies performed on 87 patients with essential tremor showed that the results obtained with a digitizing tablet were comparable to those produced by tri-axial accelerometers (45). The study also confirmed the observation by Bain and colleagues that the frequency and amplitude of essential tremor changed significantly with different tasks, with a tendency for tremor frequencies to constrict during kinetic tasks compared to a maintained posture (3,45).

VI. CONCLUSION

Essential tremors are highly complex phenomena that vary continuously with the patients' state of activity. The parameters of tremor alter from beat to beat and from minute to minute making assessment of severity a complex task. However, quantifying essential tremor severity is necessary if its natural history and the influence of treatment are to be comprehended. It is now possible to measure essential tremor and its impact on the patient in a multi-dimensional way that includes electrophysiological techniques, clinical rating scales, simple objective tests of limb function, and measures of disability, social handicap, and quality of life. Patient disability self-questionnaires provide meaningful results in terms of deciding whether or not a particular treatment has actually helped essential tremor patients with their activities of daily living, although "quality of life" or social handicap measures are perhaps the most important from the patients' perspectives. However, in spite of the importance of these measures a great deal of further research is required to produce optimal disability, social handicap and quality of life questionnaires for essential tremor patients. Similarly the design of impairment rating scales for essential tremor needs further scrutiny. The main advantage of these simple measures over physiological techniques is that statistically significant changes are likely to mean something to patients.

Selection of an optimal physiological technique to accompany the clinical methods depends critically on the component of essential tremor being assessed. The use of accelerometers is a reasonable way of quantifying the postural component of essential tremor but is less satisfactory for the intention component, which would be better captured with a three-dimensional motion analysis system, whilst a graphic digitizing tablet is a reliable and validated method for measuring the magnitude of essential tremor during drawing and writing (4,45). Long-term ambulatory EMG recordings provide a solution to the sampling problem and allow essential tremor to be recorded in the patients' normal environment. The main outcome measure of this approach is tremor

Table 7.3   Essential Tremor: Results of Three Randomized Controlled Studies of Primidone [Modified From Ref. (8)]

Studies of primidone	No. cases	Dosage mg/day	Statistical significance	Accel.	Impair. scales	Perf. tests	Disab.	Social handicap
Findley et al. 1985 (47)	22	750 mg	p < 0.01	56%	28%	24%	NA	NA
Koller et al. 1986 (48)	12	250 mg	p < 0.01	55%	NQ	0%	0%	0%
Sasso et al. 1988 (49)	13	750 mg	p < 0.05	NA	16%	9%	NA	NA

Note: NA, not assessed; NP, not published; NQ, not quantified; Accel, accelerometry; Impairm, impairment; perf, performance; disab, disability.

occurrence rate, which ultimately measures what proportion of time a tremulous muscle is active, because essential tremor is an action tremor. However, occurrence rate or averaged tremor magnitude do not describe the behavior of essential tremor when it most matters. A point that was nicely illustrated by Jager and King (46); who described a man with marked hereditary essential tremor who was able to shoot deer with a rifle at a hundred yards because he was temporarily able to suppress his tremor.

A comprehensive review of the published data on controlled therapeutic trials involving patients with essential tremor showed that the effect of medication (including primidone and propranolol) on tremor may have been over-estimated, as a 50% reduction in acceleration did not translate into a similar alleviation of disability or social handicap (8). There was a progressive decline in the apparent benefit produced by anti-essential tremor medications when the benefit was measured in terms of social handicap, disability or functional performance tests compared to electrophysiological parameters or clinical ratings of impairment (8). Table 7.3 illustrates this effect for primidone.

This fall off in efficacy as the measurement instrument becomes more realistic is termed a "detractor" effect, a term that describes the relationships between impairment (tremor) and the objective disability or social handicap that it produces (8). These relationships may have a complex shape depending on the precise behavioral characteristics of tremor. In order to more fully understand the impact of essential tremor upon patients the shapes of the detractors require further study. In the meantime clinical trials that use multi-dimensional clinical evaluations are to be strongly recommended.

REFERENCES

1. Deuschl G, Bain PG, Brin M, Ad Hoc Scientific Committee of the Movement Disorder Society. Consensus-statement of the movement disorder society on tremor. Mov Disord 1998; 13(suppl 3):2–23.

2. Cleeves L, Findley LJ. Variability in amplitude of untreated essential tremor. J Neurol Neurosurg Psychiatry 1987; 50:704–708.
3. Bain PG, Mally J, Gresty MA, Findley LJ. Assessing the impact of essential tremor on upper limb function. J Neurol 1993; 241:54–61.
4. Elble RJ, Sinha R, Higgins C. Quantification of tremor with a digitizing tablet. J Neuroscience Methods 1990; 32:193–198.
5. Deuschl G, Koster B, Scheidt C. Diagnostic criteria and clinical course of psychogenic tremors. Mov Disord 1998; 13:294–302.
6. Bain PG, Findley LJ, Thompson PD, Gresty MA, Rothwell JC, Harding AE, Marsden CD. A study of hereditary essential tremor. Brain 1994; 117:805–824.
7. Critchley M. Observations on essential (heredofamilial) tremor. Brain 1949: 72:113–139.
8. Bain PG. The effectiveness of treatments for essential tremor. The neurologist 1997; 3:305–321.
9. Hobart JC, Lamping DL, Thompson AJ. Evaluating neurological outcome measures: the bare essentials. J Neurol Neurosurg Psychiatry 1996; 60:127–130.
10. Landy FJ, Farr JL. Performance rating. Psychol Bull 1980; 87:72–107.
11. Nunnally JC. Psychometric Theory. New York: McGraw Hill, 1978:Chapter 15.
12. Bain PG, Findley LJ, Atchison P, Behari M, Vidailhet M, Gresty MA, Rothwell JC, Thompson PD, Marsden CD. Assessing tremor severity. J Neurol Neurosurg Psychiatry 1993; 56:868–873.
13. Bain PG, Findley LJ. Assessing Tremor Severity. London: Smith-Gordon, 1993.
14. Fahn S, Tolosa E, Marin C. Clinical rating scale for tremor. In: Jankovic J, Tolosa E, eds. Parkinson's Disease and Movement Disorders. Baltimore-Munich: Urban & Schwarzenberg, 1988:225–234.
15. Mally J. Aminophylline and essential tremor. Lancet 1989; 2:278–279.
16. Louis ED, Wendt KJ, Albert SM, Pullman SL, Yu Q, Andrews H. Validity of a performance-based test of function in essential tremor. Arch Neurol 1999; 56:841–846.
17. Wade DT. Measurement in Neurological rehabilitation. Oxford: Oxford University Press, 1992:171.
18. Gibson HB. The spiral maze: a psychomotor test with implications for the study of delinquency. Br J Psychol 1964; 55:219–225.
19. Morgan MH, Langton-Hewer R, Cooper R. Effect of beta adrenergic blocking agent propranolol on essential tremor. J Neurol Neurosurg Psychiatry 1973; 36:618–624.
20. Louis ED, Barnes LF, Wendt KJ, Albert SM, Pullman SL, Yu Q, Schneider FR. Validity and test-retest reliability of a disability questionnaire for essential tremor. Mov Disord 2000; 15:516–523.
21. Matsumoto JY, Dodick DW, Stevens LN, Newman RC, Caskey PE, Fjerstad W. Three-dimensional measurement of essential tremor. Mov Disord 1997; 14:288–294.
22. O'Boyle CA, Browne JP, McGee HM, Hickey A, Joyce CRB. Manual for the SEIQoL-DW. Dublin: Department of Psychology, Royal College of Surgeons of Ireland, 1996.
23. Padgaonker AJ, Krieger KW, King AI. Measurement of angular acceleration of a rigid body using linear accelerometers. J Appl Mech (Trans ASME) 1975; 42:552–556.

24. Gilbert JA, Maxwell GM, McElhaney JH, Clippinger FW. A system to measure the forces and movements at the knee and hip during level walking. J Orth Res 1984; 2:281–288.
25. Ladin Z, Flowers WC, Messner W. A quantitative comparison of a position measurement system and accelerometry. J Biomech 1989; 22:295–308.
26. Frost JD. Triaxial vector accelerometry: a method for quantitatifying tremor and ataxia. IEEE Trans Biomed Eng 1978; 25:17–27.
27. Jankovic J, Frost JD. Quantitative assessment of parkinsonian and essential tremor: clinical application of triaxial accelerometry. Neurology 1981; 31:1235–1240.
28. Bain PG. A combined clinical and neurophysiological approach to the study of patients with tremor. J Neurol Neurosurg Psychiatry 1993; 56:839–844.
29. Marsden CD. Origins of normal and pathological tremor. In: Findley LJ, Capildeo R, eds. Movement Disorders: Tremor. London: Macmillan Press, 1987:37–55.
30. Gresty MA, Findley LJ. Definition, analysis and genesis of tremor. In: Findley LJ, Capildeo R, eds. Movement Disorders: Tremor. London: Macmillan Press, 1984:15–26.
31. Basmajian JV, De Luca CJ. Muscles Alive: Their Functions Revealed by Electromyography. Baltimore: Williams and Wilkins, 1985.
32. Lippold OCJ. The relation between integrated action potentials in a human muscle and its isometric tension. J Physiol (Lond) 1952; 117:492–499.
33. Bouisset S, Maton B. Quantitative relationship between surface EMG and intramuscular electromyographic activity in voluntary movement. Am J Phys Med 1972; 51:285–295.
34. Bigland B, Lippold OCJ. Motor unit activity in voluntary contraction of human muscle. J Physiol (Lond) 1954; 125:322–335.
35. Elble RJ, Randall JE. Motor unit activity responsible for 8- to 12-Hz component of human physiological finger tremor. J Neurophysiol 1976; 39:370–383.
36. Solomonow M, Baratta R, Zhou BH. The EMG force model of electrically stimulated muscles: dependence on control strategy and predominant fiber composition. IEEE Trans Biomed Eng 1987; 34:692–703.
37. Bacher M, Scholz E, Diener HC. 24 continuous EMG tremor quantification based on EMG recording. Electroencephalogr Clin Neurophysiol 1989; 72:176–183.
38. Elble RJ, Koller WC (eds). Tremor. Baltimore and London: Johns Hopkins University Press, 1990:28–32.
39. Spieker S, Jentgens C, Boose A, Dichgans J. Reliability, specificity, and sensitivity of long-term tremor recordings. Electroencephalogr Clin Neurophysiol 1995; 97:326–331.
40. Spieker S, Strole V, Sailer A, Boose A, Dichgans J. Validity of long-term tremor electromyography in the quantification of tremor. Mov Disord 1997; 12:985–991.
41. Lanska DJ. 19th-Century American contributions to the recording of tremors. Mov Disord 2000; 720–729.
42. Findley LJ, Gresty MA, Halmagyi M. A novel method of recording arm movements. A study of common abnormalities. Arch Neurol 1981; 38:38–42.
43. Steg G, Ingvarsson PE, Johnels B, Valls M, Thorselius M. Objective measurement of motor disability in Parkinson's disease. Acta Neurol Scanda 1989; 126:67–75.

44. Tetrud J, Felsing G, Sunnarborg D, Delimeier W. Assessment of tremor using a solid-state angular rate sensor. Presented at 45th American Academy of Neurology, New York, May 1993.
45. Elble RJ, Brilliant M, Leffler K, Higgins C. Quantification of essential tremor in writing and drawing. Mov Disord 1996; 11:70–78.
46. Jager BV, King T. Hereditary tremor. Arch Int Med 1955; 95:788–793.
47. Findley LJ, Cleeves L, Calzetti S. Primidone in essential tremor of the hands and head: a double-blind controlled clinical study. J Neurol Neurosurg Psychiatry 1985; 48:911–915.
48. Koller WC, Biary N, Cone S. Disability in essential tremor. Effect of treatment. Neurology 1986; 36:1001–1004.
49. Sasso E, Perucca E, Calzetti S. Double-blind comparison of primidone and phenobarbital in essential tremor. Neurology 1988; 38:808–810.

APPENDIX 1—TREMOR SEVERITY RATING SCALE

Tremor severity rating scale designed by Bain and colleagues [modified from Ref. (12)] showing a postural tremor and intention tremor component of essential tremor affecting the patients right arm that have been scored grades 4 and 2 respectively. The tremor components in other parts of the body, for example left arm, legs, voice, and head can be scored in a similar fashion.

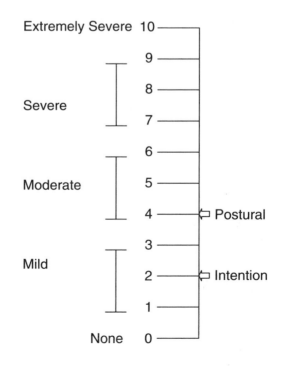

APPENDIX 2—FAHN, TOLOSA, MARIN TREMOR RATING SCALE

Fahn, Tolosa, and Marin tremor scale [modified from Ref. (14)]. Items 1–21 are all scored on a 0–4 scale (14). The maximum possible score is 144.

Part A: Tremor impairment

Tremor of:	Rest	Posture	Act/Int	Total
1 Face			xxxxx	
2 Tongue			xxxxx	
3 Voice	xxxxx	xxxxx		
4 Head			xxxxx	
5 R arm				
6 L arm				
7 Trunk			xxxxxx	
8 R leg				
9 L leg				
Subtotal A:				

Part B: Handwriting, drawing, and pouring

Handwriting:
10 A dated sample of the patient's best handwriting.

Drawings:
11-12 Draw a spiral on the figures provided, without crossing the lines, with the right and then left hand.
13 Draw straight lines on the figure provided, without crossing the lines, with the right and then left hand.

Pouring:
14 Water is poured from one cup to another.

	Right	Left	Total
10 Handwriting		dominant only	
11 Drawing A			
12 Drawing B			

	Right	Left	Total
13 Drawing C			
14 Pouring			
Subtotal B:			

Part C: Functional disabilities due to tremor

15 Speaking	
16 Eating	
17 Drinking	
18 Hygiene	
19 Dressing	
20 Writing	
21 Working	
Subtotal C:	

Global assessment by examiner:
0: no functional disability
1: mild disability   (1–24% impaired)
2: moderate disability   (25–49% impaired)
3: marked disability   (50–74% impaired)
4: severe disability   (75–100% impaired)

Global assessment by patient:
0: no functional disability
1: mild disability   (1–24% impaired)
2: moderate disability   (25–49% impaired)
3: marked disability   (50–74% impaired)
4: severe disability   (75–100% impaired)

Subjective assessment by patient compared to last visit:
+3:   marked improvement   (50–100% improved)
+2:   moderate improvement   (25–49% improved)
+1:   mild improvement   (10–24% improved)

0:	unchanged	
−1:	mild worsening	(10–24% worse)
−2:	moderate worsening	(25–49% worse)
−3:	marked worsening	(50–100% worse)

APPENDIX 3—ACTIVITIES OF DAILY LIVING QUESTIONNAIRE

Activities of Daily Living Questionnaire [Modified from Ref. (12)]

The patient is asked to put a circle around the number (from 0 to 3) that most appropriately reflects the degree of difficulty encountered with each task (6,12,13):

Key: 0   Able to do the activity without difficulty.
       1   Able to do the activity with a little effort.
       2   Able to do the activity with a lot of effort.
       3   Cannot do the activity by yourself.

Disability Questionnaire

1	Cut food with a knife and fork.	0	1	2	3
2	Use a spoon to drink soup.	0	1	2	3
3	Hold a cup of tea.	0	1	2	3
4	Pour milk from a bottle or carton.	0	1	2	3
5	Wash and dry dishes.	0	1	2	3
6	Brush your teeth	0	1	2	3
7	Use a handkerchief to blow your nose.	0	1	2	3
8	Take a bath.	0	1	2	3
9	Use the lavatory.	0	1	2	3
10	Wash your face and hands.	0	1	2	3
11	Tie up your shoelaces.	0	1	2	3
12	Do up buttons.	0	1	2	3
13	Do up a zip.	0	1	2	3
14	Write a letter.	0	1	2	3
15	Put a letter in an envelope.	0	1	2	3
16	Hold and read a newspaper.	0	1	2	3
17	Dial a telephone.	0	1	2	3
18	Make your self understood on the telephone.	0	1	2	3
19	Watch a television.	0	1	2	3
20	Pick up your change in a shop.	0	1	2	3
21	Insert an electric plug into a socket.	0	1	2	3
22	Unlock your front door with the key.	0	1	2	3
23	Walk up and down stairs.	0	1	2	3
24	Get up out of an armchair.	0	1	2	3
25	Carry a full shopping bag.	0	1	2	3

APPENDIX 4—TREMOR DISABILITY QUESTIONNAIRE

Tremor Disability Questionnaire (20)

For items 1–31, the subject is asked three questions:

a. Do you have difficulty or disability?
b. If no difficulty, then do you need to modify the way you perform this task?
c. If no difficulty, then have you experienced a loss of efficiency when performing this task?

1. Signing your name
2. Writing a letter, postcard, thank you card, or check
3. Typing
4. Placing a letter in an envelope
5. Drinking from a glass
6. Pouring milk or juice from a bottle
7. Carrying a cup of coffee
8. Using a spoon to drink soup
9. Carrying a tray of food
10. Eating in a restaurant
11. Inserting a coin in a pay telephone or a washing machine
12. Dialing a telephone
13. Holding a telephone to your ear
14. Buttoning your buttons
15. Tying your shoelaces
16. Zipping up a zipper
17. Putting on your eyeglasses
18. Putting on your contact lenses
19. Using eye drops
20. Cutting, trimming, or filing your nails
21. Putting on your watch
22. Brushing your teeth
23. Replacing a dollar bill in your wallet or purse
24. Reading a book, magazine, or newspaper
25. Unlocking door with a key
26. Threading a needle
27. Using a screwdriver
28. Screwing in a light bulb
29. Placing a plug in an electrical socket
30. Tying your necktie (males) or putting on your lipstick (females)
31. Shaving (males) or putting on your eyeliner (females)
    For Items 32–34, the subject is asked:
32. Does your voice almost always tremble when you talk?
33. Does your head often shake uncontrollably?
34. Does your tremor often embarrass you?
35. Do you have uncontrollable tremor in your legs?
36. Do you have uncontrollable tremor in your trunk?

APPENDIX 5—ASSESSMENT OF TREMOR RELATED HANDICAP

Assessment of tremor related handicap [modified from Ref. (12)]

The patient is asked to answer the following questions by putting a circle around the appropriate letter: A, B, C or D (6,12,13).

Has your tremor stopped you:

1)	Working?	A	B	C	D
2)	Applying for a job or promotion?	A	B	C	D
3)	Shopping by yourself?	A	B	C	D
4)	Doing your favorite hobby or sport?	A	B	C	D
5)	Traveling by public transport?	A	B	C	D
6)	Driving a car?	A	B	C	D
7)	Eating out?	A	B	C	D
8)	Going on holiday?	A	B	C	D
9)	Accepting a party invitation?	A	B	C	D

Key: A No

B Yes, because you are embarrassed by the tremor.

C Yes, because of the physical difficulties produced by the tremor.

D Yes, because of BOTH the physical difficulties and the embarrassment produced by tremor.

8

Impact of Essential Tremor and Its Medical and Surgical Treatment on Neuropsychological Functioning, Activities of Daily Living, and Quality of Life

Alexander I. Tröster and Karen A. Tucker

University of North Carolina School of Medicine, Chapel Hill, North Carolina, USA

I. INTRODUCTION

Essential tremor, one of the most common movement disorders associated with advanced age, has traditionally been considered benign. However, symptoms of essential tremor may range from mild tremor that does not warrant medical treatment, to more severe forms that result in disability and handicap. Severe tremor is hardly "benign" as it may affect not only the ability to carry out activities of daily living (ADLs), but social and emotional well being. Patients may withdraw from social activities due to fear of embarrassment related to such difficulties as speaking indistinctly and spilling food and beverages, potentially resulting in worsening of depressive symptoms. Recent research has also revealed cognitive changes in essential tremor that may further impair an individual's ability to function in daily life. Most theoretical models suggest a strong relationship between functional status and quality of life (QOL). For example, the model of Wilson and Cleary (1) (Fig. 8.1), which has been used to conceptualize QOL determinants in Parkinson's disease (2) posits that functional status is a function of, among other factors, physical and emotional symptoms, and that functional status is a more proximal determinant of QOL than symptoms or biological disease variables. It is reasonable to assume then that essential tremor, via its impact on cognition, emotion, and ADLs, has the potential to exert a significant and detrimental impact on QOL. By logical extension, it is probable that successful treatments of essential tremor, even if symptomatic rather than curative, would positively impact QOL. The impact of essential tremor on QOL and its treatments has been difficult to capture, probably in large part due to the lack of a disease-specific QOL instrument for essential tremor, and the only very recent and sparse use of generic QOL measures. This chapter discusses the

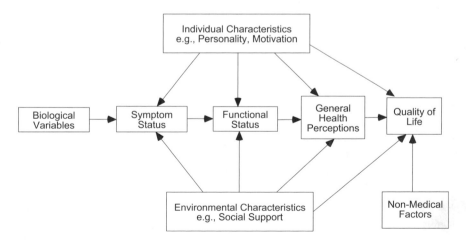

Figure 8.1 Model linking clinical variables with health-related QOL. [From Wilson and Cleary (1).]

changes in ADLs, cognitive functioning, and QOL that patients experience as a consequence of essential tremor and its treatment.

II. THE IMPACT OF ESSENTIAL TREMOR ON ACTIVITIES OF DAILY LIVING

The majority of patients with essential tremor exhibit hand tremor, but tremor may also affect other portions of the body to a significant degree. In a sample of 678 patients with essential tremor (3), tremor affected the hands in 90% of patients and the head/neck in 50% of patients. Voice tremor was observed among 30%, and leg and chin tremor among 15% of the sample. How tremor is distributed may be related to gender. In a large scale study of 450 patients with essential tremor, men were more likely than women to exhibit severe postural hand tremor, whereas women had a higher incidence and severity of head and voice tremor than men (4).

Several factors, including the severity of the tremor, contribute to whether ADLs are disrupted in patients with essential tremor. For instance, patients with unilateral rather than bilateral hand tremor have less difficulty performing ADLs (5). Daily functioning may also depend on whether the tremor affects the dominant or nondominant hand (6). Though there are typically only small to moderate differences in the amount of tremor between the hands, patients with dominant hand tremor are more likely to present for treatment. In addition to tremor severity and location, type of tremor may influence the extent to which execution of ADLs is affected. Specifically, patients with intention tremor of the hands (who also were more likely to have a gait disorder and more severe essential tremor overall) experienced greater reductions in ADLs (7). Action tremor is particularly disruptive to a patient's ability to perform tasks such as writing, drawing, and pouring (8).

In addition to the physical limitations imposed by essential tremor, daily activities may be avoided due to embarrassment or self-consciousness in public (9). Patients with essential tremor have a similar level of embarrassment while performing ADLs in social situations as patients with Parkinson's disease (10). Thus, essential tremor has the potential to affect not only an individual's independent functioning, but social activities, relationships, and emotional well being.

Another determinant of functioning and disability in essential tremor is the presence of comorbid conditions. Patients with essential tremor have an increased incidence of concomitant neurological and psychiatric disorders. Among comorbid neurological conditions, the prevalence of movement disorders is higher in essential tremor patients than in the general population. In a sample of 678 patients with essential tremor, a family history of tremor was reported in >60% (3). More than 6% of the sample had concomitant Parkinson's disease, 7% had dystonia, and 2% experienced myoclonus. Onset of tremor occurred on average at 45 years of age with a mean age of 65 years at study enrollment.

Functional disability was common and 18% of the sample reported a history of work-related impairment.

Patients with essential tremor are more likely to develop or to experience exacerbation of psychiatric disorders that may influence the ability to function. Essential tremor patients have reported significant symptoms of depression and anxiety that were similar to levels experienced by Parkinson's disease patients (11). Regardless of tremor severity, heightened symptoms of depression and anxiety are related to greater functional disability in patients with essential tremor (12). Embarrassment in social situations due to tremor may induce or worsen symptoms of social phobia (13). The combined prevalence of primary social phobia and social phobia secondary to essential tremor was 33% in a large sample of patients with essential tremor (14). The severity of social phobia was associated with disability, regardless of tremor severity.

Essential tremor patients are also more likely to have hearing difficulties than similarly aged individuals. In a study of 250 essential tremor patients, 127 Parkinson's disease patients, and 127 normal controls, patients with essential tremor had more impaired hearing than either the Parkinson's disease group or controls (15). Hearing difficulties seemed to be directly related to essential tremor since the degree of hearing loss was associated with the severity of tremor. The mechanism of this hearing loss remains to be explained, as does its functional impact.

Although tremor severity rating scales, such as that of Fahn, Tolosa, and Marin (16), often capture the impact that tremor has on functions such as pouring a liquid, these scales do not survey a broad range of ADLs. To overcome this issue, Lyons et al. (17) devised a measure to specifically assess changes in ADLs that often occur in essential tremor. The Tremor Activities of Daily Living Scale (TADLS) is based on 30 activities that are often difficult for patients with essential tremor to perform, including feeding (drinking, eating), grooming (brushing teeth, shaving), manipulating household objects (unlocking a door, using a telephone, washing dishes, using a television remote), and work-related activities (writing, typing on a computer keyboard).

III. QUALITY OF LIFE IN ESSENTIAL TREMOR

QOL is a broad concept defying universally accepted definition, but one that inarguably involves the notion of a subjective sense of well-being that is multiply determined. QOL issues that are particularly relevant to essential tremor include physical and instrumental ADLs (i.e., those activities that allow a patient to remain independent within home and community), emotional functioning, and social stigma (18). Although the changes in physical abilities and the emotional repercussions of essential tremor most likely have a significant impact on QOL, these have been difficult to quantify given the absence of a disease-specific QOL instrument. The few studies that attempted to address QOL have used either generic instruments or instruments specific to other movement disorders such as Parkinson's disease (2). Unfortunately neither of these approaches is optimal—generic measures lack sensitivity in essential tremor and fail to address the issues most relevant to essential tremor, while instruments appropriate for Parkinson's disease may lack optimal face validity and patient acceptance because the instrument also asks questions irrelevant to essential tremor. A brief, disease-specific QOL instrument for essential tremor that has patient acceptance has been developed (19). Using factor analytic techniques Tröster et al., developed a 30-item instrument that yields a total score and scores in five areas of QOL: physical, psychosocial, communication, hobbies/leisure, and work/finance. Initial validity evaluation of this instrument (the Quality of Life in Essential Tremor Questionnaire or QUEST) in a sample of 200 patients indicated that the scale had good to excellent internal consistency (an index of reliability and construct validity) ranging from 0.79 to 0.95. Furthermore, patterns of correlations among patient-rated tremor severity in various body parts and scores in different QOL domains suggested good construct and face validity. For example, communication was most strongly related to voice and head tremor, while physical aspects of QOL were most strongly related to upper extremity tremor, especially of the dominant hand. In a follow-up study with 65 patients (20), it was observed that the QUEST was sensitive to both patient- and physician-rated tremor severity. Correlation patterns among QUEST domains and tremor severity in various body parts were more congruent with expectations when patient- rather than physician-rated tremor severity was considered. An important finding too was that the QUEST Work/Finance scale tended to be most strongly associated with depressive symptoms, social support, and perceived stigma, suggesting that psychosocial factors may be better predictors of work satisfaction than objective tremor severity. Of course it remains to be determined whether tremor-related work disruption leads to depression, isolation, and stigma, or instead the psychosocial consequences of tremor lead to occupational difficulties.

IV. NEUROPSYCHOLOGICAL FUNCTIONING IN PATIENTS WITH ESSENTIAL TREMOR

Cognition is grossly intact in essential tremor patients visiting clinics, and it is probably for this reason that few systematic investigations of neuropsychological functioning in essential tremor have been undertaken. An impetus for such studies has been the resurgence of surgical treatments for movement disorders, as well as the suggestion by some that essential tremor and Parkinson's disease (which is associated with cognitive changes) might share certain pathophysiological mechanisms. Gasparini et al. (21) were the first to publish a report on neuropsychological functioning in patients with essential tremor. They compared the neuropsychological test performance of 27 patients with essential tremor to that of 15 Parkinson's disease patients and 15 healthy controls. Essential tremor patients performed significantly worse than controls on measures involving response inhibition and problem solving (Stroop Color-Word and Wisconsin Card Sorting (WCST) tests, respectively). Patients with Parkinson's disease performed significantly worse than normal controls on the same tests, but also showed deficits on measures of cognitive switching and verbal fluency (Trailmaking Test Part B and FAS, respectively). The authors further explored whether neuropsychological performance differed among the essential tremor patients as a function of family history of Parkinson's disease or essential tremor. Fifteen of the essential tremor patients had a family history of essential tremor, and 12 essential tremor patients had a family history of Parkinson's disease. A family history of Parkinson's disease was associated with worse performance in comparison to controls on the measure of verbal fluency. The authors concluded that patients with essential tremor or Parkinson's disease both experience a disruption of frontal lobe functions that may reflect a common dysregulation of dopamine pathways. Deficiencies in dopamine in both conditions could lead to a frontal subcortical pattern of neuropsychological deficits. Although this proposal may be intuitively appealing, the Gasparini et al. study did not provide information about the neuropsychological functions related to brain regions other than the frontal lobes.

Several studies evaluated a broader range of cognitive functions in essential tremor. Lombardi et al. (11) administered a battery of neuropsychological tests to 18 essential tremor and 18 Parkinson's disease patients who presented consecutively for surgical treatment of tremor. The battery of tests included measures of vocabulary, language, visuospatial processes, verbal and visual reasoning, attention/concentration, learning, memory, executive functions, and mood. The essential tremor and Parkinson's disease subjects were similar in age and overall level of cognitive impairment. They had an average age of 66 and 67 years, respectively, and average Mini-Mental State Exam (MMSE) scores of 27. In comparison to a normative sample, the essential tremor patients performed significantly worse on measures of verbal fluency (FAS, Animals) and had significantly more depressive symptoms. These symptoms did not appear to affect performance on any of the measures since there was not a significant correlation between depressive symptoms and neuropsychological test performance. In addition, the essential tremor sample obtained lower than expected scores (though scores not significantly below those of controls) on measures of object-naming (Boston Naming Test—BNT), attention/concentration (Digit Span, Letter-Number Sequencing), executive functioning, and measures of learning and memory (California Verbal Learning Test—CVLT list-learning, delayed recall and recognition). Differences between the Parkinson's disease and normative samples were significant on measures of verbal fluency (FAS, Animals), visual perception (Hooper Visual Organization Test), delayed recall (CVLT), executive functioning (WCST), and depressive symptoms. As with the essential tremor patients, severity of depressive symptoms was not significantly associated with neuropsychological test scores, but this might relate to the fact that the depression scores were restricted in range and mild. Parkinson's disease patients had lower than expected scores on measures of object-naming, facial recognition, visual perception (Picture Completion) and attention/concentration (Letter-Number Sequencing, Spatial Span). In comparison to Parkinson's disease patients, patients with essential tremor were significantly worse on tests of lexical verbal fluency and attention/concentration. Parkinson's disease patients were worse than essential tremor patients on a task requiring facial recognition. The authors concluded that the difficulties the essential tremor patients demonstrated were suggestive of frontosubcortical dysfunction. They also noted that the cognitive declines demonstrated by the essential tremor patients resembled those of patients with cerebellar lesions (e.g., deficits of working memory, executive functioning, verbal fluency).

In the largest study to date, examining 101 patients with essential tremor referred for thalamotomy or thalamic deep brain stimulation (22), the essential tremor patients had significantly lower scores than test normative samples on measures of auditory selective attention (Brief Test of Attention), response inhibition (Stroop Color-Word interference condition), manual dexterity bilaterally (Grooved Pegboard), verbal fluency (FAS, Animals), object-naming (BNT), visuoperceptual functions (Hooper Visual Organization Test, Facial Recognition Test), and learning/memory (CVLT). The average T scores on these measures were suggestive of mildly impaired attention, response inhibition, and letter fluency; moderately impaired manual dexterity; and subtle declines (below average scores) on tasks involving categorical fluency, object-naming, visuoperceptual functions, and learning/memory.

The results of Tröster et al. (22) were generally consistent with the pattern of performance noted in the earlier studies, with the exception of the WCST. The WCST was performed normally as judged by average scores in this sample, though approximately one quarter of the patients had impaired performance. Patients in the prior studies showed deficits on the WCST. This difference may be related to Tröster et al's. (22) exclusion of patients with concomitant medical conditions and depression that were not controlled well with medication. Alternatively, the absence of a finding in the current study may be related to the greater duration of illness noted in the patients in the previous studies. For example, in the Tröster et al. (22) study, though the subjects were older (72 years), the duration of illness was shorter (14 years) compared to that of patients in the Lombardi et al. (11) and Gasparini et al. (21) studies (essential tremor durations of 36 and 20 years, respectively; average ages of 66 and 68 years, respectively). It is possible that patients with essential tremor demonstrate a progression of deficits affecting motor skills, verbal fluency, and attention, that does not include executive functioning until later in the course of the disease. Additional studies are necessary to establish the independent effects of tremor severity and duration on neuropsychological functioning. Tröster et al. (22) concluded that the deficits demonstrated by the essential tremor patients were suggestive of difficulty with the "initiation and maintenance of efficient information processing strategies" that has also been observed in Parkinson's disease patients, and that some of these deficits were reminiscent of those shown by persons with cerebellar dysfunction.

The difficulties with executive functioning among patients with essential tremor were substantiated by the results of a subsequent study (23). These investigators administered a similarly extensive battery of tests to 13 patients with essential tremor being considered for surgical treatment of tremor. The essential tremor patients showed deficits on measures of executive functioning (WCST Categories; Stroop Color-Word) and figural fluency (Ruff Figural Fluency). Lower than expected scores were found in verbal fluency (FAS). However, measures of learning/memory (CVLT Total), object-naming (BNT), and categorical fluency (Animals) were within normal limits. The small sample size of the study may have yielded inadequate power to detect the wider range of deficits demonstrated in the Lombardi et al. (11) and Tröster et al. (22) studies. Overall, the currently available studies of neuropsychological functioning in essential tremor suggest that the most consistent deficits occur in verbal fluency, particularly lexical fluency. Milder declines were found in object-naming, attention/concentration, learning/memory, and executive and visuoperceptual functions.

V. IMPACT OF MEDICAL AND SURGICAL TREATMENTS ON NEUROPSYCHOLOGICAL FUNCTIONING, ADLs, AND QOL

A. Pharmacotherapy of Essential Tremor

Medications for essential tremor have been found to adequately reduce tremor in ~50% of patients (24–26). If the tremor is disabling, treatment with primidone or propranolol should be initiated. If control of tremor is inadequate with one medication, then these medications may be combined. Propranolol and benzodiazepines (e.g., clonazepam) may be used if tremor is prominent during moments of stress. Some reports suggest that topiramate and gabapentin may be helpful in the control of tremor (24,27,28). Other medications including carbonic anhydrase inhibitors, phenobarbital, nimodipine, clonidine, clozapine, and mirtazapine have variable levels of efficacy.

Many patients have reported a reduction of tremor with the use of alcohol. A recent pilot study examined the usefulness of an 8-carbon alcohol called 1-octanol in essential tremor (29). 1-Octanol significantly reduced tremor without intoxication. To date, no studies have specifically compared neuropsychological, functional or QOL changes associated with the various pharmacological treatments for essential tremor.

B. Surgical Intervention for Treatment of Essential Tremor

1. Thalamotomy

Thalamotomy and alternative surgical treatments such as deep brain stimulation (DBS) experienced a resurgence in the 1990s. Multiple reports have shown the efficacy of thalamotomy in reducing contralateral tremor (30–31). Gamma knife thalamotomy for essential tremor may be effective for patients who are unsuitable for other surgical procedures (32,33). Overall, thalamotomy appears to substantially diminish contralateral tremor in >90% of patients (34,35).

2. Changes in Neuropsychological Functioning and ADLs Associated with Thalamotomy

Modern thalamotomy in Parkinson's disease appears relatively safe from a cognitive standpoint [for reviews, see Refs. (36,37)]. Although a similar conclusion can be reached with regard to thalamotomy in essential tremor, it is clear that the procedure, especially if bilateral, is not without risk. One of the earlier studies in a more recent series of thalamotomy (38) observed one transient and one permanent "verbal cognitive deficit" among eight unilateral operations. Two studies indicated that cognitive complications are probably less common after DBS than thalamotomy. Pahwa et al. (35), in a non-randomized, small sample study, found a cognitive complication rate of 29% after thalamotomy, as opposed to one of 0% after DBS. In a similar study, though significant improvement in ADLs (Frenchay Activities Index) was found six months following thalamotomy (5), cognitive impairments were observed in one thalamotomy but no DBS patients.

3. Thalamic Deep Brain Stimulation

Several studies have demonstrated the effectiveness of thalamic DBS in the reduction of postural and action tremor in patients with essential tremor (39–44). One long term study found that tremor remains significantly ameliorated even after 6 years (43). Though head tremor may be more resistant to treatment than the limbs, improvements can be observed at 3, 6, and 12 months following implantation (45).

One study examined the effectiveness of subthalamic nucleus (STN) DBS for essential tremor (46). Significant reductions were noted in tremor affecting the upper and lower extremities as well as the head, without major complications. Further research is needed to determine whether this alternate location for surgical intervention offers any benefits over thalamic DBS in terms of tremor reduction or complications.

Though thalamic DBS is associated with fewer complications than thalamotomy, some risk for temporary or permanent adverse events remains. In a sample of 86 patients who underwent 149 DBS implants, 30% of the patients experienced at least one negative consequence ranging from mild and transient to more severe and chronic (47). These complications consisted of the following: 35% hardware-related, 31% perioperative, 31% postoperative, and 15% stimulation-related. Five percent of the sample sustained a chronic neurological deficit following surgery. The most common complications following thalamic DBS are dysarthria and disequilibrium (48). Adjusting the stimulation parameters alleviates these complications in the majority of patients. Patients undergoing bilateral DBS appear to be at greater risk for dysarthria than patients with unilateral DBS (48,49). Staging the surgeries for bilateral implantation does not appear to reduce the risk of dysarthria or gait disequilibrium, and dysarthria may worsen when both stimulators are turned on (42).

4. Changes in Activities of Daily Living and Quality of Life Following DBS

Several studies have demonstrated effective reduction of disability and significant improvements in ADLs, such as writing and pouring, following DBS in patients with essential tremor (50). Clinicians and patients have rated similar levels of improvement, ranging from 40% to 60%, on measures of ADLs such as the TADLS (17,51). Improvements of ADLs have been noted in comparisons of baseline and post surgical scores and in comparisons of stimulation turned on and off (8,51). These improvements occur after both unilateral and bilateral DBS (40). Such ADL improvements are associated with gains in QOL (18). Aspects of QOL rated as improved include perceived stigma, communication, and emotional well-being (which may be related to amelioration of anxiety).

5. Neuropsychological Changes Associated with Thalamic DBS

Very little research has focused on neuropsychological changes associated with thalamic DBS in essential tremor. One study evaluated 40 patients with essential tremor one month before and three months after unilateral DBS (18). Statistically significant, but clinically modest postoperative gains were demonstrated on measures of verbal memory (Wechsler Memory Scale-Revised: Logical Memory II; CVLT: Recognition), visual attention (Spatial Span Backwards), visual Gestalt formation (Hooper Visual Organization Test), and visual construction (Dementia Rating Scale-(DRS) Construction). Significant improvement was also noted in dominant hand dexterity (Grooved Pegboard). Overall, only one neuropsychological measure declined following surgery, namely letter fluency.

In a follow-up study, the same patients were administered neuropsychological tests 12 months following surgery, with largely similar results (52). In comparison to baseline, subjects retained improvements in delayed verbal memory, visual construction, visual perception, and dominant hand manual dexterity. They exhibited an additional improvement from baseline on a measure of verbal learning (CVLT: Immediate Recall), perhaps reflecting a practice effect. Significant increases in performance were found between the 3- and 12-month evaluations on measures of verbal learning and concept formation (DRS: Conceptualization). Twelve months following surgery, no significant declines were noted on any of the measures in comparison to baseline. However, four patients with baseline deficits in verbal fluency showed substantial further decrements following surgery. The authors concluded that individuals with poor verbal fluency prior to surgery may be more susceptible to exacerbation of this deficit following surgery.

A few studies have compared neuropsychological test performance with stimulation turned on or off. The results of one case report suggest that thalamic DBS may improve verbal fluency (53). In an 80-year-old man, scores were more than one standard deviation higher on verbal fluency and verbal recall tasks with stimulation on than in the stimulation off condition. No differences were noted in other measures of attention, verbal memory, or visual perception. Thus, there was an isolated marked improvement in verbal fluency and recall with thalamic DBS. Another study yielded contradictory findings, suggesting that thalamic DBS may disrupt verbal recall (54). Significantly more words were recalled in the stimulation off than in the stimulation on condition during a list learning task (Rey Auditory Verbal Learning Test). Since only two of the nine patients in this study had essential tremor, it is difficult to discern whether similar findings would be obtained in a larger sample of essential tremor patients.

Research has rarely examined the surgical and stimulation parameters that might predict cognitive or ADL changes after DBS in essential tremor. In one study the characteristics of 27 essential tremor patients with mild cognitive declines following surgery were compared with those of 22 patients without such declines (55). There were no significant differences between the two groups in baseline neuropsychological performance, disease, demographics, or postoperative motor functioning. However, a larger proportion of patients with cognitive declines underwent left, rather than right thalamic DBS. A significantly higher pulse width was used in the group with cognitive declines in comparison to the stable group and there was a significant association between cognitive decline and pulse width ≥ 120 μs. Onset of essential tremor after age 37 was another significant predictor of worse cognitive outcome.

Deuschl and Bain (56) sought to develop guidelines for patient selection that take into account the risks and benefits of DBS and thalamotomy. They concluded that appropriate candidates were <75 years of age, were not severely depressed, and were without dementia (defined by a cutoff of 130 on the Mattis Dementia Rating Scale). Severe brain atrophy and other life-limiting diseases were also considered negative treatment indicators. The patient's motor symptoms were also an important consideration because surgery tends to be more successful in alleviating resting and postural tremors than intention tremor.

VI. CONCLUSIONS

Symptoms of essential tremor often have a significant negative impact on ADLs and QOL. Thalamotomy and DBS provide significant reduction of tremor, however, they are not without risk, possibly leading to dysarthria or subtle cognitive changes involving disturbance of verbal fluency. Profound disturbance of neuropsychological function appears to be less common with DBS than with thalamotomy, and less frequent with unilateral than bilateral DBS. The limited number of available studies of ADLs and QOL in patients with essential tremor following DBS demonstrate promising gains in functioning and QOL.

However, much research is needed to understand the nature of these changes and how they can be maximized. Even less is known about the cognitive, functional, and QOL impact of medications used to treat essential tremor and comparisons of pharmacologic and surgical therapies remain to be carried out. The recent development of a "disease-specific" QOL measure for essential tremor may be a catalyst for such studies.

Though emotional disturbance has long been recognized as a possible concomitant of essential tremor, cognition was assumed to be intact. Recent studies consistently show that mild, perhaps in many cases subclinical decrements in verbal fluency, executive functions, and memory are seen in essential tremor. These neuropsychological alterations overlap, but are less severe, than those in Parkinsons's disease, and cerebellar and subcortical dysfunction may be underlie these cognitive changes.

REFERENCES

1. Wilson IB, Cleary PD. Linking clinical variables with health-related quality of life. A conceptual model of patient outcomes. JAMA 1995; 1273:59–65.
2. Tröster AI, Lyons KE, Straits-Tröster KA. Determinants of health-related quality of life changes in Parkinson's disease. In: Martínez Martín P, Koller WC eds. Quality of Life in Parkinson's Disease. Barcelona, Spain: Masson, 1999:55–77.
3. Koller WC, Busenbark K, Miner K. The relationship of essential tremor to other movement disorders: report on 678 patients. Essential Tremor Study Group. Ann Neurology 1994; 35:717–723.
4. Hubble JP, Busenbark KL, Pahwa R, Lyons K, Koller WC. Clinical expression of essential tremor: effects of gender and age. Mov Disord 1997; 12:969–972.
5. Schuurman PR, Bosch DA, Bossuyt PM, Bonsel GJ, van Someren EJ, de Bie RM, Merkus MP, Speelman JD. A comparison of continuous thalamic stimulation and thalamotomy for suppression of severe tremor. N Engl J Med 2000; 342:461–468.
6. Louis ED, Wendt KJ, Pullman SL, Ford B. Is essential tremor symmetric? Observational data from a community-based study of essential tremor. Arch Neurol 1998; 55:1553–1559.
7. Stolze H, Petersen G, Raethjen J, Wenzelburger R, Deuschl G. The gait disorder of advanced essential tremor. Brain 2001; 124:2278–2286.
8. Sydow O, Thobois S, Alesch F, Speelman JD. Multicentre European study of thalamic stimulation in essential tremor: a six year follow up. J Neurol Neurosurg Psychiatry 2003; 74:1387–1391.
9. Velickovic M, Gracies JM. Movement disorders: keys to identifying and treating tremor. Geriatrics 2002; 57:32–36.
10. Metzer WS. Severe essential tremor compared with Parkinson's disease in male veterans: diagnostic characteristics, treatment, and psychosocial complications. South Med J 1992; 85:825–828.
11. Lombardi WJ, Woolston DJ, Roberts JW, Gross RE. Cognitive deficits in patients with essential tremor. Neurology 2001; 57:785–790.
12. Louis ED, Barnes L, Albert SM, Cote L, Schneier FR, Pullman SL, Yu Q. Correlates of functional disability in essential tremor. Mov Disord 2001; 16:914–920.

13. George MS, Lydiard RB. Social phobia secondary to physical disability. A review of benign essential tremor (BET) and stuttering. Psychosomatics 1994; 35:520–523.
14. Schneier FR, Barnes LF, Albert SM, Louis ED. Characteristics of social phobia among persons with essential tremor. J Clin Psychiatry 2001; 62:367–372.
15. Ondo WG, Sutton L, Dat Vuong K, Lai D, Jankovic J. Hearing impairment in essential tremor. Neurology 2003; 61:1093–1097.
16. Fahn S, Tolosa E, Marin C. Clinical rating scale for tremor. In: Jankovic J, Tolosa E, eds. Parkinson's Disease and Movement Disorders. Baltimore: Williams & Wilkins, 1988:225–234.
17. Lyons KE, Pahwa R, Busenbark KL, Tröster AI, Wilkinson S, Koller WC. Improvements in daily functioning after deep brain stimulation of the thalamus for intractable tremor. Mov Disord 1998; 13:690–692.
18. Tröster AI, Fields JA, Pahwa R, Wilkinson SB, Strait-Tröster KA, Lyons K, Kieltyka J, Koller WC. Neuropsychological and quality of life outcome after thalamic stimulation for essential tremor. Neurology 1999; 53:1774–1780.
19. Tröster AI, Pahwa R, Fields JA, Tanner CM, Lyons KE. Development of the Quality of Life in Essential Tremor Questionnaire (QUEST): A 30-item disease-specific quality of life instrument. Neurology 2004; 62(suppl 5):A500–A501.
20. Tröster AI, Pahwa R, Tanner CM, Lyons KE. Validation of the Quality of Life in Essential Tremor Questionnaire (QUEST). Mov Disord 2004; 19(suppl 9):S168.
21. Gasparini M, Bonifati V, Fabrizio E, Fabbrini G. Brusa L, Lenzi GL, Meco G. Frontal lobe dysfunction in essential tremor: a preliminary study. J Neurol 2001; 248:399–402.
22. Tröster AI, Woods SP, Fields JA, Lyons KE, Pahwa R, Higginson CI, Koller WC. Neuropsychological deficits in essential tremor: an expression of cerebello-thalamo-cortical pathophysiology? Eur J Neurol 2002; 9:143–151.
23. Lacritz LH, Dewey R Jr, Giller C, Cullum CM. Cognitive functioning in individuals with "benign" essential tremor. J Int Neuropsychol Soc 2002; 8:125–129.
24. Lyons KE, Pahwa R, Comella CL, Eisa MS, Elble RJ, Fahn S, Jankovic J, Juncos JL, Koller WC, Ondo WG, Sethi KD, Stern MB, Tanner CM, Tintner R, Watts RL. Benefits and risks of pharmacological treatments for essential tremor. Drug Saf 2003; 26:461–481.
25. Chen JJ, Swope DM. Essential tremor: diagnosis and treatment. Pharmacotherapy 2003; 23:1105–1122.
26. Lambert D, Waters CH. Essential tremor. Curr Treat Options Neurol 1999; 1:6–13.
27. Pahwa R, Lyons K, Hubble JP, Busenbark K, Rienerth JD, Pahwa A, Koller WC. Double-blind controlled trial of gabapentin in essential tremor. Mov Disord 1998; 13:465–467.
28. Ondo W, Hunter C, Vuong KD, Schwartz K, Jankovic J. Gabapentin for essential tremor: a multiple-dose, double-blind, placebo-controlled trial. Mov Disord 2000; 15:678–682.
29. Bushara KO, Goldstein SR, Grimes GJ Jr, Burstein AH, Hallett M. Pilot trial of 1-octanol in essential tremor. Neurology 2004; 62:122–124.
30. Zirh A, Reich SG, Dougherty PM, Lenz FA. Stereotactic thalamotomy in the treatment of essential tremor of the upper extremity: reassessment including a blinded measure of outcome. J Neurol Neurosurg Psychiatry 1999; 66:772–775.

31. Akbostanci MC, Slavin KV, Burchiel KJ Stereotactic ventral intermedial thalamotomy for the treatment of essential tremor: results of a series of 37 patients. Stereotact Funct Neurosurg 1999; 72:174–177.
32. Young RF, Jacques S, Mark R, Kopyov O, Copcutt B, Posewitz A, Li F. Gamma knife thalamotomy for treatment of tremor: long-term results. J Neurosurg 2000; 93:S128–S135.
33. Niranjan A, Kondziolka D, Baser S, Heyman R, Lunsford LD. Functional outcomes after gamma knife thalamotomy for essential tremor and MS-related tremor. Neurology 2000; 55:443–446.
34. Pahwa R, Lyons K, Koller WC. Surgical treatment of essential tremor. Neurology 2000; 54:S39–S44.
35. Pahwa R, Lyons KE, Wilkinson SB, Tröster AI, Overman J, Kieltyka J, Koller WC. Comparison of thalamotomy to deep brain stimulation of the thalamus in essential tremor. Mov Disord 2001; 16:140–143.
36. Wilkinson SB, Tröster AI. Surgical interventions in neurodegenerative disease: impact on memory and cognition. In: Tröster AI, ed. Memory in Neurodegenerative Disease: Biological, Cognitive, and Clinical Perspectives. Cambridge, UK: Cambridge University Press, 1998:362–376.
37. Tröster AI, Fields JA. The role of neuropsychological evaluation in the neurosurgical treatment of movement disorders. In: Tarsy D, Vitek JL, Lozano AM, eds. Surgical treatment of Parkinson's Disease and Other Movement Disorders. Totowa, NJ: Humana Press, 2003:213–240.
38. Goldman MS, Ahlskog JE, Kelly PJ. The symptomatic and functional outcome of stereotactic thalamotomy for medically intractable essential tremor. J Neurosurg 1992; 76:924–928.
39. Kumar R, Lozano AM, Sime E, Lang AE. Long-term follow-up of thalamic deep brain stimulation for essential and parkinsonian tremor. Neurology 2003; 61:1601–1604.
40. Limousin P, Speelman JD, Gielen F, Janssens M. Multicentre European study of thalamic stimulation in parkinsonian and essential tremor. J Neurol Neurosurg Psychiatry 1999; 66:289–296.
41. Mobin F, De Salles AA, Behnke EJ, Frysinger R. Correlation between MRI-based stereotactic thalamic deep brain stimulation electrode placement, macroelectrode stimulation and clinical response to tremor control. Stereotact Funct Neurosurg 1999; 72:225–232.
42. Pahwa R, Lyons KL, Wilkinson SB, Carpenter MA, Tröster AI, Searl JP, Overman J, Pickering S, Koller WC. Bilateral thalamic stimulation for the treatment of essential tremor. Neurology 1999; 53:1447–1450.
43. Rehncrona S, Johnels B, Widner H, Tornqvist AL, Hariz M, Sydow O. Long-term efficacy of thalamic deep brain stimulation for tremor: double-blind assessments. Mov Disord 2003; 18:163–170.
44. Vesper J, Chabardes S, Fraix V, Sunde N, Ostergaard K and Kinetra Study Group. Dual channel deep brain stimulation system (Kinetra) for Parkinson's disease and essential tremor: a prospective multicentre open label clinical study. J Neurol Neurosurg Psychiatry 2002; 73:275–280.
45. Koller WC, Lyons KE, Wilkinson SB, Pahwa R. Efficacy of unilateral deep brain stimulation of the VIM nucleus of the thalamus for essential head tremor. Mov Disord 1999; 14:847–850.

46. Murata J, Kitagawa M, Uesugi H, Saito H, Iwasaki Y, Kikuchi S, Tashiro K, Sawamura Y. Electrical stimulation of the posterior subthalamic area for the treatment of intractable proximal tremor. J Neurosurg 2003; 99:708–715.

47. Beric A, Kelly PJ, Rezai A, Sterio D, Mogilner A, Zonenshayn M, Kopell B. Complications of deep brain stimulation surgery. Stereotact Funct Neurosurg 2001; 77:73–78.

48. Taha JM, Janszen MA, Favre J. Thalamic deep brain stimulation for the treatment of head, voice, and bilateral limb tremor. J Neurosurg 1999; 91:68–72.

49. Obwegeser AA, Uitti RJ, Witte RJ, Lucas JA, Turk MF, Wharen RE. Quantitative and qualitative outcome measures after thalamic deep brain stimulation to treat disabling tremors. Neurosurgery 2001; 48:274–281.

50. Ondo W, Jankovic J, Schwartz K, Almaguer M, Simpson RK. Unilateral thalamic deep brain stimulation for refractory essential tremor and Parkinson's disease tremor. Neurology 1998; 51:1063–1069.

51. Bryant JA, De Salles A, Cabatan C, Frysinger R, Behnke E, Bronstein J. The impact of thalamic stimulation on activities of daily living for essential tremor. Surg Neurol 2003; 59:479–485.

52. Fields JA, Tröster AI, Woods SP, Higginson CI, Wilkinson SB, Lyons KE, Koller WC, Pahwa R. Neuropsychological and quality of life outcomes 12 months after unilateral thalamic stimulation for essential tremor. J Neurol Neurosurg Psychiatry 2003; 74:305–311.

53. Lucas JA, Rippeth JD, Uitti RJ, Shuster EA, Wharen RE. Neuropsychological functioning in a patient with essential tremor with and without bilateral VIM stimulation. Brain Cogn 2000; 42:253–267.

54. Loher TJ, Gutbrod K, Fravi NL, Pohle T, Burgunder JM, Krauss JK. Thalamic stimulation for tremor. Subtle changes in episodic memory are related to stimulation per se and not to a microthalamotomy effect. J Neurol 2003; 250:707–713.

55. Woods SP, Fields JA, Lyons KE, Pahwa R, Tröster AI. Pulse width is associated with cognitive decline after thalamic stimulation for essential tremor. Parkinsonism Relat Disord 2003; 9:295–300.

56. Deuschl G, Bain P. Deep brain stimulation for tremor [correction of trauma]: patient selection and evaluation. Mov Disord 2002; 17:S102–S111.

9

Neuroimaging of Essential Tremor

Jo Ann Antenor and Joel S. Perlmutter

Washington University in St. Louis, St. Louis, Missouri, USA

I. INTRODUCTION

Essential tremor is one of the most common neurologic movement disorders with a prevalence between 0.3% and 4% in the United States (1) and may affect the limbs, head, neck, voice, or various combinations. About half of the patients have an autosomal dominant pattern of inheritance (2,3) but only two different gene loci have been linked to essential tremor in different pedigrees (4,5). The underlying pathophysiology remains elusive with no clear findings on pathologic examinations of brains (6,7). Neuroimaging, however, has provided several clues to the pathophysiology of essential tremor and mechanisms of action of therapeutic interventions.

II. ANATOMIC PATHOLOGY (CT AND MRI)

There have been no peer-reviewed reports of structural brain abnormalities in essential identified using computed tomography (CT) or magnetic resonance imaging (MRI) with the exception of a single report that found task-specific action tremor in a hand present after a frontal cortical infarct in a person with essential tremor (8). However, many investigators have reported sites of structure lesions that alleviate essential tremor. The inference is that the sites of such lesions indicate interruption of a brain circuit critical for production of essential tremor. For example, ipsilateral cerebellar infarct (9), contralateral pontine stroke (10), contralateral hemispheric stroke (11), and contralateral infarct near the thalamus (12) abolish essential tremor on one side of the body. All of these suggest that the integrity of the cerebellar-rubro-thalamo-cortico-pontine-cerebellar circuit is critical to essential tremor. These types of observations led to the placement of thalamic lesions in the region of the ventral intermediate (VIM) nucleus (target of cerebellar output) to alleviate tremor (13).

III. FUNCTIONAL IMAGING

Anatomical imaging, has provided modest insight into identification of functional alterations in specific brain regions that lead to essential tremor. Functional imaging may help fill the gap. It provides a better approach for detecting and characterizing changes in regional brain function associated with essential tremor. Most studies have utilized positron emission tomography (PET) or functional MRI (fMRI) for these investigations.

A. Resting State

Regional measurements of cerebral blood flow or metabolism are closely coupled to neuronal activity, at least under normal physiologic conditions (14,15), enabling PET measurements of flow or metabolism to be used to identify sites of brain dysfunction associated with essential tremor. For example, PET measures of [^{18}F] fluoro-2-deoxyglucose (FDG) uptake in essential tremor patients at rest (i.e., no tremor present) demonstrate significantly increased FDG uptake in the medulla and thalami, but not in the cerebellar cortex (16). The authors suggested that the inferior olivary nucleus was the main site of increased uptake although the resolution of the PET scanner did not permit specific identification of that part of the medulla with increased uptake. Since changes in flow or metabolism may reflect changes in neuronal activity in target synaptic fields, including local interneurons (17–21), increased metabolism in inferior olivary nuclei could reflect increased activity of the local interneurons within the nuclei or increased activity of inputs via the spino-olivary tract or the central tegmental tract.

In contrast, PET measures of blood flow using [^{15}O] water found that essential tremor patients compared to normals had increased flow in cerebellar hemispheres even with the limbs at rest and no tremor present (22,23). This suggests over-activity of cerebellar pathways in essential tremor patients even in the absence of tremor, which is a different conclusion from the FDG study cited above.

B. Physiologic Activation

PET measurements of blood flow or metabolism may also be used to map responses to physiological and pharmacologic stimuli (17,24–28). The underlying assumption is that a change in flow or metabolism reflects a change in neuronal activity in target synaptic fields, including local interneurons (17–21). It is important to note that higher flow or metabolism may accompany either increased excitation or inhibition since both may cost energy to maintain or change membrane gradients. The relative metabolic demands of excitation versus inhibition remain controversial (29,30). It is important to remember that changes in flow may not coincide with changes in local metabolism or neuronal activity under pathological conditions (18).

This activation strategy has been applied to essential tremor. Initial studies used the presence of involuntary tremor as the activation and compared these to the limb at rest. Using this approach, involuntary postural tremor was found to further increase flow in the region of the red nucleus, bilateral thalamus, and cerebellar vermis (22,23,31,32) but no detectable changes were identified in the inferior olive or medulla (23,32).

Functional MRI can also be used for activation studies but there are some important differences between using PET and fMRI. MR imaging relies primarily on the perturbations of the resonant frequency of water protons in tissue induced by fluctuating external magnetic fields. Image contrast depends on the specifics of the magnetic pulse sequence applied to the field of view and proton density, longitudinal (spin–lattice) relaxation time (T1), and transverse (spin–spin) relaxation time (T2) of protons in the tissue. Magnetic field inhomogeneities induced by tissue characteristics change the apparent T2 altering image contrast, called T2*. Functional MRI studies depend upon changes in the blood oxygen level-dependent (BOLD) signal between two successive scans. Changes in BOLD indicate a relative increase in local brain blood flow that is not paralleled by equivalent changes in oxygen extraction thereby producing a change in blood oxygen content in the postcapillary vasculature. Without this mismatch between flow and oxygen extraction there would be no BOLD signal change identified (33).

One fMRI study measured BOLD responses in 15 people with essential tremor during tremor of one limb; during passive wrist oscillations in these 15 and 12 controls, and during simulated wrist tremor in the controls (34). They found that tremor in essential tremor was associated with increased

BOLD activity in the contralateral sensorimotor cortex, thalamus, and pallidum as well as bilateral cerebellar hemispheres, dentate nuclei and red nuclei. These findings are similar to those of the PET blood flow studies, described above. Interestingly, passive wrist oscillation in these essential tremor patients only produced unilateral activation of the cerebellar hemispheres, dentate and red nucleus, and simulated tremor in the controls only produced ipsilateral BOLD responses in the cerebellar hemisphere and dentate nucleus; contralateral responses in the red nucleus and bilateral responses in the thalamus (34). Taken together these findings indicate that the tremor of essential tremor compared with passive tremor-like movements in essential tremor patients and simulated tremor in controls is selectively associated with activation of the ipsilateral red nucleus and contralateral pallidum, cerebellar hemisphere and dentate nucleus. One might interpret this as the tremor of essential tremor being different from either passive oscillations or voluntary movement since it is associated with bilateral rather than only contralateral activity in cerebellar-thalamo-cortico-cerebellar circuits.

Functional MRI has the advantages of permitting a large number of scans and conditions to be done and studied noninvasively as long as the movement associated with the activation paradigm does not perturb the head position during data acquisition. However, fMRI activation studies are best suited for types of activations that can be repeatedly turned on and off. For this reason, direct drug effects are best studied with PET activation, although new methods may eventually permit such studies with fMRI (35–37).

IV. NEUROIMAGING OF THERAPEUTIC INTERVENTIONS

A. Effects of Drugs

A variety of drugs such as beta-blockers, primidone or ethanol may temporarily reduce tremor (38,39) and PET activation studies have provided some insights into the mechanisms of drug effects. These studies have been primarily focused on the effects of ethanol. PET studies with normals found that ingestion of ethanol (1 g/kg) reduced cerebellar blood flow but increased flow in the right temporal and frontal areas (40), but these were intoxicating doses making it less clear how this may relate to doses used for treating essential tremor. Furthermore, a study of FDG uptake after ethanol 0.75 g/kg found whole brain reductions and normalized reductions in the occipital cortex with increases in the left temporal cortex (41). The shift in global FDG uptake raises a flag of caution in the interpretation of normalized regional responses since the absolute direction of a response may be misleading—in other words, a region may have an increased normalized response but in absolute terms have a reduced FDG uptake, although proportionally less than the global reduction. Thus, any drug activation study must first determine whether there is a global shift prior to assuming that global normalization for regional analysis is appropriate (42–44).

Another approach to investigate the effects of a drug such as alcohol is to measure its effects on blood flow responses induced by a physiologic activity, in this case by the tremor of essential tremor. One study used PET measures of blood flow to identify responses to tremor in 6 alcohol-responsive essential tremor patients and passive wrist oscillations in 6 matched normals before and after enough oral ethanol to reduce tremor in the patients (blood levels ∼33–35 mg/dL) (31). Like previous studies, tremor compared to rest was associated with increased cerebellar blood flow bilaterally in the hemispheres and vermis, as opposed to the ipsilateral activation from the passive wrist oscillations in the normals. Similar to studies in normals, ethanol decreased cerebellar flow bilaterally but absolute quantification was not done to permit assessment of global shifts. Given this caveat, increased flow was found in the region of the inferior olivary nucleus of the medulla in essential tremor patients but not in controls. The authors suggest that these findings are consistent with the notion that ethanol reduces cerebellar synaptic overactivity in essential tremor that leads to increased activity in inputs to olivary nuclei with subsequent increased blood flow in that region. It is unknown whether the same response would be found in essential tremor patients that have not been found to be alcohol responsive. Similar studies could also be done using other drugs such as propranolol to determine whether there are common mechanisms of action as identified by functional neuroimaging. This approach could then be used to help identify new therapies that produce similar brain responses.

B. Effects of Neurosurgical Lesions

Functional neuroimaging has also been used to investigate mechanisms of action of surgical interventions used to treat essential tremor. This approach was first done to study stereotaxic thalamotomy where a lesion is made in the VIM nucleus of the thalamus that may dramatically reduce contralateral tremor.

FDG PET studies have been done on essential tremor patients with the limbs at rest before and after VIM thalamotomy. After surgery, FDG uptake decreased in lateral prefrontal and parietal areas but no change was identified in primary motor or sensory cortical areas (45). The authors suggest that this indicates greater direct inputs from VIM to lateral prefrontal and parietal areas compared to inputs from VIM to primary motor areas. However, this interpretation assumes that a lack of an FDG PET identified regional change in a limited number of subjects indicates lack of effect. A more conservative interpretation would not make conclusions from lack of a finding with a study of limited power.

C. Effects of Deep Brain Stimulation

Functional neuroimaging also has been used to investigate the mechanism of deep brain stimulation (DBS) of the VIM nucleus of the thalamus. Despite a history of remarkable clinical benefit from this procedure, studies have only recently begun to clarify the mechanism of action of DBS. Neuroimaging has played an important role in these studies. The first major question was whether DBS acted by effectively increasing output from a stimulated region or vice versa. There may be a variety of specific mechanisms for producing these different net effects (46–50) but PET has been used to differentiate between the two basic alternatives—is the output from a stimulated region increased or decreased? The strategy for using PET to measure blood flow responses to DBS is described in Fig. 9.1.

The basic premise is that blood flow will increase in output areas if the neurons projecting from a site of stimulation increase their activity, no matter whether that activity is excitatory or inhibitory. Alternatively, if DBS has a net effect of reducing output from a region, then blood flow at that downstream target would either decrease or not change.

This basic approach was first taken in essential tremor with people with thalamic stimulators that had excellent control of tremor with the stimulators on. Left thalamic stimulation increased blood flow at the site of stimulation and at the supplementary motor area (SMA) as shown in Fig. 9.2(a) and (b) (51).

The key part of this study was that all of the PET scans were done with the arms at rest and no tremor was present either with the stimulators on or off. This eliminated the potential confound of an additional variable change (such as

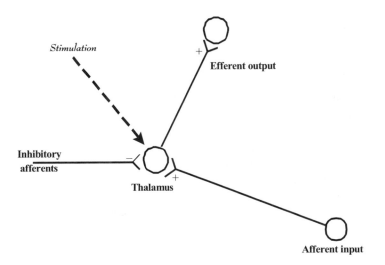

Figure 9.1 This diagram demonstrates the strategy for using PET measurements of blood flow to determine whether the net effect of deep brain stimulation in the thalamus either increases output from the thalamus to the cortex or reduces it. If it reduces it, one would expect that blood flow would either decrease or not change in targets of thalamocortical projections. Alternatively, if output from the site of thalamic stimulation increases output then blood flow would increase at these thalamocortical projection targets.

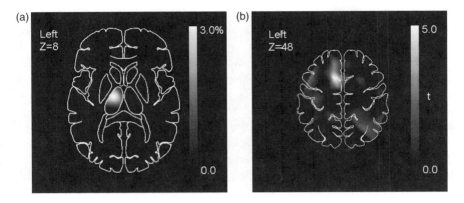

Figure 9.2 (a) Averaged regional cerebral blood flow (rCBF) response to left VIM nucleus of the thalamus DBS from 10 people with essential tremor. The image is at the level of the thalamus and the outlines are from the Talairach atlas (52). Left is on the left. This response was significant, as noted in the text. The scale is % change in rCBF. (b) This t-image shows the significant response in the left SMA from left VIM of the thalamus DBS from 10 people with essential tremor. This is a horizontal image from Talairach atlas (52) at $z = 48$ mm above the anterior-posterior commissural plane. This response is consistent with left VIM DBS increasing the activity of thalamo-cortical projections.

presence or absence of tremor) between the two conditions, thereby permitting a clear interpretation of the findings. There were no decreases in cortical areas, as one might anticipate if thalamic DBS reduced output from the thalamus. One might also expect that thalamic stimulation would produce a blood flow response in the primary motor cortex since there are direct connections from the thalamus to this area. In fact, there was a similar increase in blood flow in that area but it did not meet statistical criteria since the variance in this region was much greater than the variance in the SMA responses (51). Notably, these findings are opposite of that found with thalamotomy (45).

Identification of increased flow in SMA ipsilateral to the side of thalamic stimulation provides strong evidence about the effects of thalamic DBS. Direct outputs from the VIM nucleus of the thalamus and nearby thalamic nuclei project to this cortical region (53) suggesting that thalamic DBS produces a net increase in output from the thalamus. The relatively long time duration ($\sim$1 min) of the PET precludes determination of whether this cortical response indicates a monosynaptic connection to the site of DBS.

Other imaging studies now confirm the notion that the net effect of DBS is to produce increased output from the site of stimulation. Others have also found that VIM DBS increases flow in ipsilateral SMA (54). Subthalamic (STN) DBS in Parkinson's disease (PD) patients produces increased blood flow responses in immediate downstream targets like the pallidum and thalamus with subsequent reductions in widespread cortical areas, likely reflecting increased inhibition of thalamic projection neurons (55).

These findings seemingly contradict a PET study that DBS of the internal segment of the pallidum increases blood flow to ipsilateral premotor areas in people with PD at the same time that it reduces parkinsonian manifestations including bradykinesia, rigidity, and probably tremor (56). These findings appear consistent with reduced output from the internal pallidum to the thalamus that would increase output from the thalamus to the premotor cortex (57) Alternatively, altered motor behavior with less rigidity and possibly less tremor could reduce premotor activity. Therefore, changes in motor behavior raise a potential ambiguity in interpretation of the increased premotor blood flow—a key point when interpreting neuroimaging activation studies.

Thus, PET studies suggest that DBS increases the net output from sites of stimulation. However, it is important to consider that whether firing is increased or decreased may not be the critical factor for efficacy of DBS. The more important factor may be that driving efferent neurons interferes with transmission from the thalamus to the cortex of abnormal bursting or oscillatory neuronal firing patterns that could produce tremor by synchronously driving cortical targets (47,51).

Could fMRI of BOLD signals be used for these studies? The feasibility of this approach for thalamic stimulation, which produces clinical benefits within 30 seconds of starting stimulation has been demonstrated (58). Patients were studied with fMRI after implantation of thalamic electrodes but before surgical placement of the pulse generator. This approach does not permit an opportunity to optimize DBS programming or to let any lesion effect of surgery abate, which may substantially limit its practicality. Near infrared spectroscopy measurements found considerable variations in the blood oxygenation in the frontal cortex during either thalamic or globus pallidus interna (GPi) stimulation that raise questions about the potential for fMRI for these studies (59,60). Thorough evaluation to ensure safety must also be done prior to exposing patients to this research procedure. At least one study found that structural MRI in people with implanted DBS electrodes can be done safely (61) but others suggest that substantial caution must be exercised when doing MR scanning with active DBS electrodes in the MR field (62). Functional MRI produces larger magnitude magnetic fields that may pose additional risks for active DBS contacts and pulse generators. However, it is possible to do fMRI studies with externalized leads and pulse generators removed from the MR field (63). Finally, one must be careful during such research studies as a slightly frayed wire carries an increased risk of heating surrounding tissue.

V. FUTURE DIRECTIONS

The development and application of new neuroimaging tools promises to provide new insights into understanding the pathophysiology and treatment of essential tremor. The greatest advances may come from combining physiologic measurements with neuroimaging methods.

ACKNOWLEDGMENTS

This work has been supported by NINDS grants NS41509 and NS39821, the American Parkinson's Disease Association (APDA) Advanced Research Center for Parkinson Disease at Washington University, the Greater St. Louis Chapter of the APDA, the Barnes-Jewish Hospital Foundation (Jack Buck Fund for PD Research), the Elliot H. Stein Family Fund and the Sam & Barbara Murphy Fund.

REFERENCES

1. Rautakorpi I, Marttila R, Rinne UK. Epidemiology of essential tremor. In: Findley LJ, Capiledeo R, eds. Movement Disorders: Tremor. New York: MacMillan Publishing Co., 1984, 211–218.
2. Louis ED, Ford B, Wendt KJ, Ottman R. Validity of family history data on essential tremor. Mov Disord 1999; 14:456–461.
3. Louis ED, Ottman R. How familial is familial tremor? The genetic epidemiology of essential tremor. Neurology 1996; 46:1200–1205.
4. Gulcher JR, Jonsson P, Kong A, Kristjansson K, Frigge ML, Karason A, Einarsdottir IE, Stefansson H, Einarsdottir AS, Sigurthoardottir S, Baldursson S, Bjornsdottir S, Hrafnkelsdottir SM, Jakobsson F, Benedickz J, Stefansson K. Mapping of a familial essential tremor gene, FET1, to chromosome 3q13. Nat Genet 1997; 17:84–87.
5. Higgins JJ, Pho LT, Nee LE. A gene (ETM) for essential tremor maps to chromosome 2p22-p25. Mov Disord 1997; 12:859–864.
6. Deuschl G, Elble RJ. The pathophysiology of essential tremor. Neurology 2000; 54:S14–S20.
7. Rajput AH, Rozdilsky B, Ang L, Rajput A. Clinicopathologic observations in essential tremor: report of six cases. Neurology 1991; 41:1422–1424.
8. Kim JS, Lee MC. Writing tremor after discrete cortical infarction. Stroke 1994; 25:2280–2282.
9. Dupuis MJ, Delwaide PJ, Boucquey D, Gonsette RE. Homolateral disappearance of essential tremor after cerebellar stroke. Mov Disord 1989; 4:183–187.
10. Nagaratnam N, Kalasabail G. Contralateral abolition of essential tremor following a pontine stroke. J Neurol Sci 1997; 149:195–196.
11. Constantino AE, Louis ED. Unilateral disappearance of essential tremor after cerebral hemispheric infarct. J Neurol 2003; 250:354–355.
12. Duncan R, Bone I, Melville ID. Essential tremor cured by infarction adjacent to the thalamus. J Neurol Neurosurg Psychiatry 1988; 51:591–592.
13. Goodman SH, Wilkinson S, Overman J, Koller WC, Troster A, Pahwa R, Lyons K, Kieltyka J, Burns J, Gordon M. Lesion volume and clinical outcome in stereotactic pallidotomy and thalamotomy. Stereotact Funct Neurosurg 1998; 71:164–172.

14. Gold L, Lauritzen M. Neuronal deactivation explains decreased cerebellar blood flow in response to focal cerebral ischemia or suppressed neocortical function. Proc Natl Acad Sci USA 2002; 99:7699–7704.

15. Lauritzen M. Relationship of spikes, synaptic activity, and local changes of cerebral blood flow. J Cereb Blood Flow Metab 2001; 21:1367–1383.

16. Hallett M, Dubinsky RM. Glucose metabolism in the brain of patients with essential tremor. J Neurol Sci 1993; 114:45–48.

17. Black KJ, Gado MH, Perlmutter JS. PET measurement of dopamine D2 receptor-mediated changes in striatopallidal function. J Neurosci 1997; 17:3168–3177.

18. Jueptner M, Weiller C. Review: does measurement of regional cerebral blood flow reflect synaptic activity? Implications for PET and fMRI. Neuroimage 1995; 2:148–156.

19. McCulloch J. Mapping functional alterations in the CNS with [14C]deoxyglucose. In: Iverson LL, Iverson SD, Snyder SH, eds. Handbook of Psychopharmacology: New Techniques in Psychopharmacology. New York: Plenum, 1982; 15:321–410.

20. Raichle ME. Circulatory and metabolic correlates of brain function in normal humans. In: Plum F, ed. Handbook of Physiology: The Nervous System. Bethesda: American Physiological Society, 1987; 5(2):643–674.

21. Schwartz WJ, Smith CB, Davidsen L, Savaki H, Sokoloff L. Metabolic mapping of functional activity in the hypothalamo-neurohypophysial system of the rat. Science 1979; 205:723–725.

22. Jenkins IH, Bain PG, Colebatch JG, Thompson PD, Findley LJ, Frackowiak RS, Marsden CD, Brooks DJ. A positron emission tomography study of essential tremor: evidence for overactivity of cerebellar connections. Ann Neurol 1993; 34:82–90.

23. Wills AJ, Jenkins IH, Thompson PD, Findley LJ, Brooks DJ. Red nuclear and cerebellar but no olivary activation associated with essential tremor: a positron emission tomographic study. Ann Neurol 1994; 36:636–642.

24. Aiko Y, Shima F, Hosokawa S et al. Altered local cerebral glucose utilization induced by electrical stimulations of the thalamic sensory and parafascicular nuclei in rats. Brain Res 1987; 408:47–56.

25. Blandini F, Conti G, Martignoni E, Colangelo V, Nappi G, Di Grezia R, Orzi F. Modifications of local cerebral metabolic rates for glucose and motor behavior in rats with unilateral lesion of the subthalamic nucleus. J Cereb Blood Flow Metab 1999; 19:149–154.

26. Ceballos-Baumann AO, Boecker H, Bartensetin P, von Falkenhayn I, Riescher H, Conrad B, Moringlane JR, Alesch F. A positron emission tomographic study of subthalamic nucleus stimulation in Parkinson's disease: enhanced movement-related activity of motor-association cortex and decreased motor cortex resting activity. Arch Neurol 1999; 56:997–1003.

27. Feiwell RJ, Black KJ, McGee-Minnich LA, Snyder AZ, MacLeod A-MK, Perlmutter JS. Diminished regional cerebral blood flow response to vibration in patients with blepharospasm. Neurology 1999; 52:291–297.

28. Tempel LW, Perlmutter JS. Abnormal cortical responses in patients with writer's cramp. Neurology 1993; 43:2252–2257.

29. Chatton JY, Pellerin L, Magistretti PJ. GABA uptake into astrocytes is not associated with significant metabolic cost: implications for brain imaging of inhibitory transmission. Proc Natl Acad Sci USA 2003; 100:12456–12461.

30. Waldvogel D, van Gelderen P, Muellbacher W, Ziemann U, Immisch I, Hallett M. The relative metabolic demand of inhibition and excitation. Nature 2000; 406:995–998.

31. Boecker H, Wills AJ, Ceballos-Baumann A, Samuel M, Thompson PD, Findley LJ, Brooks DJ. The effect of ethanol on alcohol-responsive essential tremor: a positron emission tomography study. Ann Neurol 1996; 39:650–658.

32. Wills AJ, Jenkins IH, Thompson PD, Findley LJ, Brooks DJ. A positron emission tomography study of cerebral activation associated with essential and writing tremor. Arch Neurol 1995; 52:299–305.

33. Hamzei F, Knab R, Weiller C, Rother J. The influence of extra- and intracranial artery disease on the BOLD signal in fMRI. Neuroimage 2003; 20:1393–1399.

34. Bucher SF, Seelos KC, Dodel RC, Reiser M, Oertel WH. Activation mapping in essential tremor with functional magnetic resonance imaging. Ann Neurol 1997; 41:32–40.

35. Chen Q, Andersen AH, Zhang Z, Ovadia A, Gash DM, Avison MJ. Mapping drug-induced changes in cerebral R_2^* by multiple gradient recaled echo functional MRI. Magn Reson Imaging 1996; 14:469–476.

36. Chen YC, Mandeville JB, Nguyen TV, Talele A, Cavagna F, Jenkins BG. Improved mapping of pharmacologically induced neuronal activation using the IRON technique with superparamagnetic blood pool agents. J Magn Reson Imaging 2001; 14:517–524.

37. Salmeron BJ, Stein EA. Pharmacological applications of magnetic resonance imaging. Psychopharmacol Bull 2002; 36:102–129.

38. Growdon JH, Shahani BT, Young RR. The effect of alcohol on essential tremor. Neurology 1975; 25:259–262.

39. Koller WC, Biary N. Effect of alcohol on tremors: comparison with propranolol. Neurology 1984; 34:221–222.

40. Volkow ND, Mullani N, Gould L, Adler SS, Guynn RW, Overall JE, Dewey S. Effects of acute alcohol intoxication on cerebral blood flow measured with PET. Psychiatry Res 1988; 24:201–209.

41. Wang GJ, Volkow ND, Franceschi D, Fowler JS, Thanos PK, Scherbaum N, Pappas N, Wong CT, Hitzemann RJ, Felder CA. Regional brain metabolism during alcohol intoxication. Alcohol Clin Exp Res 2000; 24:822–829.

42. Hershey T, Black KJ, Carl JL, McGee-Minnich L, Snyder AZ, Perlmutter JS. Long term treatment and disease severity change brain responses to levodopa in Parkinson's disease. J Neurol Neurosurg Psychiatry 2003; 74:844–851.

43. Hershey T, Black KJ, Carl JL, Perlmutter JS. Dopa-induced blood flow responses in non-human primates. Exp Neurol 2000; 166:342–349.

44. Hershey T, Black KJ, Stambuk MK, Carl JL, McGee-Minnich LA, Perlmutter JS. Altered thalamic response to levodopa in Parkinson's patients with dopa-induced dyskinesias. Proc Natl Acad Sci USA 1998; 95:12016–12021.

45. Henselmans JM, de Jong BM, Pruim J, Staal MJ, Rutgers AW, Haaxma R. Acute effects of thalamotomy and pallidotomy on regional cerebral metabolism, evaluated by PET. Clin Neurol Neurosurg 2000; 102:84–90.

46. Benabid AL, Pollak P, Gao D, Hoffmann D, Limousin P, Gay E, Payen I, Benazzouz A. Chronic electrical stimulation of the ventralis intermedius nucleus of the thalamus as a treatment of movement disorders. J Neurosurg 1996; 84:203–214.

47. Hashimoto T, Elder CM, Okun MS, Patrick SK, Vitek JL. Stimulation of the subthalamic nucleus changes the firing pattern of pallidal neurons. J Neurosci 2003; 23:1916–1923.

48. Montgomery EB Jr, Baker LD. Mechanisms of deep brain stimulation and future technical developments. Neurol Res 2000; 22:259–266.

49. Windels F, Bruet N, Poupard A, Urbain N, Chouvet N, Couvet G, Feuerstein C, Savasta M. Effects of high frequency stimulation of subthalamic nucleus on extracellular glutamate and GABA in substantia nigra and globus pallidus in the normal rat. European Journal of Neuroscience 2000; 12:4141–4146.

50. Wu YR, Levy R, Ashby P, Tasker RR, Dostrovsky JO. Does stimulation of the GPi control dyskinesia by activating inhibitory axons? Mov Disord 2001; 16:208–216.

51. Perlmutter JS, Mink JW, Bastian AJ, Zackowski K, Hershey T, Miyawaki E, Koller W, Videen TO. Blood flow responses to deep brain stimulation of thalamus. Neurology 2002; 15:1388–1394.

52. Talairach J, Tournoux P. Co-planar stereotaxic atlas of the human brain. New York: Theime Verlag, 1988.

53. Hoover JE, Strick PL. Multiple output channels in the basal ganglia. Science 1993; 259:819–821.

54. Ceballos-Baumann AO, Boecker H, Fogel W, Alesch F, Bartenstein P, Conrad B, Diederich N, von Falkenhayn I, Moringlane JR, Schwaiger M, Tronnier VM. Thalamic stimulation for essential tremor activates motor and deactivates vestibular cortex. Neurology 2001; 56:1347–1354.

55. Hershey T, Revilla FJ, Wernle A, McGee-Minnich L, Antenor JV, Videen TO, Dowling JL, Mink JW, Perlmutter JS. Cortical and subcortical blood flow effects of subthalamic nucleus stimulation in PD. Neurology 2003; 61:816–821.

56. Davis KD, Taub E, Houle S, Lang AE, Dostrovsky JO, Tasker RR, Lozano AM. Globus pallidus stimulation activates the cortical motor system during alleviation of parkinsonian symptoms. Nat Med 1997; 3:671–674.

57. Mink JW. The basal ganglia: focused selection and inhibition of competing motor programs. Prog Neurobiol 1996; 50:381–425.

58. Rezai AR, Lozano AM, Crawley AP, Joy ML, Davis KD, Kwan CL, Dostrovsky JO, Tasker RR, Mikulis DJ. Thalamic stimulation and functional magnetic resonance imaging: localization of cortical and subcortical activation with implanted electrodes. Technical note. J Neurosurg 1999; 90:583–590.

59. Murata Y, Katayama Y, Oshima H, Kawamata T, Yamamoto T, Sakatani K, Suzuki S. Changes in cerebral blood oxygenation induced by deep brain stimulation: study by near-infrared spectroscopy (NIRS). Keio J Med 2000; 49(suppl 1):A61–A63.

60. Sakatani K, Katayama Y, Yamamoto T, Suzuki S. Changes in cerebral blood oxygenation of the frontal lobe induced by direct electrical stimulation of thalamus and globus pallidus: a near infrared spectroscopy study. J Neurol Neurosurg Psychiatry 1999; 67:769–773.

61. Uitti RJ, Tsuboi Y, Pooley RA, Putzke JD, Turk MF, Wszolek ZK, Witte RJ, Wharen RE Jr. Magnetic resonance imaging and deep brain stimulation. Neurosurgery 2002; 51:1423–1428.

62. Georgi JC, Stippich C, Tronnier VM, Heiland S. Active deep brain stimulation during MRI: A feasibility study. Magn Reson Med 2004; 51:380–388.

63. Stefurak T, Mikulis D, Mayberg H, Lang AE, Hevenor S, Pahapill P, Saint-Cyr J, Lozano A. Deep brain stimulation for Parkinson's disease dissociates mood and motor circuits: a functional MRI case study. Mov Disord 2003; 18:1508–1516.

10

Medical Treatment of Essential Tremor

Anokh Pahwa

University of Texas Medical Branch, Galveston, Texas, USA

Kelly E. Lyons and Rajesh Pahwa

University of Kansas Medical Center, Kansas City, Kansas, USA

Essential tremor is one of the most common movement disorders; however, there are currently no medications that have been developed specifically for the treatment of essential tremor. The medications that are currently used were discovered by serendipity when tremor reduction was observed after treatment for a concomitant illness. The current treatments are symptomatic and are not known to slow the progression of the disease. Treatment is generally initiated when the tremor becomes disabling and interferes with daily activities. The treatment of essential tremor can be frustrating as there are a limited number of medications available and these medications are not beneficial for all patients. Consequently, a large number of patients continue to have significant functional impairment. This chapter will discuss the medications currently used or under study for the treatment of essential tremor including beta-blockers, anticonvulsants, benzodiazepines, botulinum toxin, alcohol, and atypical antipsychotics.

I.   BETA-ADRENERGIC ANTAGONISTS

A.   Propranolol

Beta-blockers antagonize the effects of catecholamines at beta-adrenoceptors by competitively binding to the receptors. They have been used in the treatment of tremor for over 30 years (1–3), although how they exert their effect on tremor is unknown. Beta-blockers are well-absorbed after oral ingestion and tend to reach their peak concentration in 2–3 h. The most widely studied beta-blocker used in essential tremor is propranolol, a nonselective beta-adrenergic antagonist (4–8). Propranolol undergoes extensive first-pass metabolism and has a relatively low bioavailability. In addition to its beta-antagonizing effects, it may also block some serotonin receptors, although the clinical significance of this is unknown. Approximately 50% of essential tremor patients will show some benefit from propranolol for hand tremor, and the benefit can be as much as a 50–60% reduction in tremor in some patients. Multiple controlled studies have demonstrated a positive effect of propranolol on tremor based on both subjective and objective criteria (7–10), whereas others have reported a lack of benefit with propranolol (11). In a dose-response study, patients were given an escalating dose from 80 to 800 mg/day of propranolol (12). In these patients, there was no correlation between increasing serum propranolol levels and symptom control. The maximum benefit from propranolol was seen within a dose range between 160 and 320 mg/day and dosages above this provided no additional benefit.

Although propranolol has been reported to be efficacious for hand tremor, there is insufficient evidence to determine the role of propranolol in head and voice tremor (13–15). One study reported that propranolol improved head tremor at doses of 160 and 320 mg/day; however, placebo and propranolol at 80 mg/day had no benefit (13). Another double-blind, placebo-controlled study using accelerometry examined the effects of propranolol on head tremor after a single oral dose of 120 mg and following 2 weeks of sustained treatment with two different dosage regimens, 120 and 240 mg daily. When compared with placebo, a significant reduction in head tremor was observed following the single oral dose but not after sustained administration of the beta-blocker at either dosage (14). Massey and Paulson (15) reported improvement in voice tremor in 3 of 4 patients after treatment with propranolol.

A once daily long-acting preparation of propranolol, propranolol-LA, is also used in the treatment of essential tremor. Koller (16) compared long-acting propranolol with the standard preparation using a crossover study design. The long-acting preparation was preferred by the majority of patients due to convenience of once daily administration. Similar efficacy was observed between the two preparations. Similarly, in a controlled study, long-acting propranolol was as effective in reducing tremor amplitude as standard propranolol preparations (17).

Standard propranolol preparations should be started at 10–60 mg/day and slowly increased as needed with most patients achieving benefit from doses up to 120 mg/day. However, the dose can be slowly increased to 240–320 mg/day if needed and well tolerated. Propranolol-LA should be started at 60 mg/day and slowly increased to 120 mg/day if needed, higher dosages can be tried if necessary for tremor control and well tolerated by the patient. The adverse effects associated with propranolol are generally mild and do not require the discontinuation of the medication. The most commonly noted adverse effects are nausea, vomiting, diarrhea, bradycardia, hypotension, drowsiness, paresthesias, lightheadedness, weakness, fatigue, and lethargy. Other adverse effects reported include hallucinations, vivid dreams, insomnia, confusion, short-term memory loss, depression, agranulocytosis, alopecia, rashes, dry eyes, and impotence. Contraindications to the use of propranolol include severe bronchial asthma, sinus bradycardia, high-grade or complete atrioventricular block, and cardiogenic block (18). In addition, propranolol should not be used with calcium channel blockers.

Although its mechanism of action in treating tremor is unknown, both central and peripheral sites of action have been suggested. One theory suggests that propranolol has a central site of action (19). Evidence supporting this theory is the lack of effect of intravenous or intra-arterial propranolol and a delay in the effect of oral therapy. In addition, propranolol is lipophilic and readily crosses the blood–brain barrier. However, specific B2 antagonists that act predominantly peripherally are generally effective at controlling tremor. This suggests that propranolol may act peripherally (20).

B. Metoprolol

There are multiple reports of metoprolol given in divided doses of 100–200 mg/ day indicating effectiveness in the treatment of tremor (21–25). In a double-blind, controlled study of propranolol, metoprolol, and placebo (26), metoprolol and propranolol were shown to be more effective than placebo in controlling tremor. In contrast, in a controlled study of the efficacy of chronic oral administration of metoprolol, atenolol, and sotalol in essential tremor (27), only sotalol proved superior to placebo on both subjective and objective assessments.

C. Nadolol

There is very little literature on the effects of nadolol in the treatment of essential tremor. In one double-blind, placebo-controlled study (28), nadolol at 120 and 240 mg daily reduced essential tremor. The benefit was observed in patients who had previously responded to propranolol.

D. Atenolol

In a double-blind crossover study in 24 essential tremor patients, atenolol (100 mg/day) was compared with propranolol (240 mg/day) and placebo (29). Atenolol and propranolol caused a similar decrease in heart rate and also suppressed tremor intensity. There were no significant differences between the two drugs and both were significantly better than placebo. On subjective reports, the majority of the patients preferred propranolol to atenolol. In contrast, in a study of atenolol, metoprolol, and sotalol for essential tremor, atenolol was not found to be superior to placebo in controlling tremor (27).

E. Sotalol

Sotalol at doses of 75–200 mg/day has been shown to be effective in the treatment of tremor (20,27). In a double-blind, placebo-controlled trial of sotalol, metoprolol, and atenolol, only sotalol was shown to be superior to placebo in controlling tremor (27). Similarly, in a randomized, double-blind, placebo-controlled study comparing sotalol, propranolol, and atenolol for essential tremor, only sotalol was found to be comparable to propranolol in controlling tremor (20).

F. Pindolol

In a double-blind, crossover study, the effectiveness of 120 mg of propranolol and 15 mg of pindolol in controlling positional tremor was assessed in 24 essential tremor patients. Compared with placebo, tremor amplitude was reduced with propranolol and was increased with pindolol, whereas frequency remained unchanged (30).

G. Arotinolol

The effects of arotinolol on tremor were examined in 15 essential tremor patients who received 30 mg/day of arotinolol for 8 weeks (31). A reduction in both postural and action tremor was observed. In a multicenter, randomized, crossover, multiple-dose study of 175 essential tremor patients, arotinolol and propranolol were compared (32). Several dosages were evaluated: arotinolol 10, 20, and 30 mg/day and propranolol 40, 80, and 160 mg/day. Arotinolol was found to be as effective as propranolol in reducing tremor; however, motor-task performance scores revealed that arotinolol had a more significant effect than propranolol.

II. ANTICONVULSANTS

A. Primidone

The discovery that primidone has an effect on essential tremor was made serendipitously when O'Brien et al. (33) gave primidone to a patient with epilepsy. It was noted that the patient's essential tremor was unexpectedly reduced. A follow-up study (33) revealed that 12 out of 20 patients with essential tremor treated with primidone had a decrease in tremor. Multiple studies have confirmed the positive effect of primidone in treating essential tremor (34,35). The majority of the studies used primidone up to 750 mg/day. Although primidone has been reported to be effective for hand tremor, no consistent reduction in head tremor has been reported (34).

In a double-blind study, the efficacy and side effects of two dosages of primidone, 250 and 750 mg/day were compared after 1 year of treatment (36). Eighty-seven of 113 patients completed the study, 15 patients discontinued the study because of side effects, 5 had worsening of tremor, and 6 were lost to follow-up. A significantly higher percentage of patients in the 750 mg/day of primidone group discontinued the study. The patients at both doses showed a significant improvement in tremor compared with baseline; however, efficacy between the two groups was equivalent and fewer side effects were reported in the 250 mg/day group indicating that 250 mg/day of primidone is as effective as 750 mg/day with fewer side effects. Primidone has also been shown to be as effective as propranolol in controlling tremor (37). Several studies have indicated the possibility that tolerance may develop to primidone (38,39). However, one study treated 11 patients with essential tremor with primidone for 12 months and found that tremor control was still adequate after this time (40).

The mechanism of action of primidone on tremor is unknown. Primidone is metabolized to phenobarbital and phenylethylmalonamide (PEMA). As serum concentrations of primidone decrease, concentrations of phenobarbital and PEMA increase. PEMA administered alone has no effect on tremor (41). It has been proposed that both primidone and phenobarbital contribute to the anti-tremor effect (42), however, the anti-tremor effect is present when there is no detectable serum phenobarbital. In addition, the effect diminishes once serum concentrations of primidone drop (35). The current theory suggests that primidone or another unidentified metabolite of primidone is responsible for the anti-tremor effect.

Primidone should be started at 12.5–25 mg at bedtime for 1 week. After 1 week, the dose can be increased to 50 mg at bedtime and continually increased by 50 mg/week to 250 mg/day or until tremor symptoms are controlled. The frequent adverse effects associated with primidone typically resolve with continued therapy and include ataxia and vertigo. Less frequent effects include nausea, vomiting, fatigue, emotional disturbances, impotence, diplopia, polyuria, and rash (18).

B.   Topiramate

Topiramate is an anticonvulsant with several modes of action. It enhances GABAergic activity, inhibits carbonic anhydrase, antagonizes the alpha-amino-3-hydroxy-5-methyl-4-ioxazoleproprionic acid (AMPA)/kainate subtype of the glutamate receptor (43) and inhibits voltage-gate sodium and calcium channels (44). An open-label trial indicated that topiramate may be clinically useful in treating essential tremor (45). Connor (46) further assessed the efficacy of topiramate in a double-blind, placebo-controlled, crossover study. At a mean final dose of 333 mg/day, patients on topiramate demonstrated significant improvement in tremor scores, functional ability, and activities of daily living when compared with patients treated with placebo. Adverse events included weight loss, paresthesias, confusion, word-finding difficulty, dizziness, disorientation, and ataxia.

Jankovic et al. (47) conducted a multicenter, placebo-controlled, parallel study in 223 essential tremor patients. One hundred and seventeen patients received topiramate and 106 received placebo. Patients could receive one concomitant anti-tremor agent, which remained stable throughout the study. After randomization, doses were titrated over 12 weeks to the dose at which tremor resolved or the maximum tolerated dose up to 400 mg/day. The final dose was maintained for 12 weeks. Tremor was assessed with the Fahn–Tolosa–Marin Tremor Rating Scale (TRS). The mean age was 62 years and 50% were not receiving anti-tremor medication at baseline. The mean dose of topiramate was 292 mg/day administered in two doses per day. Total normalized TRS scores improved 29% from baseline with topiramate and 16% with placebo which was a significant improvement with topiramate compared with placebo. Tremor control was rated as good/very good by 72% of topiramate treated subjects. Thirty-two percent of the topiramate subjects and 10% in the placebo group discontinued use due to adverse events. The most common adverse events were paresthesias, weight loss, taste perversion, memory difficulty, fatigue, nausea, appetite decrease, and somnolence.

C. Gabapentin

Gabapentin is an amino acid that is structurally similar to GABA. Gabapentin does not act directly on the GABA receptor, but it may affect the metabolism or reuptake of GABA. Three controlled trials have assessed the efficacy of gabapentin as a treatment for essential tremor (48–50); two of the trials supported its efficacy (48,49), whereas one study failed to demonstrate any improvement (50). In the first study, Gironell et al. (48) reported gabapentin (1200 mg/day) to be superior to placebo and equal to propranolol (120 mg/day) according to observational assessments, motor tasks, global impressions, and electrophysiologic measures. A double-blind, placebo-controlled, crossover trial assessed higher-dose gabapentin (1800–3600 mg/day) as an adjunctive therapy to current anti-tremor medications in essential tremor patients (49). In this study, subjective global scores, activities of daily living scores, pouring tests, and objective tremor rating scores were significantly improved, whereas examiner global scores, spiral drawings, and accelerometry did not improve. In this study, higher doses of gabapentin were not superior to lower doses. In contrast to these mostly positive findings, Pahwa et al. (50) did not find any statistical differences between gabapentin (1800 mg/day) as an adjunctive therapy and placebo in terms of objective ratings, functional ability, or activities of daily living measures in a double-blind, placebo-controlled, crossover study. There are several possible explanations for the contradictory results seen in the various gabapentin studies. In the study by Gironell et al. (48), patients were not taking additional anti-tremor medications, whereas in the other two studies gabapentin was used as an adjunctive therapy. In addition, the patients in the Pahwa et al. (50) study had greater disability from tremor at baseline than those in the other studies, which may have affected treatment outcome. Gabapentin has a good safety profile, with adverse effects including sedation, drowsiness, fatigue, dizziness, and nausea.

D. Phenobarbital

Phenobarbital has a long history of being used to treat tremor, although studies have shown it to have little clinical benefit. Two double-blind, controlled studies have demonstrated significant improvements in tremor with phenobarbital (51,52), whereas other studies have shown no benefit in tremor with phenobarbital (35). Adverse effects include drowsiness, fatigue, and intolerable sedation. On the basis of the inconsistency of these results, phenobarbital is generally not used in the treatment of essential tremor.

III. BENZODIAZEPINES

Benzodiazepines bind to molecular components of GABA receptors in the central nervous system (CNS). Benzodiazepines potentiate GABAergic inhibition at all levels of the CNS including the spinal cord, hypothalamus, hippocampus, substantia nigra, cerebellar cortex, and cerebral cortex. This is due to an enhancement of GABA's effect, rather than a direct activation of the GABA receptor. At high doses, some benzodiazepines may also exert a negative effect on transmission at the skeletal neuromuscular junction. Their mechanism of action in decreasing tremor is unknown.

Long-term use of benzodiazepines involves a risk of habituation and addiction, whereas sudden removal of these drugs can lead to withdrawal symptoms. Common adverse effects include somnolence, dizziness, depression, fatigue, loss of co-ordination, memory loss, and confusion.

A. Clonazepam

In a double-blind, placebo-controlled study (53), clonazepam was shown to be ineffective in doses up to 4 mg/day as a treatment for essential tremor. However, it has been shown to be effective in improving kinetic tremor at a mean dose of 2.2 mg/day in 14 out of 14 patients thought to have a kinetic predominant type of essential tremor (54). Nonetheless, in clinical practice clonazepam is often used in the treatment of essential tremor and can be particularly helpful in patients with underlying anxiety.

B. Alprazolam

In a double-blind, placebo-controlled, parallel study of 24 essential tremor patients (55), alprazolam significantly reduced tremor compared with placebo. Side effects included transient fatigue and sedation. Similarly, in a double-blind, placebo-controlled, crossover study of alprazolam, primidone, and acetazolamide in 22 essential tremor patients (56), alprazolam at a mean dose of 0.75 mg/day was found to be more effective than placebo at controlling tremor and was equivalent to primidone. Mild sedation was the only adverse event reported.

C. Diazepam

There is very little information in the literature on the effects of diazepam in the treatment of essential tremor. In a double-blind, crossover study of diazepam and propranolol (6), diazepam was less effective than propranolol in controlling the symptoms of essential tremor.

IV. BOTULINUM TOXIN

Clostridium botulinum produces botulinum toxins which are potent neurotoxins. Botulinum toxins bind to presynaptic receptors and cleave SNARE proteins that are involved with vesicle fusion at neuromuscular junctions, thus blocking the release of acetylcholine from a nerve into a muscle (57,58). The muscle is essentially denervated. Botulinum toxin is not approved for the treatment of tremor but studies have shown it to be effective for tremor (59).

Jankovic et al. (60) studied botulinum toxin A in a randomized, placebo-controlled study of essential hand tremor. In this study, injections of 50 U of botulinum toxin or placebo were administered in the flexors and extensors of the wrist. A second dose of 100 U was also administered if patients failed to respond to the first dose. Objective and subjective measurements were obtained. Although accelerometry showed improvement in 9 out of 12 patients, no significant difference was observed in functional ability. All patients reported finger weakness as a side effect of the botulinum toxin A injections. In a similar study, Brin et al. (61) examined the effects of high-dose (100 U) vs. low-dose (50 U) botulinum toxin A injections when compared with placebo for the treatment of hand tremor. Again, both doses of botulinum toxin lead to decreased postural tremor, but there was no significant improvement in functional disability. Thirty percent of the patients in the low-dose group reported subjective finger weakness compared with 70% in the high-dose group, although all patients showed weakness according to grip strength measurements. Other adverse events were minor and included pain at the injection site, stiffness, rash, hematoma, and paresthesias. Both of these studies (60,61) used fixed dosages and required injection into four specified forearm muscles regardless of the patients' specific tremor. In contrast, three open-label studies (62–64) revealed improvement in functional disability and finger weakness was less common. These three studies allowed specific locations of injections to be determined by the examiner according to actual tremor location. In clinical practice, botulinum toxin has a limited role in the treatment of essential hand tremor and commonly causes hand and finger weakness.

The use of botulinum toxin for head tremor has also been examined. An open-label study of essential tremor and cervical dystonia patients reported significant improvement in head tremor on both subjective measures and accelerometry (65). Adverse effects were transient and included dysphagia, neck weakness, and pain at the injection site. In a crossover study of 10 essential tremor patients with horizontal head tremor and no dystonia, Pahwa et al. (66) found that, in general, bilateral injections of botulinum toxin A showed no significant improvement over placebo; however, 3 patients did have significant improvement. Adverse effects were reported to be frequent but transient and included neck weakness, difficulty swallowing, headache, dizziness, neck soreness, and dry skin. In clinical practice, botulinum toxin is a reasonable treatment option for essential head tremor.

There are limited data on the effect of botulinum toxin for the treatment of essential voice tremor. Open-label trials have indicated that botulinum toxin A may have some benefit for essential voice tremor (67,68). In a study of 15 patients with essential voice tremor (67), 67% of patients reported subjective improvement, whereas only 50% of patients reported objective improvement. Improvement in essential voice tremor after botulinum toxin A injections has been shown to persist for longer than 10 weeks (68). Adverse events are often transient and include a breathy voice quality and dysphagia.

V. ALCOHOL

A. Ethanol

Ethanol was discovered to reduce tremor over 50 years ago (69). The reduction in tremor caused by ethanol is short-lived (45–60 min) and is associated with a transient rebound phenomenon when the alcohol is removed. At low blood-alcohol levels, the reduction in tremor is specific to essential tremor; however, efficacy of other treatments cannot be predicted based on tremor responsiveness to ethanol (70). Unfortunately, the dose of ethanol required for significant benefit has been noted to approach intoxication, limiting alcohol's use as a therapeutic agent (71). The exact mechanism by which ethanol reduces tremor is unknown. However, a positron emission tomography study has shown alcohol to reduce the over-activity noted in the cerebellum of essential tremor patients (72). That is, alcohol may exert its action by interacting with GABA receptors in the cerebellum, thus reducing synchronized oscillations in the inferior olive.

B. Octanol

Octanol is an 8-carbon alcohol that has been shown to decrease harmiline-induced tremor in animal models of essential tremor at much lower doses than ethanol. Octanol is known to inhibit low-threshold calcium channels in inferior olive neurons, thus reducing synchronized oscillations (73,74). Octanol is approved in the US by the Food and Drug Administration (FDA) for use as a food additive with a maximum accepted daily input of 1 mg/kg of body weight. A pilot study assessed the tolerability, safety, and efficacy of octanol with a one-time dose of 1 mg/kg in 12 patients with essential tremor (75). The one-time dose was well tolerated and resulted in moderate reduction of tremor for 90 min. The only noted adverse effect was headache relieved by acetaminophen in 3 patients. There were no elevations of liver function tests, no changes in vital signs, and no signs of intoxication in any patients.

On the basis of this study, an open-label dose-escalation study of oral octanol in patients with essential tremor was performed (76). Twenty patients were started on octanol at a dose of 1 mg/kg, and the dose was escalated to 64 mg/kg over 10 days. Doses were escalated in the absence of adverse effects, and the dose endpoint was intoxication. The adverse effects noted were an unusual taste in the mouth, transient headache, nausea, dry mouth, and subjective sedation. The sedation was only noted at 64 mg/kg and was not associated with noticeable signs of intoxication. Spiral drawing, handwriting, and accelerometry showed significant reduction in tremor, with a maximum effect noted at 2 h. There was a trend towards a dose-related effect, but statistical significance was precluded by the power of the study.

These initial studies indicate that octanol may play a beneficial role in the treatment of essential tremor. Well-controlled studies are needed to further explore this possibility.

VI. CARBONIC ANHYDRASE INHIBITORS

There have been several open-label studies that have reported some degree of efficacy with carbonic anhydrase inhibitors, methazolamide and acetazolamide, in the treatment of essential tremor (77,78). These results are inconsistent with controlled studies that have reported no significant differences between methazolamide or acetazolamide and placebo in functional disability, motor tasks, tremor severity, or accelerometry (56,79). Adverse events were common and included paresthesias, drowsiness, headache, anorexia, nausea, depression, abdominal cramping, confusion, irritability, elevated creatine, altered taste, and diarrhea.

VII. CALCIUM CHANNEL ANTAGONISTS

Various calcium channel antagonists have been studied as a treatment for essential tremor; however, their use in clinical practice is limited. Nifedipine has been reported to worsen essential tremor and verapamil has been shown to have no effect on tremor (80). In a placebo-controlled study of nicardipine in essential tremor, nicardipine significantly reduced tremor compared with placebo; however, this benefit was not maintained after 1 month (81). In a crossover study of nicardipine and propranolol for essential tremor, both drugs were found to significantly reduce tremor (82). Finally, a double-blind, placebo-controlled study of nimodipine for essential tremor (83), 8 of 15 patients experienced an improvement in tremor with nimodipine when compared with placebo. Headache and heartburn were the most commonly reported side effects.

VIII. ATYPICAL ANTIPSYCHOTICS

A. Clozapine

Clozapine has been reported to be effective in the treatment of essential tremor, but its use is limited by the risk of severe adverse effects. Open-label and double-blind studies have reported significant improvement in hand tremor with clozapine (84,85). The potentially life-threatening risk of agranulocytosis is reported to occur in ~1% of patients taking clozapine and weekly blood monitoring limits the use of clozapine for essential tremor. Additional side effects can include sedation, increased salivation, tachycardia, dizziness, constipation, hypotension, headache, sweating, dry mouth, syncope, visual disturbances, seizures, and rarely fatal myocarditis.

B. Quetiapine

In an open-label study, quetiapine (up to 75 mg/day) was used as monotherapy in 10 essential tremor patients (86). Three out of 10 patients reported a >20% improvement in tremor. Adverse events included a paradoxical psychiatric reaction in 1 patient and anger in another which lead to the discontinuation of the drug and somnolence leading to a dose reduction in 2 patients. Further controlled studies are needed to assess the effectiveness of quetiapine in essential tremor.

IX. ANTIDEPRESSANTS

A. Mirtazapine

Mirtazapine is an antidepressant that acts centrally as a presynaptic A2 adrenoceptor agonist. Although there are reports of mirtazapine improving tremor (87,88), in the only double-blind, placebo-controlled study (89), no significant improvements were reported with mirtazapine. Owing to its lack of efficacy and significant adverse effects including sedation, confusion, dry mouth, polyuria, headache, and weight gain, mirtazapine is not recommended for the routine treatment of essential tremor.

X. TREATMENT SUMMARY

As there is no cure for essential tremor or is there any treatment to reduce its progression, treatment is started in patients in whom tremor is causing functional impairment. As essential tremor worsens in stressful or anxiety-provoking situations, patients with mild essential tremor may only suffer from functional disability during exposure to certain social stressors. As such, these patients can be treated with alcohol, short-acting beta-adrenergic antagonists like propranolol (10–40 mg) or benzodiazepines like alprazolam (0.25–0.5 mg) on an as needed basis. Once the tremor causes functional disability, initial therapy for patients requiring daily treatment should be beta-blockers (such as propranolol) or primidone. If tremor control is inadequate with either of these two medications, a combination of these drugs can be tried. If tremor cannot be adequately controlled with these medications or the patient cannot tolerate these medications, topiramate or gabapentin may be tried. In addition, benzodiazepines may be an option especially if the patient has associated anxiety. In patients with head or voice tremor, botulinum toxin might be tried. If the tremor continues to be disabling after trials of these medications, surgery such as deep brain stimulation of the thalamus may be the next treatment option.

REFERENCES

1. Marshall J. Tremor. In: Vinken PK, Bruyn GW, eds. Handbook of Clinical Neurology. Vol. 6. Amsterdam: North-Holland Publishing Co., 1968:809–825.
2. Winkler GF, Young RR. Efficacy of chronic propranolol therapy in action tremors of the familial, senile, or essential varieties. N Engl J Med 1974; 290:984–988.
3. Sevitt I. The effect of adrenergic beta-receptor blocking drugs on tremor. Practitioner 1971; 207:677–678.

4. Winkler GF, Young RR. The control of essential tremor by propranolol. Trans Am Neurol Assoc 1971; 96:66–68.
5. Tolosa ES, Loewenson RB. Essential tremor: treatment with propranolol. Neurology 1975; 25:1041–1044.
6. Murray TJ. Long-term therapy of essential tremor with propranolol. Can Med Assoc J 1976; 115:892–894.
7. Dupont E, Hansen HJ, Dalby MA. Treatment of benign essential tremor with propranolol: a controlled clinical trial. Acta Neurol Scand 1973; 69:75–84.
8. Teravainen H, Fogelholm R, Larsen A. Effect of propranolol on essential tremor. Neurology 1976; 26:27–30.
9. Calzetti S, Findley LJ, Gresty MA et al. Effect of a single dose of propranolol on essential tremor: a double-blind controlled study. Ann Neurol 1983; 13:165–171.
10. Calzetti S, Findley LJ, Perucca E et al. The response of essential tremor to propranolol: evaluation of clinical variables governing the efficacy of prolonged administration. J Neurol Neurosurg Psychiatry 1983; 46:393–398.
11. Sweet RD, Blumberg J, Lee LJ et al. Propranolol treatment of essential tremor. Neurology 1974; 24:64–67.
12. Koller WC. Dose response relationship of propranolol in essential tremor. Arch Neurol 1986; 35:42–43.
13. Koller WC. Propranolol therapy for essential tremor of the head. J Neurol 1984; 34:1077–1079.
14. Calzetti S, Sasso E, Negrotti A et al. Effect of propranolol in head tremor: quantitative study following single dose and sustained drug administration. Clin Neuropharmacol 1992; 15:470–476.
15. Massey EW, Paulson GW. Essential vocal tremor: clinical characteristics and response to therapy. South Med J 1985; 78:316–317.
16. Koller WC. Long-acting propranolol in essential tremor. Neurology 1985; 36:108–110.
17. Cleeves L, Findley L. Propranolol and propranolol-LA in essential tremor: a double-blind comparative study. J Neurol Neurosurg Psychiatry 1988; 51:379–384.
18. Physician's Desk Reference. 58th ed. Montvale, NJ: Thompson PDR, 2004.
19. Young RR. Essential-familial tremor and other action tremors. Semin Neurol 1982; 2:386–391.
20. Jefferson D, Jenner P, Marsden CD. Beta-adrenoreceptor antagonists in essential tremor. J Neurol Neurosurg Psychiatry 1979; 42:904–909.
21. Britt CR, Peters BH. Metoprolol for essential tremor. N Engl J Med 1979; 301:331.
22. Ljung O. Treatment of essential tremor with metoprolol. N Engl J Med 1979; 301:1005.
23. Newman RP, Jacobs L. Metoprolol in essential tremor. Arch Neurol 1980; 37:596–597.
24. Riley T, Pleet AB. Metoprolol tartrate for essential tremor. N Engl J Med 1979; 301:663.
25. Turnbull DM, Shaw DA. Metoprolol in essential tremor. Lancet 1980; 1:95.
26. Calzetti S, Findley LJ, Gresty MA et al. Metropolol and propranolol in essential tremor: a double-blind controlled study. J Neurol Neurosurg Psychiatry 1981; 44:814–819.
27. Leigh PN, Jefferson D, Twomey A, Marsden CD. Beta-adrenoreceptor mechanisms in essential tremor; a double-blind placebo controlled trial of metoprolol, sotalol and atenolol. J Neurol Neurosurg Psychiatry 1983; 46:710–715.
28. Koller WC. Nadolol in essential tremor. Neurology 1983; 33:1076–1077.

29. Larsen TA, Teravainen H, Calne DB. Atenolol vs. propranolol in essential tremor. A controlled, quantitative study. Acta Neurol Scand 1982; 66:547–554.

30. Teravainen H, Larsen A, Fogelholm R. Comparison between the effects of pindolol and propranolol on essential tremor. Neurology 1977; 27:439–442.

31. Kuroda Y, Kakigi R, Shibasaki H. Treatment of essential tremor with arotinolol. Neurology 1988; 38:650–652.

32. Lee KS, Kim JS, Kim JW, Lee WY, Jeon BS, Kim D. A multicenter randomized crossover multiple-dose comparison study of arotinolol and propranolol in essential tremor. Parkinsonism Relat Disord 2003; 9:341–347.

33. O'Brien MD, Upton AR, Toseland PA. Benign familial tremor treated with primidone. Br Med J 1981; 282:178–180.

34. Findley LJ, Cleeves L, Calzetti S. Primidone in essential tremor of the hands and head: a double-blind controlled clinical study. J Neurol Neurosurg Psychiatry 1985; 481:911–915.

35. Koller WC, Royse V. Efficacy of primidone in essential tremor. Neurology 1986; 36:121–124.

36. Serrano-Duenas M. Use of primidone in low doses (250 mg/day) versus high doses (750 mg/day) in the management of essential tremor. Double-blind comparative study with one-year follow-up. Parkinsonism Relat Disord 2003; 10:29–33.

37. Gorman WP, Cooper R, Pocock P et al. A comparison of primidone, propranolol, and placebo in essential tremor using quantitative analysis. J Neurol Neurosurg Psychiatry 1986; 491:64–68.

38. Crystal HA. Duration of effectiveness of primidone in essential tremor. Neurology 1986; 36:1543.

39. Shale H, Fahn S. Response to essential tremor to treatment with primidone [abstract]. Neurology 1987; 37:123.

40. Sasso E, Perucca E, Fava N et al. Primidone in the long-term treatment of essential tremor: a prospective study with computerized quantitative analysis. Clin Neuropharmacol 1990; 13:67–76.

41. Calzetti S, Findley L, Risani F et al. Phenylethylmalonamide in essential tremor. J Neurol Neurosurg Psychiatry 1981; 44:932–934.

42. Findley LJ, Calzetti S. Double-blind controlled study of primidone in essential tremor: preliminary results. Br Med J 1982; 285:608.

43. Glauser TA. Topiramate. Epilepsia 1999; 40(suppl 5):S71–S80.

44. Kawasaki, Tancredi V, D'Arcangelo G et al. Multiple actions of the novel anticonvulsant drug topiramate in the rat subiculum *in vitro*. Brain Res 1998; 807:125–134.

45. Connor GS. Topiramate as a novel treatment for essential tremor [abstract]. Mov Disord 1999; 14:908.

46. Connor GS. A randomized double-blind placebo controlled trial of topiramate treatment for essential tremor. Neurology 2002; 59:132–134.

47. Jankovic J, Ondo WG, Stacy MA et al. A multicenter, double-blind, placebo-controlled trial of topiramate in essential tremor [abstract]. Mov Disord 2004; 19(suppl 9):S448–S449.

48. Gironell A, Barbanoj M, Kulisevsky J et al. A randomized placebo controlled comparative trial of gabapentin and propranolol in essential tremor. Arch Neurol 1999; 56:475–480.

49. Ondo WG, Hunter C, Schwartz K et al. High dose gabapentin for essential tremor: a double-blind, placebo-controlled, crossover trial. Mov Disord 2000; 15:678–682.
50. Pahwa R, Lyons K, Hubble J et al. Double-blind controlled trial of gabapentin in essential tremor. Mov Disord 1998; 13:465–467.
51. Baruzzi A, Procaceranti G, Martinelle P. Phenobarbitol and propranolol in essential tremor: a double-blind controlled clinical trial. Neurology 1983; 33:296–300.
52. Findley LK, Cleeves L. Phenobarbitol in essential tremor. Neurology 1985; 35:1784–1787.
53. Thompson C, Lang A, Pareks JD et al. A double-blind trial of clonazepam in benign essential tremor. Clin Neuroparmacol 1984; 7:83–88.
54. Biary N, Koller W. Kinetic predominant essential tremor: successful treatment with clonazepam. Neurology 1987; 37:471–474.
55. Huber SJ, Paulsen GW. Efficacy of alprazolam for essential tremor. Neurology 1988; 38:241–243.
56. Gunal DI, Afsar N, Bekiroglu N et al. New alternative agents in essential tremor therapy; double-blind, placebo-controlled study of alprazolam and acetazolamide. Neurol Sci 2000; 21:315–317.
57. Montecucco C, Shiavo G, Rossetto O. The mechanism of action of tetanus and botulinum neurotoxins. Arch Toxicol Suppl 1996; 18:342–354.
58. Catsicas S, Grenningloh G, Pcij EM. Nerve-terminal proteins: to fuse to learn. Trends Neurosci 1994; 17:368–373.
59. Jost WH, Kohl A. Botulinum toxin: evidence-based medicine criteria in rare conditions. J Neurol 2000; 248(suppl 1):139–144.
60. Jankovic J, Schwartz K, Clemence W et al. A randomized, double-blind, placebo-controlled study to evaluate botulinum toxin A in essential hand tremor. Mov Disord 1996; 11:250–256.
61. Brin MF, Lyons KE, Doucette J et al. A randomized, double-masked, controlled trial of botulinum toxin type A in essential hand tremor. Neurology 2001; 56:1523–1528.
62. Pacchetti C, Mancini F, Bulgheroni M et al. Botulinum toxin treatment for functional disability induced by essential tremor. Neurol Sci 2000; 21:349–353.
63. Trosch RM, Pullman SL. Botulinum toxin A injections for the treatment of hand tremors. Mov Disord 1994; 9:601–609.
64. Henderson JM, Ghika JA, Van Melle G et al. Botulinum toxin A in non-dystonic tremors. Eur Neurol 1996; 36:29–35.
65. Wissel J, Mashur F, Schelosky L et al. Quantitative assessment of botulinum toxin treatment in 43 patients with head tremor. Mov Disord 1997; 12:722–726.
66. Pahwa R, Busenbark K, Swanson-Hyland EF et al. Botulinum toxin treatment of essential head tremor. Neurology 1995; 45:822–824.
67. Hertegard S, Granqvist S, Lindestad PA. Botulinum toxin injections for essential voice tremor. Ann Otol Rhinol Laryngol 2000; 109:204–209.
68. Warrick P. The treatment of essential voice tremor with botulinum toxin A: a longitudinal case report. J Voice 2000; 14:410–421.
69. Critchley M. Observations on essential tremor. Brain 1949; 72:113–139.
70. Koller WC, Biary N. Effect of alcohol on tremors: comparison with propranolol. Neurology 1984; 34:221–223.
71. Sinclair JG, Lo GF, Harris DP. Ethanol effects on the olivocerebellar system. Can J Physiol Pharmacol 1982; 60:610–614.

72. Boecker H, Wills AJ, Ceballos-Bauman A et al. The effect of ethanol on alcohol-responsive essential tremor: a positron emission tomography study. Ann Neurol 1996; 39:650–658.
73. Sinton CM, Krosser BI, Walton KD, Llinas RR. The effectiveness of different isomers of octanol as blockers of harmaline-induced tremor. Pflugers Arch 1989; 414:31–36.
74. McCreery MJ, Hunt WA. Physio-chemical correlates of alcohol intoxication. Neuropharmacology 1977; 17:451–461.
75. Bushara KO, Goldstein SR, Grimes GJ et al. Pilot trial of 1-octanol in essential tremor. Neurology 2004; 62:122–124.
76. Shill HA, Bushara KO, Mari Z et al. Open-label dose-escalation study of oral 1-octanol in patients with essential tremor. Neurology 2004; 62:2320–2322.
77. Muenter MD, Daube JR, Caviness JN et al. Treatment of essential tremor with methazolamide. Mayo Clinic Proc 1991; 66:991–997.
78. Busenbark K, Pahwa R, Hubble J et al. The effect of acetazolamide on essential tremor: an open-label trial. Neurology 1992; 42:1394–1395.
79. Busenbark K, Pahwa R, Hubble J et al. Double-blind controlled study of methazolamide in the treatment of essential tremor. Neurology 1993; 43:104–107.
80. Topaktas S, Onur R, Dalkara T. Calcium channel blockers and essential tremor. Eur Neurol 1987; 27:114–119.
81. Garcia-Ruiz PJ, Garcia de Yenebes Prous J, Jiminez-Jiminez J. Effect of nicardipine on essential tremor: brief report. Clin Neuropharmacol 1993; 16:456–459.
82. Jiminez-Jiminez FJ, Garcia-Ruiz PJ, Cabrera-Valdivia F. Nicardipine versus propranolol in essential tremor. Acta Neurol 1994; 16:184–188.
83. Biary N, Bahou Y, Sofia MA et al. The effect of nimodipine on essential tremor. Neurology 1995; 45:1523–1525.
84. Pakkenberg H, Pakkenberg B. Clozapine in the treatment of tremor. Acta Neurol Scand 1986; 73:295–297.
85. Ceravolo R, Salvetti S, Piccini P et al. Acute and chronic effects of clozapine in essential tremor. Mov Disord 1999; 14:468–472.
86. Micheli F, Cersosimo MG, Raina G, Gatto E. Quetiapine and essential tremor. Clin Neuropharmacol 2002; 25:303–306.
87. Pact V, Giduz T. Mirtazapine treats resting tremor, essential tremor, and levodopa induced dyskinesias. Neurology 1999; 53:1154.
88. Ertan S, Koksal A, Ozemecki S. Clinical efficacy of mirtazapine in essential tremor [abstract]. Mov Disord 2000; 15(suppl 3):102.
89. Pahwa R, Lyons KE. Mirtazapine in essential tremor: a double-blind, placebo-controlled pilot study. Mov Disord 2003; 18:584–587.

11

Surgical Treatment of Tremor

Yasuhiko Baba and Ryan J. Uitti

*Mayo Clinic, Jacksonville,
Florida, USA*

I. INTRODUCTION

Tremor is a common involuntary movement disorder, and can arise from various etiologies (1), with essential tremor being the most common (prevalence between 0.05% and 5.5%) (2). Many patients with tremor syndromes live with substantial inconvenience before eventually seeking medical advice. The management of tremor was fairly nihilistic until the 1950–60s at which time both pharmacological treatments and stereotactic neurosurgeries were first commonly employed. In the late 1950s, the ventrolateral thalamus replaced the globus pallidus as a main surgical target for tremor of various types (3,4). In the 1960s, microelectrode recording techniques, employed during the course of functional stereotactic surgery in order to better delineate surgical targets, were introduced by Albe-Fessard et al. (5) and others. These electrophysiologic studies helped to determine the ventral intermediate (VIM) nucleus of the thalamus as the optimal lesioning target for treatment of tremor. Such techniques were commonly used and thousands of thalamotomies were carried out during the 1950–60s for tremor from Parkinson's disease (PD) and essential tremor (6–8). Major limitations encountered with surgical treatments in the first half of the 20th century included inconsistent targeting and surgical complications.

With the introduction of anti-tremor pharmacological agents, including β-blockers, primidone and levodopa in the 1960s, the use of surgical therapy for tremor declined substantially (9). However, despite advances in pharmacotherapy for tremor, many patients do not receive substantial benefit (10). This has led to a resurgence of interest in the surgical treatment of tremor.

While thalamotomy became increasingly used to treat severe, unilateral tremor in the 1980s, it was noted that thalamic stimulation, used for localization purposes intraoperatively, could itself alleviate tremor (11). This led to further exploration of deep brain stimulation (DBS) for the treatment of tremor. Studies have focused on the optimal location and size of permanent or "functional" lesions as they relate to minimizing movement disorder symptoms.

Improvements in radiology [computed tomography (CT) and magnetic resonance imaging (MRI)] and stereotactic software guidance systems have dramatically reduced the frequency of adverse effects and increased the reliability of outcomes. Additionally, the development of pathophysiological models of tremor disorders has contributed to advancements in functional surgery for movement disorders. However, as with all forms of surgery, the safety and efficacy of treatment may vary substantially on the basis of available equipment, expertise and experience, not to mention patient selection.

II. PATHOPHYSIOLOGY OF TREMOR

Individual basal ganglia and thalamo-cortical circuits originate in different somatotopically-organized cortical areas and project to the striatum, globus pallidus, subthalamic nucleus (STN), and thalamus, with other tracts completing the loop in returning to cortex (12). Output of the basal ganglia is directed, via the thalamus, to the motor and supplementary motor cortices, and the dorsal cingulate region. Major output from the basal ganglia includes the globus pallidus interna (GPi) and substantia nigra pars reticulata (SNr), which have been postulated to function via an indirect and a direct pathway (13,14). Activation of the direct pathway normally inhibits GPi neurons, while that of the indirect pathway stimulates GPi neurons, which in turn act upon thalamic nuclei (13). Normally, the direct pathway provides positive feedback, and the indirect pathway provides negative feedback to the precentral motor fields (13).

In animal studies, the administration of harmaline, a β-carboline drug, produces an essential tremor-like tremor. It is also well known that excessive catecholamines can exacerbate physiological tremor. It is believed that oscillations in the olivocerebellar circuit are crucial to the pathogenesis of essential tremor (15–17). The fact that lesions in the cerebellum (18), pons (19), and thalamus (20) greatly minimize or abolish tremor in essential tremor suggest that abnormal oscillations are transmitted to the motor cortex via the cerebellum and its projections to the ventrolateral thalamus (cerebellocortical loop) (21). Positron emission tomography (PET) studies in essential tremor have also shown increased activation in the cerebellum, red nucleus, striatum, thalamus, and sensorimotor cortex coincident with tremor (22,23).

Elble and others have suggested that central oscillations in the cortico-basal ganglia-thalamo-cortical loop play an important role in the production of tremor (21). Based on primate models of PD, loss of dopamine results in increased output from the GPi as a result of excessive excitatory drive from the STN (24). Intermittent oscillations are also detected in the motor cortex (25), ventrolateral thalamus (26), GPi (27) and STN (28) in PD patients with tremor.

Cerebellar tremor, a term which is clinically often used synonymously with intention tremor, is produced by lesions or dysfunction in the cerebellar nuclei (dentate and globose-emboliform) or cerebellar outflow tract to the contralateral ventrolateral thalamus (brachium conjunctivum) (21). In animal models, tremor-related activity is present in the motor and somatosensory cortex and globose-emboliform nucleus (29). Cerebellar tremor seems associated with oscillation of sensorimotor feedback loops between the limbs and motor cortex. This oscillation is probably enhanced by reverberation in the thalamocortical loop or some other central pathway with a natural tendency to oscillate (21,30).

"Holmes" tremor, which has also been termed "rubral tremor," "midbrain tremor," and "thalamic tremor," arises from lesions in various cerebellar outflow pathways surrounding the red nucleus (31,32). Pathological and PET studies in cerebellar outflow tremor states have shown lesions in both nigrostriatal and cerebellothalamic (brachium conjunctivum) pathways (33,34).

The pathogenesis of tremor associated with various etiologies remains unclear. However, previous pathophysiological and neuroradiological studies provide the evidence that the ventrolateral thalamus is one of the most effective targets for functional neurosurgery aimed at minimizing or eliminating tremor, regardless of etiology. The ventrolateral nucleus of the thalamus is divided into the ventralis oralis posterior (VOP) nucleus and ventralis intermedius nucleus (VIM). The VIM receives input from somatosensory pathways and deep cerebellar nuclei, and projects to the motor cortex (9). Oscillations in the nervous system may be routed through the VIM, resulting in pathological tremor (9). It is also possible that the VIM itself is the generator of oscillations that drive tremor (35). Others propose that tremor originates in the globus pallidus based on the fact that tremor lessens when probes are introduced into the pallidum during pallidotomy (36). These theories require further exploration, and a full understanding of why thalamotomy and pallidotomy improve the symptoms of essential tremor or PD, while not causing involuntary movements, remains to be explained (37).

III. SURGICAL OPTIONS AND INDICATIONS

Patients with disabling tremor, on account of functional or cosmetic incapacity, may be candidates for surgery. The definition of "disabling" may vary significantly between patients. Trials with pharmacotherapy at appropriate dosages are warranted for all patients with disabling tremor. Essential tremor patients who continue to have disability, despite trials with a non-selective beta-blocker such as propranolol and a trial of primidone, without major psychiatric or medical problems, may be candidates for surgery.

It is convenient to subdivide surgery for tremor into two groups, ablation/ lesioning and DBS. Targets for these forms of treatment are generally shared between ablative and stimulation surgeries, although these modalities may well operate with different mechanisms. The two main forms of surgery will be discussed sequentially followed by conclusions regarding implementation and selection of specific procedures for individual tremor patients.

IV. THALAMOTOMY

VIM thalamotomy is useful for treatment of medically intractable tremor from not only essential tremor, but also parkinsonian, cerebellar, post-traumatic, and poststroke tremor (38–41). Thalamotomy has also been employed for treatment of other hyperkinetic disorders such as dystonia, hemiballism, and dyskinesias with various etiologies (42,43). Tremor induced by toluene abuse, presumably on the basis of cerebellar outflow dysfunction, has been successfully treated by thalamotomy (44). Similar to traditional thalamotomy, treatment with gamma knife lesioning has been performed for patients with action tremor and tremor due to PD who are unable to tolerate standard neurosurgical procedures (45–47).

Marked to complete relief of tremor is made by lesions as small as 2 mm located within the VIM nucleus. Tremor cells within the VIM may be identified by neuronal firing at frequencies that coincide with electromyographic (EMG) tremor activity (48), although tremor relief can occur even in the absence of tremor cells being identified. This form of treatment may be indicated in patients with essential tremor and those with parkinsonism in whom tremor overshadows other signs. Additionally, thalamotomy may be particularly appropriate for patients with distinctly asymmetric tremor, as bilateral thalamotomy is associated with a particularly high risk of irreversible dysarthria (49). Patients who would not be able to return to the medical center for stimulator programming would also be potential candidates for thalamotomy.

V. THALAMIC STIMULATION

In the 1960s, shortly after the introduction thalamotomy, it was recognized that high-frequency stimulation of the VIM nucleus of the thalamus produced relief of tremor (50,51). In the late 1980s, Benabid et al. (52) reintroduced high-frequency VIM stimulation as a surgical procedure for parkinsonian and essential tremor with similar efficacy to thalamotomy and fewer complications. Thalamic stimulation is recommended as a treatment for medically refractory disabling tremor in PD and essential tremor (53). Thalamic stimulation is generally preferable to thalamotomy for tremor suppression because of reversibility of side effects, comparable efficacy to thalamotomy, potential for modifying stimulation parameters over time for worsening tremor, potential for bilateral treatment, and reversibility (53,54). Occasional patients with primary writing tremor (55,56), children with choreiform movements (57), those with painful dystonic posturing resulting from paroxysmal nonkinesigenic dyskinesia (58), and patients with "thalamic hand" syndrome (poststroke thalamic central pain and dystonia) (59,60) have also been treated and had good results with thalamic stimulation. Thalamic stimulation, produces reversible changes and does not cause damage to adjacent brain parenchyma (61). Because of lower risk for dysphasia and dysarthria, thalamic DBS is also practical to perform bilaterally (62). Additionally, thalamic stimulation may be advantageous over lesioning, as treatment can be modified over time. On the other hand, DBS procedures may carry a higher risk for infection and hardware malfunction, as well as greater equipment costs and need for periodic pulse generator replacement.

It is assumed that high frequency stimulation alters abnormal brain activity by one or more of the following mechanisms: (1) depolarizing block, (2) "jamming" of neural activity, (3) channel blocking, (4) neuronal energy depletion, (5) synaptic failure, (6) antero- and retrograde effects, (7) activation of inhibitory and inactivation of excitatory neurotransmission, (8) effects on non-neuronal cells, and (9) effects on local concentration of iron or neuroactive molecules (63). However, the specific mechanism of action of DBS is not fully understood. Ceballos-Baumann et al. (64) investigated the functional effect of VIM DBS, and found that VIM DBS is associated with increased regional cerebral blood flow (rCBF) in the ipsilateral motor cortex. They suggested that the beneficial effect of VIM DBS correlates with increased synaptic activity in the motor cortex, probably occurring as a result of activation of thalamocortical projections, or frequency-dependent neuroinhibition that overrides the abnormal periodic neuronal pattern underlying tremor. Perlmutter et al. (65) also found increased blood flow in the ipsilateral supplementary motor area, which is a terminal field of thalamocortical projections, in patients with VIM DBS.

VI. SUBTHALAMIC STIMULATION

Bergman et al. (66) reported two 1-methyl-4-phenyl-1,2,3,6-tetrahydropyridine (MPTP)-treated monkeys that showed improvements of contralateral tremor, rigidity and akinesia after ibotenic acid injection in the ipsilateral STN. On the basis of this and other evidence, the subthalamic nucleus became a target for functional surgery in movement disorders (67,68). It has been reported that stimulation of the posteromedial subthalamic area remarkably improves both distal and proximal symptoms in essential tremor (69). The efficacy associated with this target also extends to axial tremor. Stimulation of a similar target, including the zona incerta, may also be effective in reducing proximal tremor in various types of patients who are refractory to VIM thalamotomy (70).

VII. METHODOLOGY

A. Selection of Patients and Surgical Types

Appropriate patient selection is the most important key to obtain a favorable outcome from any surgical procedure. Thorough neurological, neuropsychological, pharmaceutical, radiological, and systematic medical evaluations are best comprehensively performed by a dedicated team including a neurologist, neurosurgeon, neuroradiologist, neuropsychologist, and nurse.

The risks and potential benefits of brain surgery dictate that essential tremor patients are best treated initially with pharmacological agents with surgery reserved for circumstances in which medication fails to provide consistent or substantial benefit. Relative contraindications for all surgery include major psychiatric disturbances (major depression, psychosis) and dementia. Thalamotomy can result in postoperative dysarthria and dysphagia, especially when performed bilaterally (71). Therefore, significant abnormalities of speech and swallowing are relative contraindications particularly for lesioning operations (72). Chronic anticoagulation is not an absolute surgical contraindication, but careful perioperative management is required. The presence of severe hypertension, brain atrophy and white matter signal changes, may increase the occurrence of intracerebral hemorrhage. Additionally, the presence of intracranial lesions on MRI or CT may compromise accurate radiological target determination (72). Patients with other severe medical illnesses are generally not surgical candidates because of higher risk for the surgical procedure and limited life span. Patients with cardiac pacemakers/defibrillators or spinal cord stimulators initially were generally not treated with DBS. However, several patients treated with DBS have subsequently been successfully treated with cardiac pacemakers/defibrillators when required (73) and therefore these devices are not absolute contraindications for DBS.

Selection of the target and surgical type must be determined by virtue of each patient's needs. Consequently, it is essential to delineate the patient's current and potential future needs that most influence daily life. While DBS can be performed with less neurologic complications than a lesioning procedure, it does require potentially frequent adjustments in stimulation parameters and occasional pulse generator replacements, as well as carrying potential risk for infection and delayed complications with hardware. On the other hand, lesioning procedures are performed relatively easily without high cost. While some patients have had DBS contralateral to lesioning procedures, it remains to be seen whether such a practice offers substantial benefits.

B. Operative Methodology

CT or MRI of the brain is obtained prior to and generally following the procedure to assess for hematoma and edema and to verify lesion/electrode placement. Prior to surgery, cerebral angiography may rarely be performed to delineate surrounding blood vessels in the target area, although high quality MR imaging usually obviates the need for angiography.

Stereotactic surgery was developed in order to better determine the relationship of the surgical target to nearby structures, which can be visualized radiographically, and then to direct an electrode or other probe, to the target with minimal damage to surrounding structures (74). The optimal means for targeting continues to be a subject of debate (75), but always includes neural imaging. Initial targeting is guided by integration of CT or MRI imaging, with frames for stereotactic surgery being formulated via specially designed computer software (72).

Small statistical differences in MRI versus CT-derived targets have been identified and although direct comparison with clinical outcomes has not been made, most institutions have concluded that MRI-based target localization is superior to CT (76). Comparisons of MRI-guided and ventriculography-based stereotactic surgery for PD have concluded that each results in similar clinical outcomes, concerning efficacy and complications (77). Lesions in thalamotomy are made using stereotactic radiofrequency ablation, often following electrophysiological recordings and stimulation procedures. It has been determined that electrophysiologic recording typically leads to final placement of lesions within 2–3 mm of MRI targets, with the actual lesion overlapping the MRI theoretical target in 40–50% of patients (78). Occasionally DBS electrodes themselves are employed in the process of placing permanent lesions (79).

Surgical techniques vary between centers. This discussion provides descriptions of only some of the techniques commonly used. Ablative and DBS procedures are performed under local anesthesia so that the patient can be monitored with clinical outcome criteria intraoperatively (36,80). Usually after the stereotactic frame is placed under local anesthesia, CT or MRI is performed to locate the coordinates of the anterior commissure (AC) and posterior commissure (PC). Computer programs allow for subsequent simulation of surgical tracts with the patient's MRI, disclosing the precise trajectory and distance to target from the burr hole and lead guiding apparatus. Stereotactic devices are subsequently fixed to the frame and microelectrode recording/stimulation ensues. Electrophysiological assessments of the activity of the target are frequently employed to ensure proper targeting and placement of the electrode. The sensorimotor region of various targets is delineated by recording increases in neuronal discharge coincident with passive manipulation of the limbs, during active movement, and with sensory stimulation (usually over the first three digits of the hand or at the corner of the mouth contralateral to microelectrode recording in the VOP-thalamus, and several millimeters posterior to the ideal VIM target). Within VIM, microelectrode recording may also disclose tremor cells firing coincident to tremor seen in the contralateral limbs. In the STN, the arm and face are in the most lateral region and the leg is slightly more medial. The reverse is the case for the VIM, where the leg is lateral to the arm (81).

After localization of the target by electrophysiological recording, in ablative procedures, radiofrequency lesioning is performed along the trajectory, following a test lesion (reversible, with lower temperatures being employed). In DBS procedures, electrode implantation is performed with the electrode array straddling the greatest extent of the sensorimotor region of each target nucleus. The electrode is placed into the intended target with X-ray confirmation followed by intraoperative stimulation and characterization of stimulation effects (Fig. 11.1).

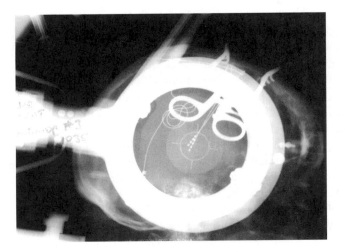

Figure 11.1 Implantation of thalamic deep brain stimulation electrode. Electrode positioning following MRI targeting is confirmed with intraoperative lateral X-ray of the head.

In thalamotomy, a burr hole is made and, based on previously delineated coordinates; a monopolar microelectrode is advanced to identify somatotopy in the thalamic somatosensory nucleus, ventralis posterior. Moving anteriorly to sensory recordings made following tactile stimulation of the contralateral hand or face, leads to stimulation of the VIM nucleus, which has a characteristic spontaneous discharge coincident with tremor activity (74). A separate, monopolar, stimulating electrode may subsequently be used, noting tremor suppression once the correct area is reached (74). The operation is monitored clinically in terms of speech, manual and foot dexterity, sensation, tone and tremor, and electrically, in response to proprioceptive, kinesthetic, and electrical stimulation of the involved limb (35,72,82). Once the appropriate coordinates are determined, a lesion is made with a semi-microelectrode (74,82). This electrode is hollow, allowing the insertion of a thermocouple device, and uses a radiofrequency current to create heat and a consequent lesion (74).

According to a survey of current practice (pallidotomy) in North America (83), lesions are typically made employing a median temperature of 75°C for one minute. Microelectrode recording was performed by 50% of the centers surveyed, with the main target defining criteria being (1) the firing pattern of spontaneous neuronal discharge and (2) the response to passive manipulation of a limb. Proponents for microelectrode recordings indicate that such recordings altered the final target in almost every instance, with one of nine targets being >4 mm from the image-guided site (84).

Microvascular doppler evaluation, performed in order to identify intracerebral vessels in proximity to targets for thermocoagulation (in thalamotomy or pallidotomy), has been described as a means to minimize risk of vascular injury. A prominent vascular sound was identified in 3 of 13 cases in one series (85). It is unclear whether use of this technique significantly impacts on safety in these lesioning operations and this evaluation is rarely performed.

In thalamic stimulation, placement of the stimulating quadripolar lead is performed under local anesthesia with subsequent implantation of an external, programmable stimulator being placed under general anesthesia (11). Contrast ventriculography is used by some to allow advancement of the electrode through a burrhole towards the VIM nucleus target (11). Most centers employ MRI or CT-guided software to prepare a surgical targeting trajectory for placement of the stimulation lead. Electrophysiological confirmation of the target proceeds as with thalamotomy. When stimulation through the quadripolar lead suppresses tremor, the electrode is implanted and connected to a percutaneous lead that is tunneled to the implanted pulse generator (11). A similar technique is used for placement of the stimulator for pallidal and STN stimulation (86). Microelectrode recordings in the STN suggest a somatotopic arrangement that may aid in electrode placement (87).

The effects of intravenous anesthesia with propofol on intraoperative electrophysiologic monitoring were studied in patients during thalamotomy. Infusion of this agent needed to be reduced to detect neural noise levels required for targeting, as well as clinical confirmation of outcomes with stimulation. The rapid onset of action and clearing of action make propofol a useful anesthetic agent during functional neurosurgery (88).

VIII. FOLLOW-UP CARE

Evaluation after surgery is important and careful follow-up is required to identify neurological deficits or procedure-related complications, as well as to modify pharmacological and stimulation treatment. CT or MRI examination may be performed to confirm lesioning or implanted electrode site location, and to identify procedure-related complications (Fig. 11.2). In DBS procedures, pulse generators may be turned "on" to delineate clinical effects and determine need for programming adjustment. Most patients require evaluation every 1–3 months immediately after surgery and thereafter at yearly intervals.

DBS-related complications or side effects may occur at various times following implantation and stimulation. These include disturbances in consciousness, seizures, confusion, bradyphrenia, and cerebral hemorrhage. Infection, skin erosion and malfunction of the hardware may occur as a later complication. External magnetic devices and other electronic tools may cause inadvertent turning "off" of a pulse generator. Rarely, patients who suddenly lose stimulation may show sudden neurological deterioration, requiring immediate treatment (89). One patient with STN DBS was left in a vegetative state from permanent brainstem lesioning after receiving pulsatile radiofrequency diathermy for a dental condition (90). As such, all surgically invasive and therapeutic procedures

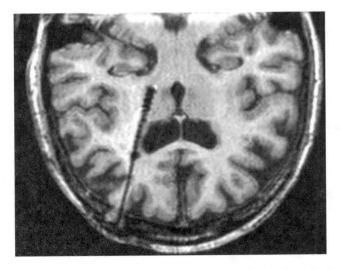

Figure 11.2 MRI findings of unilateral thalamic deep brain stimulation electrode implant. T1 weighted axial imaging of unilateral thalamic stimulation.

making use of power devices are best carried out only after consultation with the DBS device manufacturer.

IX. OUTCOME

A. Thalamotomy

The number of reports of essential tremor patients who have undergone thalamotomy is relatively small compared with those of PD. However, many of the previous studies describe the usefulness of thalamotomy in minimizing tremor from either essential tremor or PD. VIM (38,91–95), VL (96) or zona incerta (ZI) (97) have all served as effective ablative targets within the thalamus in essential tremor patients. In long-term follow-up studies, persistent efficacy results in 60–100% of patients (91–94,96,97). In the largest study with substantial follow-up (mean follow-up period: 8.6 years; $n = 65$), Mohadjer and colleagues reported complete and marked tremor relief in 68.7% of patients following ZI thalamotomy. Interestingly, improvement of tremor in the limbs ipsilateral to the thalamotomy was also revealed in 8.5% of the patients.

There is no significant difference in efficacy of tremor reduction solely based on lesioning volume, comparing minimal ($\sim$40 mm^3) lesioning with large lesioning volumes (91). In most essential tremor patients, a small thalamotomy ($\sim$40 mm^3) in the VIM produces an adequate response (98).

Gamma knife thalamotomy for essential tremor has been reported (45,99,100). In general, although there is no apparent improvement of tremor for the first few months after gamma knife surgery (99), complete or marked relief of tremor is seen in over 80% of essential tremor patients one year after gamma knife thalamotomy (99,100). In a study reporting tremor rating scale (TRS) scores (101), tremor severity improved 85%, specific motor tasks by 78%, and functional ability by 73% (100). Also, at four years postgamma knife thalamotomy, complete or marked relief of tremor was seen in nearly 90% of essential tremor patients (100). Complications reported by centers performing gamma knife thalamotomy include mild contralateral paresthesia in the face and upper extremity, mild contralateral limb weakness, and dysarthria (100,102). Delayed complications such as progressive, complex, disabling movement disorders, and stroke due to radiation vasculopathy after gamma knife surgery, have also been reported (103,104). Additional studies of gamma knife surgery outcome are required.

Adverse effects in essential tremor patients after unilateral thalamotomy include dysarthria, bradykinesia, hypotonia, weakness in the contralateral limbs, gait disturbance, and dysdiadochokinesis (93,97). Akbostanci et al. (93) reported that the overall incidence of complications in essential tremor patients occurred with 49% of the procedures, and 13.9% of patients permanently experienced an adverse effect such as dysarthria, mild contralateral weakness, and gait disturbance. Mohadjer et al. (97) reported that motor disturbance in the contralateral limbs, as a permanent adverse effect associated with thalamotomy, was seen in 5% of essential tremor patients (incoordination in 3%, and speech disturbance in 1%). On the other hand, Goldman and Kelly (96) reported that there was no severe persistent morbidity. Incidence of morbidity and mortality associated with thalamotomy may also relate to specific diagnoses. In PD patients, immediate postoperative complications consist of contralateral weakness (34–42%) (105,106), dysarthria (13–66%) (105–108) and cognitive impairment (10–23%) (105–107,109). Most of these complications are generally resolved spontaneously within a few months after surgery, but persistent postoperative complications including contralateral hemiparesis, paresthesia, seizure, ataxia, apraxia, hypotonia, and gait disturbance are seen in 0.5–26% of patients (106).

Hemorrhagic complications may accompany the procedure causing serious or lethal morbidity in 1–2% of patients. Nevertheless, the benefits from surgery usually far outweigh the potential risk for complications at experienced surgical centers. Bilateral thalamotomy has a high incidence of complications including dysarthria, dysphagia and hypophonia (71). The mortality risk for thalamotomy in PD is <0.3% (110). Causes of death include hemorrhage in deep gray matter, postoperative infection, and pulmonary embolism.

B.   Thalamic Stimulation

Studies of thalamic DBS for the treatment of essential tremor have indicated consistent benefit, whereas the degree of efficacy is variable (see Table 11.1) (11,111–118). The VIM nucleus is the ideal target for tremor relief. The mechanism for tremor reduction by high-frequency stimulation in the VIM is still unknown. However, the findings of not only reduced tremor amplitude but also decreased regularity and rate that accompany VIM stimulation are indicative of the neurophysiological alterations which mirror clinical efficacy from this procedure (119).

Benabid et al. (11) reported that 61% of VIM DBS procedures showed complete or marked abolishment of tremor in the contralateral limb six months after implantation. Koller et al. (111) also reported that 79% of essential tremor patients showed complete or marked relief of tremor in the contralateral limb at three months after the procedure, and 31% of the patients had total tremor resolution one year after implantation.

Ondo et al. (112) reported that unilateral VIM DBS provided tremor relief of 81.8% in the contralateral upper limb, 83.3% in the contralateral lower limb, and improvement of 57.6% in ADL scores. One-year follow-up studies of Hariz et al. (113), Limousin et al. (114), and Fields et al. (116) have reported that unilateral VIM DBS showed improvements of 48.4–56.3% in tremor scores, 58.3–80.3% in ADL scores, and 38.6–43.9% in hand function scores, and improved tremor in the contralateral upper limb by 80.5% from baseline scores. Koller et al. (120) reported that after 40.2 months follow-up after VIM DBS, 64% of essential tremor patients were taking no medication for tremor. Recent long-term studies by Rehncrona et al. (117) and Sydow et al. (118) reported that VIM DBS procedures

Table 11.1 Selected Studies of Thalamic Stimulation for Essential Tremor

Author (Year)	Total cases (Bilateral)	Mean age at implant (Year)	Mean disease duration (Year)	Follow-up	Implanted site	% Improvement from baseline in TRS with stimulation-on	Adverse effects
Benabid, 1996 (11)	20 (13)	NA	NA	6 M	VIM	61% of procedures: complete or marked relief	30%: hemorrhagic 25%: skin erosion
Koller, 1997 (111)	29	66.8	34.9	3 M	VIM	79% of patients: complete or marked relief	None
Ondo, 1998 (112)	14	72.3	NA	3 M	VIM	55.5 in head tremor score, 57.6 in ADL score, 81.8 in UE, 83.3 in LE	50%: overall
Hariz, 1999 (113)	36	66	18	1 Y	VIM	48.4 in tremor score, 58.3 in ADL score, 38.6 in hand function score	8.6%: hardware-related complication (5.2% fracture of electrode, 1.7% dislocation of electrode, and 1.7%: skin erosion)
Limousin, 1999 (114)	37 (9)	63.1	26.6	1 Y	VIM	55.0 in tremor score, 80.3 in ADL score, 43.9 in hand function score, 80.5 in UE	4%: hemorrhagic

(continued)

Table 11.1 *Continued*

Author (Year)	Total cases (Bilateral)	Mean age at implant (Year)	Mean disease duration (Year)	Follow-up	Implanted site	% Improvement from baseline in TRS with stimulation-on	Adverse effects
Obwegeser, 2000 (115)	27 (13)	73	27	11 M	VIM	82.1 in UE, 60.3 in midline tremor	4%: seizure, 15%: dysarthria, 12%: disequilibrium, 10%: paresthesia, 29%: dysarthria in BS
Koller, 2001 (120)	25	72.3	33.3	40.2 M	VIM	78.5 in UE	16%: overall
Fields, 2003 (116)	40	71.7	18.1	11 M	VIM	56.3 in tremor score	None
Rehncrona, 2003 (117)	13 (1)	NA	NA	6–7 Y	VIM	47.1 in tremor score, 71.4 in hand function score, 66.7 in UE PT, 50.0 in UE AT	No complication
Sydow, 2003 (118)	19 (4)	61.8	37.7	6.5 Y	VIM	41.0 in tremor score, 58.3 in head tremor score, 38.7 in ADL score, 37.2 in hand function score, 70.0 in UE PT, 50.0 in UE AT, 75.0 in LE PT	84.2%: overall

Note: ADL: activity of daily living; AT: action tremor; BS: bilateral stimulation; TRS: Tremor Rating Scale; LE: lower extremity; M: months; NA: not available; PT: postural tremor; UE: upper extremity; VIM: ventral intermediate nucleus; Y: year(s).

provided improvements of 41.0–47.1% in tremor scores, 37.2–71.4% in hand function, and 38.7% in ADL scores. Action tremor in the contralateral upper limb, postural tremor in the contralateral upper limb, lower limb improved by 50.0%, 66.7–70.0%, and 75.0%, respectively from baseline scores.

Essential tremor patients with bilateral thalamic stimulation can obtain further efficacy for tremor suppression (115,121,122). The study of staged bilateral VIM DBS by Pahwa et al. (121) reported that total tremor scores, tremor motor score, and tremor ADL scores improved by 57%, 63%, and 57%, respectively when baseline evaluations were compared with those obtained 12 months after the second surgery. There was a 35% improvement in total tremor scores from before the first surgery to those obtained before the second surgery, and a further improvement of 40% occurred 6 months after the second surgery compared to scores immediately prior to the second surgery. Ondo et al. (122) suggested that efficacy of bilateral thalamic stimulation to the overall functional disability is higher in essential tremor patients than in PD patients, who frequently have more difficulties and adverse effects, especially balance problems with bilateral procedures.

Unilateral thalamic stimulation also improves disabling essential head tremor (112,123). Obwegeser et al. (115) reported that bilateral VIM DBS provides more robust efficacy for midline tremor and limb tremor, and improved head-posture by 95.2%, voice by 83.3%, tongue-posture, face and trunk-posture by 100%.

Disability and health-related quality of life in essential tremor patients is also improved by thalamic stimulation. Hariz et al. (124) reported that, in evaluations 1 year after surgery, eating, drinking, grooming, communication, cooking, and shopping in an ADL taxonomy scale, and emotional reactions and household management, social life, and interests/hobbies in the Nottingham health profile were significantly improved by thalamic DBS.

Unilateral VIM DBS provides significant improvements in visuoconstructional function, aspects of visual attention, visuoperceptual gestalt formation, dominant-hand fine visuomotor coordination, and aspects of verbal memory and delayed prose recall with short-term follow-up, and most of these cognitive improvements are maintained one year after the surgery (8,125). However, verbal fluency is modestly worsened by unilateral thalamic stimulation (8,125). Fields et al. (116) have suggested that preoperative poor verbal fluency may contribute to a greater risk for fluency declines after thalamic DBS. Similarly, Woods et al. (126) reported that tremor onset after age 37 years was one of the strongest predictors of cognitive decline in essential tremor patients after thalamic stimulation.

Adequately programming stimulation parameters including voltage, frequency, pulse width, and polarity configuration is important for optimal tremor control without adverse effects. In bipolar electrode stimulation, thalamic stimulation at 90 µs, 130 Hz, adjusting the voltage up to 3 V, tend to be effective for tremor suppression in most patients (127). With monopolar electrode stimulation, tremor tends to be suppressed with lower voltages, and side effects such as paresthesia, speech disturbance, and weakness, become more common at 3 or 4 V (127). Woods et al. (126) reported that higher pulse width settings ($\geq$120 μs) were the strongest predictors of cognitive decline in essential tremor patients after thalamic DBS.

Thalamic stimulation may lead to some adverse effects that are commonly mild and acceptable to patients. Overall, complications accompanying thalamic stimulation vary widely in reported series: none (117), 16% (120), 50% (112), and 84.2% (118) of patients. Dysarthria is the most common adverse effect, especially in bilateral procedures, and occurs in 20–29% of patients (62,115,121). Other adverse effects include paresthesia (10–79%), disequilibrium (9–12%), headache (11%), paresis in the contralateral limb (8%), gait disturbance (6%), and dystonia (6%) (111,115). Hemorrhagic complications related to surgery generally range from 2–4% (114,115).

C.   Thalamotomy vs. Thalamic Stimulation

Tasker et al. (128) reported that in comparison of outcome in thalamotomy and thalamic DBS, complete tremor resolution occurred in 42% in both groups, marked abolition in 79% of patients with thalamic DBS and 69% of patients with thalamotomy. Recurrent tremor occurred in 5% of patients with thalamic DBS and 15% of patients with thalamotomy. Adverse effects, including dysarthria, ataxia, and gait disturbance, were more common in patients with thalamotomy (42%) than those with thalamic stimulation (26%).

A randomized comparative study of Schuurman et al. (53) reported effects of thalamotomy and thalamic stimulation on functional abilities in patients with severe tremor due to PD, essential tremor, and multiple sclerosis. After two years of follow-up, thalamotomy and thalamic stimulation showed equal efficacy for tremor suppression, but thalamic stimulation was associated with significantly fewer adverse effects than thalamotomy and DBS resulted in greater functional improvement.

Pahwa et al. (129) also reported that there were no significant differences in clinical efficacy between essential tremor patients undergoing thalamotomy compared to those with thalamic DBS; total tremor scores improved by 49% in the thalamotomy group and by 50% in the thalamic DBS group. Motor tremor scores improved by 46% and the ADL scores improved by 70% in the thalamotomy group and by 50% and 64%, respectively, with thalamic DBS. This study also disclosed the fact that many patients with thalamic DBS require repeat surgery due to hardware complications. However, the frequency of overall adverse effects was higher for the thalamotomy group compared to the thalamic DBS group.

Schuurman et al. (95) demonstrated that thalamotomy and thalamic stimulation are associated with a small overall risk of cognitive deterioration. A comparable degree and frequency of worsening of verbal and reading tasks occurred after left-sided surgery in both thalamic procedures.

Thalamic DBS is possibly useful not only for essential tremor patients with medically refractory tremor but also those who have lost efficacy of tremor suppression after thalamotomy (130). On the other hand, tremor control with thalamotomy following failed thalamic DBS has also been reported (131).

D. Subthalamic Stimulation

Only two case reports and one study have been reported, but stimulation of the subthalamic area including ZI may improve not only distal but also proximal tremor in essential tremor patients (69,70). Kitagawa et al. (70) first reported the efficacy of subthalamic white matter (ZI) stimulation in tremor patients. One case was an essential tremor patient with a severe and refractory proximal tremor despite a prior left thalamotomy. His severe postural tremor in the contralateral limb was relieved completely by subthalamic stimulation. Another case was a severe tremor patient with dystonia, dysarthria, and gait disturbance. Subthalamic stimulation provided not only resolution of her postural tremor but also improvement in other symptoms. Murata et al. (69) studied the clinical efficacy of subthalamic DBS in eight patients with severe essential tremor involving the proximal limbs reporting that both distal and proximal tremor in the contralateral limb were suppressed markedly by subthalamic white matter stimulation including the prelemniscal radiation, ZI, and fasciculus Q. Total tremor scores were improved by 81%, ranging from 65–100%, and voice, neck, and orthostatic axial tremor were also improved.

Patel et al. (132) reported that combined stimulation of the dorsolateral and pallidofugal fibers (H2 field of Forel)/ZI is particularly effective for parkinsonism and dyskinesia. These observations suggest that subthalamic white matter stimulation has potential for tremor suppression in essential tremor patients and tremor patients with dyskinesia. Further studies of subthalamic stimulation for essential tremor patients are required to demonstrate relative clinical benefit.

X. CONCLUSION

In summary, DBS of the VIM thalamus is the most frequently employed surgical procedure for treatment of tremor. This form of therapy maintains clinical benefit chronically and is associated with a low risk of immediate and chronic side effects. Further studies are required to delineate whether other basal ganglionic targets are equally efficacious in the treatment of tremor. Additional surgical forms of treatment may develop in the future with improved understanding of mechanisms leading to pathological tremor disorders.

REFERENCES

1. Habib ur R. Diagnosis and management of tremor. Arch Intern Med 2000; 160:2438–2444.

2. Rajput AH, Offord KP, Beard CM, Kurland LT. Essential tremor in Rochester, Minnesota: a 45-year study. J Neurol Neurosurg Psychiatry 1984; 47:466–470.
3. Guridi J, Lozano AM. A brief history of pallidotomy. Neurosurgery 1997; 41:1169–1180; discussion 1180–1163.
4. Speelman JD, Bosch DA. Resurgence of functional neurosurgery for Parkinson's disease: a historical perspective. Mov Disord 1998; 13:582–588.
5. Albe-Fessard D, Arfel G, Guiot G, Hardy J, Vourch'e G, Hertzog E, Alconard P, Derome P. Derivations d'activites spontanees et evoquees dans les structures cerebrales profondes de l'homme. Rev Neurol 1962; 106:89.
6. Ohye C, Narabayashi H. Physiological study of presumed ventralis intermedius neurons in the human thalamus. J Neurosurg 1979; 50:290–297.
7. Narabayashi H, Maeda T, Yokochi F. Long-term follow-up study of nucleus ventralis intermedius and ventrolateralis thalamotomy using a microelectrode technique in parkinsonism. Appl Neurophysiol 1987; 50:330–337.
8. Hariz MI. From functional neurosurgery to "interventional" neurology: survey of publications on thalamotomy, pallidotomy, and deep brain stimulation for Parkinson's disease from 1966 to 2001. Mov Disord 2003; 18:845–853.
9. Elble RJ, Koller WC. Tremor. The Johns Hopkins series in contemporary medicine and public health. Baltimore: Johns Hopkins University Press, 1990:204 p.
10. Chen JJ, Swope DM. Essential tremor: diagnosis and treatment. Pharmacotherapy 2003; 23:1105–1122.
11. Benabid AL, Pollak P, Gao D, Hoffmann D, Limousin P, Gay E, Payen I, Benazzouz A. Chronic electrical stimulation of the ventralis intermedius nucleus of the thalamus as a treatment of movement disorders. J Neurosurg 1996; 84:203–214.
12. Alexander GE, DeLong MR, Strick PL. Parallel organization of functionally segregated circuits linking basal ganglia and cortex. Annu Rev Neurosci 1986; 9:357–381.
13. DeLong MR. Primate models of movement disorders of basal ganglia origin. Trends Neurosci 1990; 13:281–285.
14. Guridi J, Luquin MR, Herrero MT, Obeso JA. The subthalamic nucleus: a possible target for stereotaxic surgery in Parkinson's disease. Mov Disord 1993; 8:421–429.
15. Lamarre Y. Animal models of physiological, essential, and parkinsonian-like tremors. In: Findley LJ, Capildeo R, eds. Movement Disorders Tremor. New York: Oxford University Press, 1984:183–194.
16. Llinás RR. Rebound excitation as the physiological basis for tremor: a biophysical study of the oscillatory properties of mammalian central neurons *in vitro*. In: Findley LJ, Capildeo R, eds. Movement Disorders, Tremor. New York: Oxford University Press, 1984:165–182.
17. Elble RJ. Central mechanisms of tremor. J Clin Neurophysiol 1996; 13:133–144.
18. Dupuis MJ, Delwaide PJ, Boucquey D, Gonsette RE. Homolateral disappearance of essential tremor after cerebellar stroke. Mov Disord 1989; 4:183–187.
19. Nagaratnam N, Kalasabail G. Contralateral abolition of essential tremor following a pontine stroke. J Neurol Sci 1997; 149:195–196.
20. Duncan R, Bone I, Melville ID. Essential tremor cured by infarction adjacent to the thalamus. J Neurol Neurosurg Psychiatry 1988; 51:591–592.
21. Elble RJ. Origins of tremor. Lancet 2000; 355:1113–1114.
22. Jenkins IH, Bain PG, Colebatch JG, Thompson PD, Findley LJ, Frackowiak RS, Marsden CD, Brooks DJ. A positron emission tomography study of essential

tremor: evidence for overactivity of cerebellar connections. Ann Neurol 1993; 34:82–90.

23. Boecker H, Brooks DJ. Functional imaging of tremor. Mov Disord 1998; 13(suppl 3):64–72.

24. Bakay RA, DeLong MR, Vitek JL. Posteroventral pallidotomy for Parkinson's disease. J Neurosurg 1992; 77:487–488.

25. Volkmann J, Joliot M, Mogilner A, Ioannides AA, Lado F, Fazzini E, Ribary U, Llinas R. Central motor loop oscillations in parkinsonian resting tremor revealed by magnetoencephalography. Neurology 1996; 46:1359–1370.

26. Hua S, Reich SG, Zirh AT, Perry V, Dougherty PM, Lenz FA. The role of the thalamus and basal ganglia in parkinsonian tremor. Mov Disord 1998; 13(suppl 3):40–42.

27. Lemstra AW, Verhagen Metman L, Lee JI, Dougherty PM, Lenz FA. Tremor-frequency (3–6 Hz) activity in the sensorimotor arm representation of the internal segment of the globus pallidus in patients with Parkinson's disease. Neurosci Lett 1999; 267:129–132.

28. Krack P, Benazzouz A, Pollak P, Limousin P, Piallat B, Hoffmann D, Xie J, Benabid AL. Treatment of tremor in Parkinson's disease by subthalamic nucleus stimulation. Mov Disord 1998; 13:907–914.

29. Elble RJ, Schieber MH, Thach WT Jr. Activity of muscle spindles, motor cortex and cerebellar nuclei during action tremor. Brain Res 1984; 323:330–334.

30. Elble RJ. Animal models of action tremor. Mov Disord 1998; 13(suppl 3):35–39.

31. Bain PG. The management of tremor. J Neurol Neurosurg Psychiatry 2002; 72(suppl 1):I3–I9.

32. Pahwa R, Lyons KE. Essential tremor: differential diagnosis and current therapy. Am J Med 2003; 115:134–142.

33. Masucci EF, Kurtzke JF, Saini N. Myorhythmia: a widespread movement disorder. Clinicopathological correlations. Brain 1984; 107(pt 1):53–79.

34. Remy P, de Recondo A, Defer G, Loc'h C, Amarenco P, Plante-Bordeneuve V, Dao-Castellana MH, Bendriem B, Crouzel C, Clanet M et al. Peduncular "rubral" tremor and dopaminergic denervation: a PET study. Neurology 1995; 45:472–477.

35. Narabayashi H. Stereotaxic Vim thalamotomy for treatment of tremor. Eur Neurol 1989; 29(suppl 1):29–32.

36. Laitinen LV. Pallidotomy for Parkinson's disease. Neurosurg Clin N Am 1995; 6:105–112.

37. Marsden CD, Obeso JA. The functions of the basal ganglia and the paradox of stereotaxic surgery in Parkinson's disease. Brain 1994; 117(pt 4):877–897.

38. Ohye C, Hirai T, Miyazaki M, Shibazaki T, Nakajima H. VIM thalamotomy for the treatment of various kinds of tremor. Appl Neurophysiol 1982; 45:275–280.

39. Shahzadi S, Tasker RR, Lozano A. Thalamotomy for essential and cerebellar tremor. Stereotact Funct Neurosurg 1995; 65:11–17.

40. Kim MC, Son BC, Miyagi Y, Kang JK. VIM thalamotomy for Holmes' tremor secondary to midbrain tumour. J Neurol Neurosurg Psychiatry 2002; 73:453–455.

41. Speelman JD, Schuurman R, de Bie RM, Esselink RA, Bosch DA. Stereotactic neurosurgery for tremor. Mov Disord 2002; 17(suppl 3):S84–S88.

42. Cardoso F, Jankovic J, Grossman RG, Hamilton WJ. Outcome after stereotactic thalamotomy for dystonia and hemiballismus. Neurosurgery 1995; 36:501–507; discussion 507–508.

43. Ohye C, Shibazaki T. Lesioning the thalamus for dyskinesia. Stereotact Funct Neurosurg 2001; 77:33–39.
44. Miyagi Y, Shima F, Ishido K, Yasutake T, Kamikaseda K. Tremor induced by toluene misuse successfully treated by a VIM thalamotomy. J Neurol Neurosurg Psychiatry 1999; 66:794–796.
45. Ohye C, Shibazaki T, Hirato M, Inoue H, Andou Y. Gamma thalamotomy for parkinsonian and other kinds of tremor. Stereotact Funct Neurosurg 1996; 66(suppl 1):333–342.
46. Pan L, Dai JZ, Wang BJ, Xu WM, Zhou LF, Chen XR. Stereotactic gamma thalamotomy for the treatment of parkinsonism. Stereotact Funct Neurosurg 1996; 66(suppl 1):329–332.
47. Pollak P, Benabid AL, Limousin P, Krack P. Treatment of Parkinson's disease. New surgical treatment strategies. Eur Neurol 1996; 36:400–404.
48. Lenz FA, Normand SL, Kwan HC, Andrews D, Rowland LH, Jones MW, Seike M, Lin YC, Tasker RR, Dostrovsky JO et al. Statistical prediction of the optimal site for thalamotomy in parkinsonian tremor. Mov Disord 1995; 10:318–328.
49. Babel TB, Warnke PC, Ostertag CB. Immediate and long term outcome after infra-thalamic and thalamic lesioning for intractable Tourette's syndrome. J Neurol Neurosurg Psychiatry 2001; 70:666–671.
50. Hassler R, Riechert T, Mundinger F, Umbach W, Ganglberger JA. Physiological observations in stereotaxic operations in extrapyramidal motor disturbances. Brain 1960; 83:337–350.
51. Ohye C, Kubota K, Hongo T, Nagao T, Narabayashi H. Ventrolateral and Subven-trolateral Thalamic Stimulation. Motor Effects. Arch Neurol 1964; 11:427–434.
52. Benabid AL, Pollak P, Louveau A, Henry S, de Rougemont J. Combined (thalamot-omy and stimulation) stereotactic surgery of the VIM thalamic nucleus for bilateral Parkinson disease. Appl Neurophysiol 1987; 50:344–346.
53. Schuurman PR, Bosch DA, Bossuyt PM, Bonsel GJ, van Someren EJ, de Bie RM, Merkus MP, Speelman JD. A comparison of continuous thalamic stimulation and thalamotomy for suppression of severe tremor. N Engl J Med 2000; 342:461–468.
54. Koller WC, Pahwa PR, Lyons KE, Wilkinson SB. Deep brain stimulation of the VIM nucleus of the thalamus for the treatment of tremor. Neurology 2000; 55:S29–S33.
55. Minguez-Castellanos A, Carnero-Pardo C, Gomez-Camello A, Ortega-Moreno A, Garcia-Gomez T, Arjona V, Martin-Linares JM. Primary writing tremor treated by chronic thalamic stimulation. Mov Disord 1999; 14:1030–1033.
56. Racette BA, Dowling J, Randle J, Mink JW. Thalamic stimulation for primary writing tremor. J Neurol 2001; 248:380–382.
57. Thompson TP, Kondziolka D, Albright AL. Thalamic stimulation for choreiform movement disorders in children. Report of two cases. J Neurosurg 2000; 92:718–721.
58. Loher TJ, Krauss JK, Burgunder JM, Taub E, Siegfried J. Chronic thalamic stimu-lation for treatment of dystonic paroxysmal nonkinesigenic dyskinesia. Neurology 2001; 56:268–270.
59. Franzini A, Ferroli P, Servello D, Broggi G. Reversal of thalamic hand syndrome by long-term motor cortex stimulation. J Neurosurg 2000; 93:873–875.
60. Katayama Y, Yamamoto T, Kobayashi K, Oshima H, Fukaya C. Deep brain and motor cortex stimulation for post-stroke movement disorders and post-stroke pain. Acta Neurochir Suppl 2003; 87:121–123.

61. Haberler C, Alesch F, Mazal PR, Pilz P, Jellinger K, Pinter MM, Hainfellner JA, Budka H. No tissue damage by chronic deep brain stimulation in Parkinson's disease. Ann Neurol 2000; 48:372–376.
62. Benabid AL, Pollak P, Gervason C, Hoffmann D, Gao DM, Hommel M, Perret JE, de Rougemont J. Long-term suppression of tremor by chronic stimulation of the ventral intermediate thalamic nucleus. Lancet 1991; 337:403–406.
63. Lozano AM, Dostrovsky J, Chen R, Ashby P. Deep brain stimulation for Parkinson's disease: disrupting the disruption. Lancet Neurol 2002; 1:225–231.
64. Ceballos-Baumann AO, Boecker H, Fogel W, Alesch F, Bartenstein P, Conrad B, Diederich N, von Falkenhayn I, Moringlane JR, Schwaiger M, Tronnier VM. Thalamic stimulation for essential tremor activates motor and deactivates vestibular cortex. Neurology 2001; 56:1347–1354.
65. Perlmutter JS, Mink JW, Bastian AJ, Zackowski K, Hershey T, Miyawaki E, Koller W, Videen TO. Blood flow responses to deep brain stimulation of thalamus. Neurology 2002; 58:1388–1394.
66. Bergman H, Wichmann T, DeLong MR. Reversal of experimental parkinsonism by lesions of the subthalamic nucleus. Science 1990; 249:1436–1438.
67. Limousin P, Krack P, Pollak P, Benazzouz A, Ardouin C, Hoffmann D, Benabid AL. Electrical stimulation of the subthalamic nucleus in advanced Parkinson's disease. N Engl J Med 1998; 339:1105–1111.
68. Moro E, Scerrati M, Romito LM, Roselli R, Tonali P, Albanese A. Chronic subthalamic nucleus stimulation reduces medication requirements in Parkinson's disease. Neurology 1999; 53:85–90.
69. Murata J, Kitagawa M, Uesugi H, Saito H, Iwasaki Y, Kikuchi S, Tashiro K, Sawamura Y. Electrical stimulation of the posterior subthalamic area for the treatment of intractable proximal tremor. J Neurosurg 2003; 99:708–715.
70. Kitagawa M, Murata J, Kikuchi S, Sawamura Y, Saito H, Sasaki H, Tashiro K. Deep brain stimulation of subthalamic area for severe proximal tremor. Neurology 2000; 55:114–116.
71. Kelly PJ, Gillingham FJ. The long-term results of stereotaxic surgery and L-dopa therapy in patients with Parkinson's disease. A 10-year follow-up study. J Neurosurg 1980; 53:332–337.
72. Tasker RR. Thalamotomy. Neurosurg Clin N Am 1990; 1:841–864.
73. Obwegeser AA, Uitti RJ, Turk MF, Wszolek UM, Flipse TR, Smallridge RC, Witte RJ, Wharen RE Jr. Simultaneous thalamic deep brain stimulation and implantable cardioverter-defibrillator. Mayo Clin Proc 2001; 76:87–89.
74. Andrew J. Surgical treatment of tumor. In: Findley LJ, Capildeo R, eds. Movement Disorders, Tremor. New York: Oxford University Press, 1984:339–351.
75. Zonenshayn M, Rezai AR, Mogilner AY, Beric A, Sterio D, Kelly PJ. Comparison of anatomic and neurophysiological methods for subthalamic nucleus targeting. Neurosurgery 2000; 47:282–292; discussion 292–294.
76. Holtzheimer PE, 3rd, Roberts DW, Darcey TM. Magnetic resonance imaging versus computed tomography for target localization in functional stereotactic neurosurgery. Neurosurgery 1999; 45:290–297; discussion 297–298.
77. Meneses MS, Arruda WO, Hunhevicz SC, Ramina R, Pedrozo AA, Tsubouchi MH. Comparison of MRI-guided and ventriculography-based stereotactic surgery for Parkinson's disease. Arq Neuropsiquiatr 1997; 55:547–552.

78. Guridi J, Gorospe A, Ramos E, Linazasoro G, Rodriguez MC, Obeso JA. Stereotactic targeting of the globus pallidus internus in Parkinson's disease: imaging versus electrophysiological mapping. Neurosurgery 1999; 45:278–287; discussion 287–279.

79. Oh MY, Hodaie M, Kim SH, Alkhani A, Lang AE, Lozano AM. Deep brain stimulator electrodes used for lesioning: proof of principle. Neurosurgery 2001; 49:363–367; discussion 367–369.

80. Vitek JL, Bakay RA, Hashimoto T, Kaneoke Y, Mewes K, Zhang JY, Rye D, Starr P, Baron M, Turner R, DeLong MR. Microelectrode-guided pallidotomy: technical approach and its application in medically intractable Parkinson's disease. J Neurosurg 1998; 88:1027–1043.

81. Guridi J, Rodriguez-Oroz MC, Lozano AM, Moro E, Albanese A, Nuttin B, Gybels J, Ramos E, Obeso JA. Targeting the basal ganglia for deep brain stimulation in Parkinson's disease. Neurology 2000; 55:S21–S28.

82. Kelly PJ, Ahlskog JE, Goerss SJ, Daube JR, Duffy JR, Kall BA. Computer-assisted stereotactic ventralis lateralis thalamotomy with microelectrode recording control in patients with Parkinson's disease. Mayo Clin Proc 1987; 62:655–664.

83. Favre J, Taha JM, Nguyen TT, Gildenberg PL, Burchiel KJ. Pallidotomy: a survey of current practice in North America. Neurosurgery 1996; 39:883–890; discussion 890–882.

84. Alterman RL, Sterio D, Beric A, Kelly PJ. Microelectrode recording during posteroventral pallidotomy: impact on target selection and complications. Neurosurgery 1999; 44:315–321; discussion 321–313.

85. Kamiryo T, Laws ER Jr. Identification and localization of intracerebral vessels by microvascular doppler in stereotactic pallidotomy and thalamotomy: technical note. Neurosurgery 1997; 40:877–878; discussion 878–879.

86. Limousin P, Pollak P, Benazzouz A, Hoffmann D, Broussolle E, Perret JE, Benabid AL. Bilateral subthalamic nucleus stimulation for severe Parkinson's disease. Mov Disord 1995; 10:672–674.

87. Rodriguez-Oroz MC, Rodriguez M, Guridi J, Mewes K, Chockkman V, Vitek J, DeLong MR, Obeso JA. The subthalamic nucleus in Parkinson's disease: somatotopic organization and physiological characteristics. Brain 2001; 124:1777–1790.

88. Fukuda M, Kameyama S, Noguchi R, Tanaka R. Intraoperative monitoring for functional neurosurgery during intravenous anesthesia with propofol. No Shinkei Geka 1997; 25:231–237.

89. Hariz MI, Johansson F. Hardware failure in parkinsonian patients with chronic subthalamic nucleus stimulation is a medical emergency. Mov Disord 2001; 16:166–168.

90. Nutt JG, Anderson VC, Peacock JH, Hammerstad JP, Burchiel KJ. DBS and diathermy interaction induces severe CNS damage. Neurology 2001; 56:1384–1386.

91. Nagaseki Y, Shibazaki T, Hirai T, Kawashima Y, Hirato M, Wada H, Miyazaki M, Ohye C. Long-term follow-up results of selective VIM-thalamotomy. J Neurosurg 1986; 65:296–302.

92. Jankovic J, Cardoso F, Grossman RG, Hamilton WJ. Outcome after stereotactic thalamotomy for parkinsonian, essential, and other types of tremor. Neurosurgery 1995; 37:680–686; discussion 686–687.

93. Akbostanci MC, Slavin KV, Burchiel KJ. Stereotactic ventral intermedial thalamotomy for the treatment of essential tremor: results of a series of 37 patients. Stereotact Funct Neurosurg 1999; 72:174–177.

94. Zirh A, Reich SG, Dougherty PM, Lenz FA. Stereotactic thalamotomy in the treatment of essential tremor of the upper extremity: reassessment including a blinded measure of outcome. J Neurol Neurosurg Psychiatry 1999; 66:772–775.
95. Schuurman PR, Bruins J, Merkus MP, Bosch DA, Speelman JD. A comparison of neuropsychological effects of thalamotomy and thalamic stimulation. Neurology 2002; 59:1232–1239.
96. Goldman MS, Kelly PJ. Symptomatic and functional outcome of stereotactic ventralis lateralis thalamotomy for intention tremor. J Neurosurg 1992; 77:223–229.
97. Mohadjer M, Goerke H, Milios E, Etou A, Mundinger F. Long-term results of stereotaxy in the treatment of essential tremor. Stereotact Funct Neurosurg 1990; 54–55:125–129.
98. Hirai T, Miyazaki M, Nakajima H, Shibazaki T, Ohye C. The correlation between tremor characteristics and the predicted volume of effective lesions in stereotaxic nucleus ventralis intermedius thalamotomy. Brain 1983; 106(pt 4): 1001–1018.
99. Ohye C, Shibazaki T, Zhang J, Andou Y. Thalamic lesions produced by gamma thalamotomy for movement disorders. J Neurosurg 2002; 97:600–606.
100. Young RF, Jacques S, Mark R, Kopyov O, Copcutt B, Posewitz A, Li F. Gamma knife thalamotomy for treatment of tremor: long-term results. J Neurosurg 2000; 93(suppl 3):128–135.
101. Fahn S, Tolosa E, Marin C. Clinical rating scale for tremor. In: Jankovic J, Tolosa E, eds. Parkinson's Disease and Movement Disorders. Baltimore: Williams & Wilkins, 1993:271–280.
102. Niranjan A, Kondziolka D, Baser S, Heyman R, Lunsford LD. Functional outcomes after gamma knife thalamotomy for essential tremor and MS-related tremor. Neurology 2000; 55:443–446.
103. Siderowf A, Gollump SM, Stern MB, Baltuch GH, Riina HA. Emergence of complex, involuntary movements after gamma knife radiosurgery for essential tremor. Mov Disord 2001; 16:965–967.
104. Friedman JH, Fernandez HH, Sikirica M, Stopa E, Friehs G. Stroke induced by gamma knife pallidotomy: autopsy result. Neurology 2002; 58:1695–1697.
105. Fox MW, Ahlskog JE, Kelly PJ. Stereotactic ventrolateralis thalamotomy for medically refractory tremor in post-levodopa era Parkinson's disease patients. J Neurosurg 1991; 75:723–730.
106. Olanow CW. Surgical therapy for Parkinson's disease. Eur J Neurol 2002; 9(suppl 3):31–39.
107. Waltz JM, Riklan M, Stellar S, Cooper IS. Cryothalamectomy for Parkinson's disease. A statistical analysis. Neurology 1966; 16:994–1002 passim.
108. Bell DS. Speech functions of the thalamus inferred from the effects of thalamotomy. Brain 1968; 91:619–638.
109. Shapiro DY, Sadowsky DA, Henderson WG, Van Buren JM. An assessment of cognitive function in postthalamotomy Parkinson patients. Confin Neurol 1973; 35:144–166.
110. Selby G. Stereotactic surgery. In: Koller WC, ed. Handbook of Parkinson's Disease. New York: M. Dekker, 1987:421.
111. Koller W, Pahwa R, Busenbark K, Hubble J, Wilkinson S, Lang A, Tuite P, Sime E, Lazano A, Hauser R, Malapira T, Smith D, Tarsy D, Miyawaki E, Norregaard T,

Kormos T, Olanow CW. High-frequency unilateral thalamic stimulation in the treatment of essential and parkinsonian tremor. Ann Neurol 1997; 42:292–299.

112. Ondo W, Jankovic J, Schwartz K, Almaguer M, Simpson RK. Unilateral thalamic deep brain stimulation for refractory essential tremor and Parkinson's disease tremor. Neurology 1998; 51:1063–1069.

113. Hariz MI, Shamsgovara P, Johansson F, Hariz G, Fodstad H. Tolerance and tremor rebound following long-term chronic thalamic stimulation for Parkinsonian and essential tremor. Stereotact Funct Neurosurg 1999; 72:208–218.

114. Limousin P, Speelman JD, Gielen F, Janssens M. Multicentre European study of thalamic stimulation in parkinsonian and essential tremor. J Neurol Neurosurg Psychiatry 1999; 66:289–296.

115. Obwegeser AA, Uitti RJ, Turk MF, Strongosky AJ, Wharen RE. Thalamic stimulation for the treatment of midline tremors in essential tremor patients. Neurology 2000; 54:2342–2344.

116. Fields JA, Troster AI, Woods SP, Higginson CI, Wilkinson SB, Lyons KE, Koller WC, Pahwa R. Neuropsychological and quality of life outcomes 12 months after unilateral thalamic stimulation for essential tremor. J Neurol Neurosurg Psychiatry 2003; 74:305–311.

117. Rehncrona S, Johnels B, Widner H, Tornqvist AL, Hariz M, Sydow O. Long-term efficacy of thalamic deep brain stimulation for tremor: double-blind assessments. Mov Disord 2003; 18:163–170.

118. Sydow O, Thobois S, Alesch F, Speelman JD. Multicentre European study of thalamic stimulation in essential tremor: a six year follow up. J Neurol Neurosurg Psychiatry 2003; 74:1387–1391.

119. Vaillancourt DE, Sturman MM, Verhagen Metman L, Bakay RA, Corcos DM. Deep brain stimulation of the VIM thalamic nucleus modifies several features of essential tremor. Neurology 2003; 61:919–925.

120. Koller WC, Lyons KE, Wilkinson SB, Troster AI, Pahwa R. Long-term safety and efficacy of unilateral deep brain stimulation of the thalamus in essential tremor. Mov Disord 2001; 16:464–468.

121. Pahwa R, Lyons KL, Wilkinson SB, Carpenter MA, Troster AI, Searl JP, Overman J, Pickering S, Koller WC. Bilateral thalamic stimulation for the treatment of essential tremor. Neurology 1999; 53:1447–1450.

122. Ondo W, Almaguer M, Jankovic J, Simpson RK. Thalamic deep brain stimulation: comparison between unilateral and bilateral placement. Arch Neurol 2001; 58:218–222.

123. Koller WC, Lyons KE, Wilkinson SB, Pahwa R. Efficacy of unilateral deep brain stimulation of the VIM nucleus of the thalamus for essential head tremor. Mov Disord 1999; 14:847–850.

124. Hariz GM, Lindberg M, Bergenheim AT. Impact of thalamic deep brain stimulation on disability and health-related quality of life in patients with essential tremor. J Neurol Neurosurg Psychiatry 2002; 72:47–52.

125. Tröster AI, Fields JA, Pahwa R, Wilkinson SB, Strait-Troster KA, Lyons K, Kieltyka J, Koller WC. Neuropsychological and quality of life outcome after thalamic stimulation for essential tremor. Neurology 1999; 53:1774–1780.

126. Woods SP, Fields JA, Lyons KE, Pahwa R, Troster AI. Pulse width is associated with cognitive decline after thalamic stimulation for essential tremor. Parkinsonism Relat Disord 2003; 9:295–300.

127. O'Suilleabhain PE, Frawley W, Giller C, Dewey RB Jr. Tremor response to polarity, voltage, pulsewidth and frequency of thalamic stimulation. Neurology 2003; 60:786–790.
128. Tasker RR. Deep brain stimulation is preferable to thalamotomy for tremor suppression. Surg Neurol 1998; 49:145–153; discussion 153–144.
129. Pahwa R, Lyons KE, Wilkinson SB, Troster AI. Overman J, Kieltyka J, Koller WC. Comparison of thalamotomy to deep brain stimulation of the thalamus in essential tremor. Mov Disord 2001; 16:140–143.
130. Racette BA, Rich KM, Randle J, Mink JW. Ipsilateral thalamic stimulation after thalamotomy for essential tremor. A case report. Stereotact Funct Neurosurg 2000; 75:155–159.
131. Giller CA, Dewey RB Jr. Ventralis intermedius thalamotomy can succeed when ventralis intermedius thalamic stimulation fails: report of 2 cases for tremor. Stereotact Funct Neurosurg 2002; 79:51–56.
132. Patel NK, Heywood P, O'Sullivan K, McCarter R, Love S, Gill SS. Unilateral subthalamotomy in the treatment of Parkinson's disease. Brain 2003; 126: 1136–1145.

12

Occupational Therapy, Physical Therapy and Alternative Therapies for Essential Tremor

Tanya Simuni

Northwestern University Feinberg School of Medicine, Chicago, Illinois, USA

Essential tremor is one of the most common adult movement disorders (1). The reported prevalence of essential tremor varies from 1% to 22% (2) though based on the most recent data of a door-to-door survey it is estimated to be 4% (3). The incidence of essential tremor increases with age (4). The etiology of essential tremor remains unknown though genetic factors play a clear role (2). The pathophysiology of essential tremor is also not completely understood though it is believed that essential tremor is a centrally mediated disease with the disturbance of olivocerebellar pathways implicated as the cause of the clinical symptoms (5). Essential tremor is characterized by postural and action tremor that typically involves the upper extremities but also can affect the voice and head. The success of available pharmacological treatments of essential tremor ranges between 40% and 65% (6). Frequently use of pharmacological agents can be limited by the low tolerance of the medications or presence of comorbidity especially in elderly patients restricting use of the medications. Surgical treatments of essential tremor either by ablative lesioning procedures like thalamotomy, or by placing a deep brain stimulator (DBS) in the ventral intermediate nucleus (VIM) of the thalamus are very effective and provide on average 80% tremor suppression (7).

Limitations of available pharmacological therapy warrant evaluation of non-pharmacological treatment options of essential tremor. The severity of essential tremor can be variable. The degree of essential tremor related physical disability is proportional to the severity of tremor, which usually increases with age (8). Essential tremor is frequently referred to as a "benign" condition however it can be disabling for a number of patients (9). Disability stems not only from the degree of physical limitations caused by the inability to perform daily tasks (writing, drinking liquids, etc.) but to a large extent from the social embarrassment associated with tremor. Voice tremor if present can contribute to the disease burden. There are very limited published data on the role of non-pharmacological and non-surgical treatment options for essential tremor.

The first step in the decision process regarding utility and choice of non-pharmacological treatment modalities for essential tremor should be an objective evaluation of essential tremor related disability. That can be best accomplished by asking the patients to complete a self-reported disability questionnaire. Louis et al. (10) developed a 31-item 10 minutes validated tremor disability questionnaire that was demonstrated to have good test-retest reliability (10,11) (Table 12.1). Alternatively all clinical tremor rating scales have a section that addresses the level of impact of tremor on ability to perform activities of daily living (ADLs). A number of scales exist; however, the one most widely used is the Clinical Tremor Rating Scale developed by Fahn et al. (12). The scale consists of three parts: evaluation of tremor location and severity, specific motor task and function rating, and functional disability resulting from tremor. Each item is rated on a 0–4 scale with 0 being an absence of symptoms and 4 being the highest degree of symptom-related disability. The scale provides comprehensive tremor assessment and allows physicians to focus on the symptoms interfering with functional ability.

Patients with essential tremor whose symptoms impact ADLs can benefit from occupational therapy. While there are no prospective studies that looked at the role of occupational therapy for essential tremor, the occupational therapist has an important role in multidisciplinary essential tremor management. An occupational therapist can perform an in-depth functional limitations assessment. Patients with impairment of ability to handle utensils can benefit from using heavy utensils to "dampen" tremor. Patients with impaired handwriting due to essential tremor can try to use heavy pens with a large pen handle, again to "dampen" the severity of tremor. Patients with asymmetric tremor can be retrained to use the non-dominant hand to write/use utensils if that hand is less affected. Some patients can benefit from wearing wrist weights to decrease the amplitude of tremor. An occupational therapist can adjust the size and shape of utensils, design special cup holders or other devices to compensate for the tremor. The occupational therapist can evaluate the patient in the home or work environment and provide recommendations on how to adjust the space to best compensate for the essential tremor related disability. One study demonstrated a beneficial effect of rearranging the physical environment during meals to reduce eating dependency even in very old and cognitively impaired patients with essential tremor (13). Severe essential tremor symptoms especially in elderly patients can lead to decreased oral intake and malnourishment. Such patients should be instructed on the use of "finger" food. A nutritional consult can be appropriate to assure adequate calorie intake.

Table 12.1 Tremor Disability Questionnaire (26)

For each of the 31 items listed below, the subject is asked three questions:
(a) Do you have difficulty or disability?
(b) If no difficulty, then do you need to modify the way you perform this task?
(c) If no difficulty, then have you experienced a loss of efficiency when performing this task?
   1. Signing your name
   2. Writing a letter, postcard, thank you card or check
   3. Typing
   4. Placing a letter in an envelope
   5. Drinking from a glass
   6. Pouring milk or juice from a bottle
   7. Carrying a cup of coffee
   8. Using a spoon to drink soup
   9. Carrying a tray of food
   10. Eating in a restaurant
   11. Inserting a coin in a pay telephone or a washing machine
   12. Dialing a telephone
   13. Holding a telephone to your ear
   14. Buttoning your buttons
   15. Tying your shoelaces
   16. Zipping up a zipper
   17. Putting on your eyeglasses
   18. Putting on your contact lenses
   19. Using eye drops
   20. Cutting, trimming or filing your nails
   21. Putting on your watch
   22. Brushing your teeth
   23. Replacing a dollar bill in your wallet or purse
   24. Reading a book, magazine or newspaper
   25. Unlocking door with a key
   26. Threading a needle
   27. Using a screwdriver
   28. Screwing in a light bulb
   29. Placing a plug in an electrical socket
   30. Tying your necktie (males) or putting on your lipstick (females)
   31. Shaving (males) or putting on your eyeliner (females)

Note: To score, if answer to question (a) is yes, score = 2 and skip questions (b) and (c). If answer to question (b) or (c) is yes, score = 1. If answers to questions (b) and (c) are yes, score = 2. The maximum score for each numeric item is 2. The maximum total score for the 31 items is 62.

Strength training has been demonstrated to improve limb steadiness in patients with essential tremor (14). Patients with predominantly upper extremity essential tremor were instructed on a set of strength-training exercises with weights attached to the index finger. Subjects who performed training with a heavy weight load demonstrated improvement in limb steadiness compared with those who trained either with light weights or to controls as measured by electromyography (EMG) and accelerometry. However, improvement was not evident on functional tremor measurements like ADLs or ability to draw a spiral. Potentially, a strength training paradigm that targets larger weight bearing muscle groups could result in functionally meaningful improvement.

Physical therapy is considered to have a limited role in essential tremor. Based on the definition of the disease, essential tremor is viewed as a monosymptomatic disorder manifested by predominantly limb tremor (15). However, it is becoming apparent that patients with essential tremor can have balance impairment, and subtle parkinsonian features (15,16). Postural impairment is specifically prominent in patients with orthostatic tremor (17). Patients with impairment of balance, gait or postural control should be referred to physical therapy for balance evaluation and gait training.

Voice tremor can be a significant part of essential tremor disability specifically in the female population (18). It is believed that voice and head tremor are more refractory to pharmacological therapy. Botulinum toxin injections can be offered to patients with voice tremor (19). Patients with medication refractory voice tremor may benefit from speech therapy.

The degree of essential tremor severity in a given patient can vary significantly based on a number of factors. The impact of emotional status on tremor is a well known phenomenon. In 1887, Dana (20) noted that "everything that produces excitement or nervousness" can increase tremor. Tremor can be very sensitive to such factors as fatigue, temperature fluctuations, sexual arousal, diurnal fluctuations in catecholamine levels, and central nervous system stimulants. Counseling and patient education can help to ameliorate anxiety. There are a few studies that evaluated the role of behavioral treatment on essential tremor severity based on emotional status (21,22). The most widely used technique is behavioral relaxation training (BRT). BRT consists of a series of behavioral relaxation sessions followed by training in the development of coping skills by exposure to stressful situations. Some authors used auditory EMG biofeedback from the muscles involved in a particular task (like writing or eating) as part of the relaxation training (21). Decreased EMG activity correlates with decreased tremor. As patients learn relaxation strategies the feedback threshold is gradually reduced. At the end of the session the patient performs the self-regulation trial of the task with no feedback. Most BRT studies are in the case report format, include a small number of patients, do not have a control group and are not blinded (21). However, Lundervold et al. (21,23) and Chung et al. (24) reported a beneficial effect of behavioral relaxation training in a number of patients, including very elderly individuals with essential tremor measured by clinician and patient-rated tremor severity and an ADL disability scale. Other relaxation strategies like yoga could potentially be of benefit but no literature is available.

Essential tremor can be associated with a significant degree of social embarrassment along with physical disability. Patients with essential tremor frequently avoid public places especially situations requiring eating, drinking, writing, and meeting new people. This can lead to social isolation, dysphoria, and depression. Social phobia is reported as a frequent essential tremor comorbidity (25). The prevalence of social phobia in essential tremor is reported to be 32% (25). Interestingly a number of essential tremor patients were diagnosed with primary social phobia that preceded the onset of the symptoms of essential tremor (25). Severity of social phobia and tremor independently contributed to disability. Physicians treating patients with essential tremor should be sensitive to the social aspects of the disease and offer referral for psychological counseling when necessary.

In conclusion, essential tremor is a common movement disorder which can be functionally disabling. In the absence of effective pharmacological therapy physicians should evaluate the role of multidisciplinary treatment in order to maximize the functional performance and quality of life of patients with essential tremor.

REFERENCES

1. Deuschl G, Koller WC. Introduction. Essential tremor. Neurology 2000; 54(11 suppl 4):S1.
2. Findley LJ. Epidemiology and genetics of essential tremor. Neurology 2000; 54(11 suppl 4):S8–S13.
3. Dogu O et al. Prevalence of essential tremor: door-to-door neurologic exams in Mersin Province, Turkey. Neurology 2003; 61(12):1804–1806.
4. Louis ED, Jurewicz EC, Watner D. Community-based data on associations of disease duration and age with severity of essential tremor: implications for disease pathophysiology. Mov Disord 2003; 18(1):90–93.
5. Deuschl G, Elble RJ. The pathophysiology of essential tremor. Neurology 2000; 54(11 suppl 4):S14–S20.
6. Lou JS. Essential tremor: clinical correlates in 350 patients. [See comment.]
7. Lyons KE, Pahwa R. Deep brain stimulation and essential tremor. J Clin Neurophysiol 2004; 21:2–5.
8. Louis ED et al. Correlates of functional disability in essential tremor. Mov Disord 2001; 16(5):914–920.
9. Busenbark KL et al. Is essential tremor benign? Neurology 1991; 41(12):1982–1983.
10. Louis ED et al. Validity and test-retest reliability of a disability questionnaire for essential tremor. Mov Disord 2000; 15(3):516–523.
11. Wendt KJ, Ford B, Louis ED. Validity and test-retest reliability of a disability questionnaire for essential tremor. Gerontology 2000; 46(1):12–16.
12. Fahn S, Tolosa E, Martin C. Clinical rating scale for tremor. In: Jankovic J, Tolosa E, eds. Parkinson's Disease and Movement Disorders. Baltimore: Urban & Schwarzenberg, 1988.
13. Lewin LM, Lindervold D, Saslow M, Thompson S. Reducing eating dependency in nursing home patients: the effect of prompting, reinforcement, food preference and environmental design. J Clin Exper Gerontology 1989; (11):47–63.
14. Bilodeau M, Keen DA, Sweeney PJ, Shields RW. Strength training can improve steadiness in persons with essential tremor. Muscle Nerve 2000; 23(5):771–778.

15. Elble RJ. Diagnostic criteria for essential tremor and differential diagnosis. Neurology 2000; 54(11 suppl 4):S2–S6.
16. Cohen O et al. Rest tremor in patients with essential tremor: prevalence, clinical correlates, and electrophysiologic characteristics. Arch Neurol 2003; 60(3):405–410.
17. Gates P, Thyagarajan D. Orthostatic tremor: a cause of postural instability in the elderly. Medical Journal of Australia 1990; 152(7):373.
18. Louis ED, Ford B, Frucht S. Factors associated with increased risk of head tremor in essential tremor: a community-based study in northern Manhattan. Mov Disord 2003; 18(4):432–436.
19. Koller WC, Hristova A, Brin M. Pharmacologic treatment of essential tremor. Neurology 2000; 54(11 suppl 4):S30–S38.
20. Dana CL. Hereditary tremor, a hitherto undescribed form of motor neurosis. Am J Med Sci 1887; 94:386–393.
21. Lundervold DA et al. Reduction of tremor severity and disability following behavioral relaxation training. J Behav Ther Exper Psychiatry 1999; 30(2):119–135.
22. Milligan B et al. Treatment of essential tremor by behavior therapy. Use of Jacobson's progressive relaxation method (author's transl). Neurosurgery 2000; 46(3):613–622; discussion 622–624.
23. Lundervold DA, Poppen R. Biobehavioral rehabilitation for older adults with essential tremor. Gerontologist 1995; 35(4):556–559.
24. Chung W, Poppen R, Lundervold DA. Behavioral relaxation training for tremor disorders in older adults. Biofeedback & Self Regulation 1995; 20(2):123–135.
25. Schneier FR et al. Characteristics of social phobia among persons with essential tremor. J Clin Psychiatry 2001; 62(5):367–372.
26. Wendt KJ, Albert S, Schneier F, Louis ED. The Columbia University assessment of disability in essential tremor (CADET): methodological issues in essential tremor research. Parkinsonism Rel Disord 2000; (6):17–23.

II. Other Tremor Disorders

13

Parkinsonian Tremor

Anthony E. Lang and Cindy Zadikoff
Toronto Western Hospital, Toronto, Canada

I. INTRODUCTION

In 1817, James Parkinson described what is now known as Parkinson's disease (PD) in a monograph entitled "An Essay on the Shaking Palsy (1)." In it he commented on "involuntary tremulous motion, with lessened muscular power, in parts not in action and even when supported." This is now recognized as the classic resting tremor of PD. Resting tremor is one of the cardinal symptoms of PD along with bradykinesia, rigidity, and postural instability and can often be the presenting feature of PD. When looking at large series of patients with autopsy proven PD, it is the most specific sign of idiopathic PD compared to the other cardinal symptoms (2). Though rest tremor may be absent in patients with idiopathic PD, it is much more often lacking in the "Parkinson-plus" syndromes.

When rest tremor is a major or predominant feature of PD, the term tremor dominant PD is often applied. Numerous studies evaluating predictors of decline in PD have confirmed that tremor dominant patients have a less severe prognosis and clinical course than patients with predominant postural instability and gait dysfunction, and that absence of tremor at presentation is a poor prognostic indicator (3–5).

Much progress has been made in understanding the pathophysiological basis of resting tremor, but many unresolved questions remain. This chapter will attempt to review the clinical aspects, various theories regarding the location of the generator of PD tremor, animal models of the tremor, and both medical and surgical management of PD tremor.

II. CLINICAL FEATURES OF PD

The classic resting tremor of PD is a rhythmic 4–6 Hz [although early in the disease frequencies as high as 9 Hz have been observed (6)] pill rolling finger movement superimposed upon rhythmic extension and flexion movement of the wrist and pronation/supination movement of the forearm. It may be intermittent early on, often present only in stressful situations. Eventually it becomes constant and is increased by mental stress. Voluntary muscle contraction typically suppresses the tremor, at least temporarily (7). Some patients manifest an isolated longstanding unilateral resting tremor. When this persists for 2 years without any other signs and symptoms of PD, it is called monosymptomatic resting tremor (7). The tremor more commonly presents unilaterally in a hand and then spreads to involve the ipsilateral leg and then contralateral arm/leg and jaw, although onset and spread can occur in any combination. Rajput et al. retrospectively reviewed 613 PD patients followed over 22 years and found that 11%, including a small percentage with resting tremor prominent in one lower limb and contralateral upper limb, presented with anomalous asymmetrical signs (8).

In the limb, distal muscles are affected more than proximal. Conduction of prominent limb tremor often accounts for trunk or head shaking. A pure head tremor is rarely a feature of PD and is more typical of essential tremor, cervical dystonia or cerebellar disease (e.g., multiple system atrophy). More typical of PD is a resting tremor of the jaw with involvement of lower facial muscles (e.g., lips and chin) and tongue (either at rest or on protrusion) in some patients. Occasionally, involvement of the perinasal and perioral region causes a tremor similar to the "rabbit syndrome" more often seen as a complication of neuroleptic drug therapy.

The classic resting tremor is present when the limb or affected body part is at rest or in complete repose and subsides with any voluntary muscle activation. During the course of a movement the tremor is typically suppressed and reemerges, often after a brief delay, once the limb returns to the resting state. Since the tremor experienced by many patients is predominantly this classic type, disability from resting tremor may not be a major problem. The clinical presentation of the "rest" tremor is not uniform. A common variant presents or behaves more as a postural tremor (7). In the typical combination of resting and postural/kinetic tremor in PD, the two have the same frequency. This tremor is largely inhibited during movement (especially during the transition from rest to posture) but can reoccur with the same frequency after a variable latency (from <1 second to several seconds) when adopting a new posture. Sometimes the more severe tremors will persist during movement of the limb although the amplitude typically dampens considerably. Jankovic et al. (9) reported that among PD patients with both resting and postural tremor two thirds had this type of "postural tremor" with a mean latency from taking on a new posture to onset of tremor of 9.37 seconds and similar postural and resting frequencies. They referred to this as a "re-emergent" tremor (9), although it can be argued that this simply represents one of the characteristic features of classic resting tremor and therefore does not require a separate designation.

In some patients, however, the frequencies of the resting and postural/kinetic components differ. When these differ by >1.5 Hz the postural/kinetic tremor has a higher frequency and is non-harmonically related to the frequency of the resting tremor. There is some debate as to whether this type of tremor represents a combination of essential tremor and PD (10). Positron emission tomography (PET) (11), neuropathology (12), and epidemiological data (13) have failed to confirm such a relationship. It is likely that in most PD patients with a higher frequency postural tremor that this is a symptom of their disease. Patients with a longstanding isolated postural and action tremor for many years or decades before the onset of typical parkinsonian symptoms, often with a family history of tremor, probably represent examples of essential tremor and PD. This may be no more than the coincidental association of two common neurological disorders. Theoretically it might be possible that an underlying tremor diathesis could influence the presentation of parkinsonian features such that having ET or a family history of ET could make it more likely that such a person developing PD would have a tremor-dominant form. This possibility is supported by a recent study that found a significantly higher family history of tremor in PD patients with a tremor predominant presentation than in those with a postural instability gait disorder (PIGD) form (14).

Finally, isolated postural and kinetic tremors do occur in PD, typically in the akinetic rigid variant of PD. In these patients a higher frequency (7–12 Hz) kinetic tremor, sometimes called "rippling tremor," accompanies and may impair movement (10).

Though resting tremor is one of the most specific signs of idiopathic PD, tremor frequency and amplitude are poor criteria for distinguishing PD tremors from other tremors (15). The pattern of activation in antagonistic muscles is mostly reciprocal alternation, however co-contraction is also known to occur and in 10–15% there may be a synchronous pattern during action but a reciprocal pattern during rest (16). Therefore, the pattern of activation is also not a reliable discriminator between PD and other tremor disorders (17,18).

A variety of electrophysiologic tools can be used to show differences between PD tremor and other tremors, but currently there is no technique that can unequivocally distinguish between these tremors. Table 13.1 lists some of these techniques and how data derived from them can further help interpret parkinsonian tremor.

III. ETIOLOGY OF TREMOR

A. Pathological Data

The location of the resting tremor generator as well as the metabolic substrates underlying it are not completely understood. Patients with isolated rest tremor who do not develop bradykinesia for many years have a significant loss of putaminal 18-F dopa uptake similar to more typical PD (11). Furthermore, although dopaminergic neuronal loss in the substantia nigra pars compacta (SNc) resulting in striatal dopaminergic denervation is the major pathologic feature of PD, in contrast to bradykinesia and rigidity, tremor severity correlates poorly with nigrostriatal dopaminergic deficit (19–22). The severity of tremor and bradykinesia are often dissociated and may have a differential response to antiparkinson medication suggesting that the pathology underlying each of these may be in part, distinct (3,23,24). Pathology studies suggest that tremor may result from the loss of particular subgroups of mesencephalic dopaminergic neurons. Typically PD first affects the ventrolateral group of SNc neurons and then progresses to involve the ventromedial group and finally the dorsal tier of neurons (25,26). It has been suggested that retrorubral area A8 is more severely affected by dopamine cell degeneration in the tremor dominant form than in the akinetic rigid variant, where more severe damage is found in the lateral substantia nigra, area A9 (27,28).

B. Functional Imaging

In PD, PET has been used to map the cerebral metabolic rate of glucose (CMRglc) using [18F]-fluro-2-deoxyglucose (FDG-PET) during task performance and in the resting state. CMRglc, a marker of local synaptic activity, is sensitive to both direct neuronal/synaptic damage as well as secondary disruption at sites distant from the primary location of pathology (29). Early studies using FDG-PET in PD revealed mild but persistent increases in the resting CMRglc in the lenticular nucleus, especially the globus pallidus (30,31). As a result of nigrostriatal dopaminergic (DA) denervation (32), one might expect such an

Table 13.1 Electrophysiologic Tools to Aid in the Interpretation of Tremor in PD

Technique	Data analysis	Interpretation
Accelerometer applied to various body parts, often recorded in conjunction with surface electromyography (EMG) Other techniques to record movement include: *Goniometers* *Digitizing tablets* *Ultrasound* *Infrared/magnetic tracking devices*	Amplitude—using Fast Fourier Transformation (FFT) of the accelerometer and the digitally filtered EMG, the total power in the frequency range between 2 and 25 Hz is measured.	Quite variable. Mainly helpful in distinguishing normal from pathologic tremor. Amplitude typically greatest at rest in PD.
	Frequency—using FFT of the accelerometer and the digitally filtered EMG, peak frequency is measured.	In PD, usually a 4–6 Hz resting tremor, though action and postural tremor do occur and frequencies as high as 9 Hz have been recorded (6)
	Waveform analysis—detects more subtle differences of the shape of tremor curves using mathematical time series analysis	Results reflect nonlinearities of the tremor curves and can distinguish between PD and ET (157)
	Loading of limb leads to minimal reduction of amplitude and frequency in resting tremor in PD (35,36)	This implies only a minimal role of a peripheral origin in PD tremor.
EMG—using surface electrodes; commonly evaluated muscles include flexors and extensors of the wrist, fingers, elbows, knee and ankle. This is often recorded in conjunction with accelerometry	Pattern of bursts is used to determine whether antagonistic muscles are contracting alternately or synchronously	Mainly reciprocal alternation in antagonistic muscles in PD rest tremor, but co-contraction does occur (16).
	Coherence analysis of different muscles in affected tremulous limbs has shown coherence between muscles of a single limb, but often not between limbs (91).	This suggests topographical organization and functional segregation of the tremor generator

(continued)

Table 13.1 *Continued*

Technique	Data analysis	Interpretation
Electroencephalogram (EEG)	Simultaneous recordings taken from EEG and EMG show coherence between EMG tremor recordings and EEG with maximal coherence over the contralateral motor cortex (158)	This supports the role for central mechanisms and the network hypothesis in tremor generation.
Magnetoencephalogram (MEG)	Simultaneous surface EMG of hand muscles and MEG recordings show coherence between EMG and brain areas including the contralateral primary motor cortex, supplementary motor cortex, and diencephalon (159)	This suggests a large neural network in tremor generation.
Peripheral resetting techniques used in conjunction with EMG/accelerometer: – Peripheral stimulation applied to median or peroneal nerve – vibration to tendons	Mechanical displacement of wrist joint has little effect on tremor (36,39). Electrical stimulation of median nerve has little effect on tremor (40).	This implies a minimal role of peripheral generators or reflex pathways in generating PD tremor.
Central resetting techniques used in conjunction with EMG/accelerometer: – Transcranial Magnetic Stimulation (TMS)	Magnetic stimulation applied to contralateral motor cortex with simultaneous tremor recordings leads to resetting of tremor (41,42)	This suggests a role for central mechanisms and the network hypothesis in tremor generation.

increase in striatopallidal synaptic terminal activity. Subsequently, Eidelberg et al. using FDG-PET described a metabolic profile of parkinsonism that consisted of relative hypermetabolism of the lentiform nucleus, thalamus, and pons with relative hypometabolism of the lateral frontal cortex (21,33). The correlation of this profile with the severity of bradykinesia but not tremor may indicate that it is a metabolic consequence of nigrostriatal dopamine deficiency. Antonini et al. (22) compared the FDG-PET metabolic profiles of PD patients with and without tremor matched for bradykinesia and rigidity. In the tremor group there was a relative hypermetabolism of the pons, thalamus, and premotor cortical regions. In many of these studies, patients have been chronically exposed to dopaminergic medication and it is not clear how this might interfere with the imaging findings.

The role of serotonin in the generation of parkinsonian rest tremor has been postulated. A PET study demonstrated reduced midbrain 5-HT1A binding that correlated with tremor severity but not rigidity or bradykinesia. Further studies are warranted, including trials of novel serotonergic agents in the management of rest tremor (34).

IV. CENTRAL vs. PERIPHERAL TREMOR GENERATORS

A. Peripheral Generator

Some tremors are generated centrally, while others are thought to have a peripheral origin involving reflex spinal pathways or a combination of central and peripheral components. Tremors originating peripherally are much more susceptible to the influences of external mechanical factors. In the parkinsonian resting tremor, the role of mechanical factors in generating tremor is negligible. Several studies have shown little or no frequency reduction in response to weight loading of the affected limb (15,35,36). Although some studies have shown that electrical stimulation of the muscle can reset resting tremor (37,38), the majority of studies have failed to confirm this response. Several attempts combining different stimuli such as mechanical perturbations (36,39), electrical stimulation of the median nerve (40), and transcranial magnetic stimulation (TMS) of the motor cortex (41,42) have demonstrated that only the latter consistently results in resetting of the tremor (42). Attempts to treat tremor have involved sectioning the dorsal roots. This successfully reduced the amplitude of the tremor but only changed the frequency slightly (43). Furthermore, studies that involved the injection of anesthetic into muscles until rigidity and stretch reflexes were diminished failed to show a reduction in tremor (44). Therefore a peripheral location is unlikely for the primary tremor generator.

B. Central Generator

Clinical data in both primates and in humans point to a central oscillator, however the exact location remains a mystery. Lesions or perturbations in a number of sites in the central nervous system (CNS) can suppress parkinsonian tremor. For instance, removing the motor cortex or lesioning the internal capsule can suppress tremor but at the cost of unacceptable side effects (45,46). Thermocoagulation lesions (46,47) as well as chronic high frequency electrical deep brain stimulation (DBS) of the ventral intermediate (VIM) nucleus of the thalamus (48), the subthalamic nucleus (STN) (49,50) or the globus pallidus interna (GPi) (51,52) can have profound ameliorative effects on PD tremor.

1. Possible Locations of the Central Oscillator

Cerebellum: Some have suggested a role for the cerebellum in generating the parkinsonian rest tremor. Indeed, almost all tremors show cerebellar hyperactivity. PET activation studies have shown cerebellar overactivity in PD tremor. Duffau et al. (53) reported an increase in the regional cerebral blood flow (rCBF) in the cerebellar vermis in PD patients with tremor in the off state compared to the on state without tremor.

The VIM thalamus largely receives cerebellar afferents and projects mainly to the primary motor cortex (54,55). FDG-PET studies in patients treated with deep brain stimulation (DBS) of the VIM have consistently shown that effective stimulation reduces cerebellar regional blood flow compared with ineffective stimulation, whereas cortical blood flow is not significantly influenced (56). However, such changes could be entirely secondary to altered somatosensory input given the preferential activation of the cerebellum by peripheral afferents.

Rest tremor does not disappear when the cerebellum is removed. Furthermore, a patient with a prior cerebellectomy who subsequently developed PD demonstrated a prominent atypical rest tremor, with prominent postural and kinetic components (57). This experience strongly argues that the cerebellum cannot be the primary tremor generator. In fact, it has been suggested that rather than having a causal role in tremor generation, the cerebellum may actually prevent tremor from spilling over into voluntary activity (57). The hyper activity of the cerebellum could then be due to this compensatory role in actively limiting rhythmical activity produced by the basal ganglia.

Thalamus: Some studies have implicated the thalamus as the central oscillator. Llinas and colleagues proposed that central tremors are due to specific oscillating properties of thalamic cells (58,59). These cells can be activated in two ways. The first is the "relay mode" with normal summation of post-synaptic potentials at the membrane until the firing threshold is reached. The second is the "oscillatory mode." Calcium dependent changes of the membrane potential drives this mode which leads to a rebound calcium spike that then causes the next spike of a particular cell. The oscillatory mode is driven by hyperpolarization of cells. Because the GPi is overactive in PD, its inhibitory input to the thalamus could hyperpolarize the thalamic cells. Other *in vitro* experiments trying to determine the relation between the pallidum and thalamus have shown that for some frequencies of pallidal neuronal firing, the thalamus does have specific filter properties. For instance, 12–15 Hz pallidal input is transformed into a 4–6 Hz pattern due to specific membrane properties of thalamic target nuclei (60). However, there are both animal and human data showing that most pallidal tremor cells (cells firing at the typical tremor frequency often in synchrony with a visible tremor) are already firing at a low frequency (61–63) and the 12–15 Hz range of single cell oscillations does not seem to be more frequent in PD patients or 1-methyl-4-phenyl-1,2,3,6-tetrahydropyridine (MPTP) treated primates (61,64,65). Although tremor cells are numerous in the thalamus, and Lenz et al. (66) did show that some thalamic neurons fire in advance of the tremor (suggesting a role in "driving" the tremor), the important observations demonstrating that several nuclei upstream in the basal ganglia contain tremor cells make it unlikely that the thalamus is the primary generator. Furthermore, although hyperpolarization of the oscillating cells described above has been shown in animals (67), this has been demonstrated in only a minority of recordings in humans with PD (68).

Pallidum: Because the primary locus of pathology of PD is in the basal ganglia, it seems natural to assume that a large proportion of the symptoms of PD are due to abnormalities in the basal ganglia. Certainly the beneficial effects of pallidotomy (69,70) and pallidal DBS (51,52) suggest that the pallidum is involved in tremor. Different cell types in the pallidum can be separated based on their firing patterns (71–73). In one study of 3 patients with PD tremor undergoing microelectrode exploration of the globus pallidus prior to pallidotomy, 12.3% of the cells were found to fire at the frequency of the patients' rest tremor. All of these cells were found in the ventral portion of the GPi, whereas no tremor cells were found in the external segment of the globus pallidus (GPe) (61). In electrophysiologic studies of parkinsonian patients and MPTP treated monkeys, the discharge rate in STN and GPi is increased and dopaminergic therapy reduces this firing rate (74–77). In normal monkeys only a few pallidal cells show significant oscillations whereas after MPTP therapy 40% showed oscillations (65). However, in a study by Lemstra et al. (62) only one out of eleven tremor cells exhibited coherence with the periphery as determined by electromyography (EMG). Therefore, although there are certainly data pointing to overactivity of the GPi as the potential cause of tremor generation, the evidence remains inconclusive.

Subthalamic nucleus: Just as lesions or DBS in the GPi and VIM in humans implicate these targets as generators, so too does the striking and reliable ameliorative effect of STN stimulation on rest tremor implicate the STN as the central generator (50,78–80).

Electrophysiological studies have demonstrated three types of cells in the STN of PD patients: 1) tonic cells that fire at a mean frequency of 4–9 Hz and are modified by passive and voluntary movement, 2) pause cells (most frequent) that discharge irregularly at high firing rates with intervening pauses, and 3) tremor cells that fire with a burst pattern of 4–5 Hz. These account for <20%

of cells recorded in the STN of PD patients and are sensitive to kinesthetic stimulation and are somatotopically organized (81). In primates, neurons with oscillatory discharges are found in controls, but this number increases dramatically (90%) in MPTP treated parkinsonian animals (64). Levy et al. (82) found a high degree of synchronization in the STN of PD patients with resting tremor compared to those without tremor. Moreover, this synchronization often occurred at frequencies ranging from 15 to 30 Hz. In patients without tremor, only one neuron out of 84 examined showed high-frequency oscillatory activity and there was no synchronous high-frequency oscillatory activity (82). Dopaminergic medication decreased the incidence of synchronized high-frequency oscillations in the STN neuron pairs concurrent with a reduction in firing rate and limb tremor (83). In addition, lesioning of the STN reduces or abolishes tremor in both MPTP treated monkeys (84) as well as humans with PD (85,86). Finally, Plenz and Kital (87) showed that the STN and GPe form a feedback system with synchronized oscillatory bursting. Pallidal lesions abolished this bursting whereas cortical lesions favored bursting. This, too, supports the hypothesis that there is a central oscillator, perhaps an STN-GPe pacemaker, which is responsible for synchronized oscillatory activity in the dopamine depleted basal ganglia.

Network hypothesis: Although it appears that a central generator (possibly more than one) does exist within the cortical-basal ganglia-thalamo-cortical loop, tremor suppression is achieved not only by blockade of this loop, but also by blockade of the cerebello-thalamo-cortical loop. The beneficial effect then of stereotactic surgery involving the VIM would have to be secondary to an interaction between these two loops. This interaction would have to take place at the cortical level because the two projections are believed to be segregated until the cortex (88,89). Timmerman et al. (90) simultaneously recorded surface EMG of the hand muscles and brain activity using magnetoencephalography (MEG) in six PD patients off medications. The tremor was associated with a strong coherence between the EMG of the forearm muscles and activity in the contralateral primary motor cortex at tremor frequency and at double tremor frequency. There was also coherence between the primary motor cortex and the supplementary motor cortex, lateral premotor cortex, diencephalon, secondary somatosensory cortex, posterior parietal cortex and contralateral cerebellum (90). Using functional imaging, Parker et al. (55) measured rCBF in seven patients undergoing thalamic DBS for parkinsonian tremor. They were also able to demonstrate activation of the sensory motor cortex as well as supplementary motor cortex and cortico-cerebellar pathways in the presence of tremor. This suggests a larger cerebral network with abnormal coupling in a cerebello-diencephalic-cortical loop.

Clinically it appears that different muscle groups involved in PD tremor are "driven" in concert. However, using coherence analysis techniques, it is clear that the tremor in different body parts is not necessarily coherent and although the muscles in one body part are mostly coherent, the rhythms differ between different extremities, and in fact, are almost never coherent (91). One would then need to consider whether there are distinct oscillators for each extremity. More likely, the tremor is generated through a network involving the basal ganglia and its connections. Although tremor cells have been found in the STN, GPi and thalamus perhaps no single nucleus is responsible alone, but rather they are part of an unstable oscillating network. The lack of coherence of tremor in different body parts would mean that the oscillating systems within the basal ganglia are topographically organized and functionally segregated (well recognized characteristics of the normal basal ganglia) and that the channels for each extremity are uncoupled as well. The paradox, however, is that dopamine depletion leads to an "unfocusing" in which more neurons are responsive to multiple joint input. This argues for loss of functional segregation leading to hypersynchronization. The equally good response possible with GPi, thalamic, and STN lesions or DBS could be due to a blockade or stimulation-induced desynchronization of rhythmic activity within the oscillating loops (92).

Finally, although the classical model of PD holds that dopamine depletion is the primary pathologic hallmark, other neurotransmitters are also affected. Post mortem studies have shown widespread extranigral involvement including the locus coeruleus, serotonergic dorsal and median raphe, cholinergic brainstem nuclei, mesocortical dopaminergic system, dorsal motor vagal nucleus and a variety of other areas (28,93–95). As such, non-dopaminergic mechanisms could also play a role in tremor generation. For example, Doder et al. (34) found evidence for reduced raphe 5-HT1A binding in PD that correlated with tremor but not rigidity or bradykinesia.

V. ANIMAL MODELS

A variety of animal models have been used in an attempt to further our understanding of PD (96). Ultimately what has borne out of these models is that it is much easier to produce postural and action tremors than it is the resting tremor of PD. Selective lesioning in animal models has thus far failed to elicit a single locus that is capable of producing a resting tremor, but rather, multiple lesions are necessary. Destruction of three structures seems crucial for the induction of rest tremor in primates: parvocellular division of the red nucleus, cerebellothalamic fibers, and nigrostriatal fibers (97). The best tremor model is the MPTP primate model, and yet this is also far from ideal. First of all, animals do not develop a progressive disorder as in PD. Next, not all species develop a tremor and rarely do they display the classic resting tremor. Rhesus monkeys develop a low amplitude, high frequency 10–12 Hz action tremor that resembles the kinetic tremor of PD (96,98,99) whereas vervet monkeys develop a high amplitude, low frequency resting tremor more typical of the resting tremor of PD (96). There are many factors that could account for the lack of resting tremor in MPTP-treated primates. Whereas there seems to be a predilection for area A8 dopaminergic depletion in PD patients with resting tremor, in MPTP primates the pattern of neuronal loss varies from homogeneous loss of dopamine in the caudate and putamen with no gradient (100,101) and central and medial predominant loss of SNc neurons (102) to a more pronounced loss of dopamine in the putamen with a rostral-caudal gradient and predominant lateral SNc neuronal loss (103–105). Even in humans with MPTP-induced parkinsonism only four of seven patients had a 4–6 Hz rest tremor (106). Other factors that could account for the inconsistent ability of MPTP to produce tremor include the route of administration (intracarotid vs. systemic), the dose used, and the chronicity and distribution of the lesion. The physical characteristics of monkeys, such as arm length and finger position, could also influence the nature of the tremor. It may also be that the age of the animals when exposed to MPTP alters phenomenology (107). Older animals have more symptoms than younger ones. Also, the length of survival might affect the phenomenology of the tremor (96). In one human exposed to MPTP a rest tremor only developed several years after the original exposure (108).

Despite its shortcomings, the MPTP-treated monkey is a useful model that has clearly advanced our understanding of the pathogenesis of the rest tremor of PD. Single unit recording of activity in pairs of cells within the internal pallidum has demonstrated correlated activity in such monkeys with tremor but not in monkeys lacking tremor. This, along with data from humans, has led to the hypothesis discussed earlier that perhaps in pathologic tremor there is a loss of segregation or abnormal synchronization of neuronal activity within basal ganglia loops subserving different topographic regions (109). This provides both an anatomic and physiologic basis for the separation of the oscillating activity for the different extremities and also the basis for multiple oscillators within a single oscillating loop.

VI. THERAPY

A. Medical

Although the response of bradykinesia and rigidity to levodopa is quite predictable, no drug has proven to be consistently effective in treating resting tremor. Part of the problem with the response to therapy is the tendency for tremor to fluctuate in response to stress, emotion, and mental distraction (see Table 13.2).

For many years *anticholinergic drugs* were the only useful treatment of tremor. Ordenstein discovered the antitremor benefits of anticholinergics when he administered derivatives of belladonna alkaloids to ameliorate sialorrhea (110). In the 1960s Duvoisin demonstrated that the cholinesterase inhibitor physostigmine consistently increased the severity of parkinsonian symptoms and that these effects could be lessened by the administration of anticholinergic drugs such as benztropine or scopolamine (111). The most commonly used drugs include trihexyphenidyl, benztropine, and ethopropazine. The mechanism of

Table 13.2 Common Drug Therapy for Tremor in Parkinson's Disease

Drug	Typical dosages	Common side effects
Anticholinergic agents		
Trihexyphenidyl	1 mg tid–slowly titrate up to 12–18 mg/day (rarely >6 mg/day)	Confusion, dry mouth, urinary retention, constipation, blurred vision, increased intraocular pressure
Benztropine	0.5 mg up to 6 mg/day	
Ethopropazine	50 mg qd up to 500 mg/day (rarely)	
Amantadine	100 mg up to 100 mg tid	Confusion, peripheral edema, insomnia
Selegiline	5 mg qd up to 5 mg bid	Nausea, dizziness
Dopamine agonists		All dopamine agonists can cause confusion, hallucinations, peripheral edema, somnolence, nausea, and orthostatic hypotension. Cardiac valvulopathy and serositis are rare side effects of all ergot—derived agonists
Pergolide (ergot)	0.05 mg qhs up to 5 mg/d	
Ropinirole (non-ergot)	0.25 mg tid up to 24 mg/d	
Pramipexole (non-ergot)	0.125 mg tid up to 4.5 mg/d	
Carbidopa/levodopa	25/100 tid titrated to effect	Dyskinesias, hallucinations, nausea, orthostatic hypotension.
Clozapine	12.5 mg up to 75 mg (or more) daily	Rare risk of agranulocytosis requires weekly complete blood counts for the first 6 months and biweekly thereafter
Propranolol	40 mg bid up to 200 mg daily	Bradycardia, dyspnea, depression
Mirtazapine	15 mg up to 45 mg daily	weight gain, somnolence, constipation, alanine ALT elevation, rarely agranulocytosis and seizures

Note: CBC, complete blood count; ALT, alanine aminotransferase.

action of the anticholinergics remains unclear. Although distributed widely throughout the CNS, the striatum appears to have the largest concentration of acetylcholine, choline acetyltransferase and cholinesterase (112). In the normal basal ganglia the nigral dopaminergic neurons exert a tonic inhibitory effect on striatal cholinergic interneurons. It is believed that anticholinergics restore the balance between striatal dopamine and acetylcholine activities and this is the basis for anticholinergic efficacy in the treatment of parkinsonian symptoms. These agents are generally considered more effective for tremor and rigidity than bradykinesia (113,114). There is a great deal of variability in the selectivity of each drug for the muscarinic receptors (M1 and M2) (115) and some, like benztropine, have the ability to block dopamine uptake in central dopaminergic neurons (116). Although this could provide some insight into the pathophysiology underlying the different parkinsonian symptoms, there are no controlled studies that convincingly demonstrate selective clinical actions of one drug compared with another (117,118).

Using the Unified Parkinson's Disease Rating Scale (UPDRS) to assess response of resting tremor to medications, most studies have found that levodopa and anticholinergics produce a 30–50% mean reduction in resting tremor scores (118,119). Koller compared trihexyphenidyl with levodopa and amantadine and demonstrated that the two former drugs were equally effective in reducing tremor amplitude by 50% compared with a 25% reduction with amantadine, however, tremor frequency was unchanged (118). If used, anticholinergics are initiated early in the disease when symptoms are modest and tremor is the dominant manifestation. There are little data on the interactions between levodopa and anticholinergics. Delayed gastric emptying caused by anticholinergics likely delays levodopa absorption (120) and chronic levodopa therapy may contribute to cholinergic hypersensitivity (121).

Side effects are often the limiting factor in anticholinergic therapy. Confusion is a well known side effect, and often the most troublesome. These agents must be used with caution, and are essentially contraindicated in the elderly and those with prior cognitive impairment. One sometimes beneficial side effect is dry mouth, which can be helpful in alleviating sialorrhea in PD patients, although often patients find this side effect intolerable. Rarely anticholinergics can cause dyskinesia (122) as well as enhance levodopa-induced dyskinesia (123).

Amantadine is less effective for tremor than either levodopa or trihexyphenidyl (118). On occasion a patient with a mild tremor in the early stages of disease will respond to *selegiline* as monotherapy. In a double-blind cross-over trial of selegiline 10 mg/day as adjunctive therapy to levodopa in those with mild to moderate PD, Sivertsen et al. (124) found a 26% improvement in tremor scores as well as a reduction in the daily dose of levodopa.

Dopamine agonists can be used as monotherapy or adjunctive to levodopa. A reduction in tremor scores comparable to that obtained with levodopa and anticholinergics can be achieved with dopamine agonists. In one study comparing ropinirole (mean dose of 9.7 mg/day) to levodopa (mean dose 464 mg/day), the reduction in UPDRS resting tremor score (item #20) was 32% and 35% respectively, but with no change in action tremor (item #21) (125). Each dopamine agonist has a slightly different profile of activity at different receptors and although each of these drugs has been shown to be better than placebo in at least one double-blind, placebo-controlled trial, none has been proven to be superior in the treatment of tremor (126). Studies have compared ropinirole, pramipexole, and pergolide to bromocriptine. Ropinirole (mean dose 8.3 mg daily) and bromocriptine (16.8 mg daily) showed similar (39% and 30%) reductions in tremor scores (127). Dopamine agonists have also been shown to be effective in reducing tremor not only as monotherapy but also when given as adjuvant therapy with levodopa. Kunig et al. (128) evaluated the efficacy of pramipexole in patients with advanced PD and severe resting tremor and found a 61% reduction in tremor over baseline in the patients receiving pramipexole. A follow-up study of pramipexole as adjuvant therapy in 84 patients with resting tremor found a 48% improvement in the UPDRS tremor scores with pramipexole vs. 13% improvement with placebo (129).

Levodopa remains the most effective therapy for the treatment of all major features of PD. However, a "levodopa-resistant tremor" is not an uncommon problem. In some patients this is simply a dose-related phenomenon; increasing the drug to very high doses may eventually result in marked tremor suppression. In some patients, tremor does seem to be truly levodopa-resistant and there is no explanation for why seemingly identical tremors can respond so differently to dopamine replacement therapy.

A number of other second-line medications may be considered either as adjunctive therapy or as monotherapy. *Clozapine* may be effective in treating resting tremor. There have been several open label studies supporting the efficacy of low dose clozapine for PD tremor (130–132). A double-blind cross-over study comparing clozapine and benztropine showed that they were equally effective with a mean 33% reduction in UPDRS tremor score (119). Bonuccelli et al. (133) studied single doses (12.5 mg) of clozapine for resting and postural tremor in a double-blind placebo-controlled manner. Fifteen of 17 patients had a reduction in tremor after receiving clozapine but not placebo. There was no statistically significant difference between the effects on resting and postural components. The pharmacological explanation of the anti-tremor effect of clozapine is poorly understood; in addition to being a D4 dopamine receptor antagonist it has antimuscarinic effects *in vitro* and also is a central antagonist of serotonergic 5-HT 1, 5-HT 2, and 5-HT 3 receptors.

For many years it has been recognized that *propranolol* has a beneficial effect on parkinsonian tremors. Koller and Herbster (134) found that long-acting propranolol at doses ranging between 60 and 160 mg produced a 70% reduction in resting tremor and a 50% reduction in postural tremor. In that same study, primidone and clonazepam had no effect. *Gabapentin* 400 mg tid vs. placebo was studied in a double-blind cross-over manner and was ineffective in the treatment of resting tremor (135). *Mirtazapine* is an alpha-2 central antagonist that is used as an antidepressant. When mirtazapine was prescribed for sleep or depression, it was noted that tremor decreased (136). This was followed by a small one month, open-label, prospective trial in PD. According to UPDRS tremor scores there was an average improvement of 7% (137).

B. Surgical Therapy

Thalamotomy has been used in the management of parkinsonian tremor for over 40 years. The usual target is the VIM nucleus and a good effect on contralateral resting tremor is reported in 75–85% of patients (138). This benefit is also sustained for many years following thalamotomy (139). Bilateral thalamotomy results in a much greater incidence of adverse events particularly profound dysarthria.

With Laitinen's reintroduction of Leksell's ventroposterolateral (VPL) pallidotomy (140) and with the basal ganglia model emphasizing overactivity of the GPi, pallidotomy was resurrected. Lozano et al. reported 40 patients with advanced PD who underwent pallidotomy for off period immobility and disabling dyskinesias with immediate improvement in off periods and contralateral tremors (69). One year after surgery, improvement in the mean total tremor score was 52% with a 67% improvement in contralateral tremor (69). Variable results have been reported in other studies with the most notable and consistent improvements in contralateral drug induced-dyskinesias (70,73,141,142). In contrast, Vitek and his colleagues (143) have reported that the maximum effect of pallidotomy on tremor may be delayed as long as one year after the procedure. However, pallidotomy is not without risk. Neighboring structures such as the optic tract and internal capsule may be injured and so surgical complications can include visual field cuts and hemiparesis. Furthermore, as with thalamotomy, bilateral pallidotomy carries a much greater risk of speech disturbances and cognitive dysfunction than a unilateral procedure (144–146).

Deep brain stimulation has been a major advance in the management of advanced PD and the complications of its treatment. The major advantages of DBS are that no permanent lesion is established, the results are titratable via adjusting stimulus parameters, and it does not preclude further neurosurgical procedures. The exact mechanism is not yet understood. One theory is that it causes desynchronization of neuronal activity that occurs in PD (147).

Although thalamic DBS is quite effective in treating parkinsonian tremor (48,148–150), like thalamotomy, it has little effect on other often more disabling parkinsonian symptoms, and so it is now rarely used as a primary surgical target in PD patients. Selected patients with disabling tremor with little or no evidence of bradykinesia might still be considered appropriate candidates for thalamic surgery.

The two most common DBS targets in PD are the GPi and STN. GPi stimulation, is most effective at controlling contralateral dyskinesia although it also ameliorates tremor, rigidity, and bradykinesia (51,52,151,152). Pallidal stimulation can have striking beneficial effects but these seem to be more variable than with STN stimulation (possibly due to the larger size of the GPi) and some patients responding initially may lose their original benefit over the subsequent 1–3 years (152–154). Although it is purported to have fewer side effects than pallidotomy, cognitive decline can occur as well (155).

Benabid and colleagues attempted STN DBS in hopes of improving the disabling features that were not ameliorated by thalamic DBS. All primary features of off-period parkinsonism, especially tremor, as well as the motor complications of levodopa including dyskinesia and motor fluctuations are improved with STN DBS (50,78,79). Kleiner-Fisman et al. (80) reported two year follow-up of 25 patients who had received bilateral STN DBS. Marked improvements in tremor scores were noted at both one and two year follow-up. Patients with a higher initial tremor score had particularly marked improvements in their motor function following surgery. This is presumably due to the strong benefit to tremor. Krack et al. (156) published their long term experience with STN DBS with five year follow-up data available for 42 patients. DBS markedly improved tremor at the one, three, and five year follow-up and the benefit at one year and five years was similar.

VII. CONCLUSION

There are many unanswered questions related to the etiology and pathophysiology of the classic parkinsonian resting tremor, including the site or sites of the primary tremor generator and the role of non-dopaminergic systems in tremor production. Many medical therapies are available, but none is entirely successful in ameliorating tremor in all patients. Surgical therapies, yield excellent results but these are best reserved for those who fail medical therapy. It is hoped that newer therapies will provide both greater efficacy than those available currently and a better understanding of the pathogenesis of the disorder.

REFERENCES

1. Parkinson J. The shaking palsy. London, Sherwood, Neely and Jones, 2003:1817.
2. Hughes AJ, Daniel SE, Blankson S, Lees AJ. A clinicopathologic study of 100 cases of Parkinson's disease. Arch Neurol 1993; 50:140–148.
3. Jankovic J, McDermott M, Carter J, Gauthier S, Goetz C. Variable expression of Parkinson's disease: a base-line analysis of the DATATOP cohort. Neurology 1990; 40:1529–1534.
4. Rajput AH, Pahwa R, Pahwa P, Rajput A. Prognostic significance of the onset mode in parkinsonism. Neurology 1993; 43(4):829–830.
5. Marras C, Rochon P, Lang AE. Predicting motor decline and disability in Parkinson disease—A systematic review. Arch Neurol 2002; 59(11):1724–1728.
6. Koller WC, Vetere-Overfield B, Barter R. Tremors in early Parkinson's disease. Clin Neuropharmacol 1989; 12(4):293–297.

7. Deuschl G, Bain P, Brin M, Ad Hoc Scientific Committee. Consensus statement of the Movement Disorder Society on tremor. Mov Disord 1998; 13:2–23.
8. Toth C, Rajput M, Rajput AH. Anomalies of asymmetry of clinical signs in parkinsonism. Mov Disord 2004; 19(2):151–157.
9. Jankovic J, Schwartz KS, Ondo W. Re-emergent tremor of Parkinson's disease. J Neurol Neurosurg Psychiatry 1999; 67(5):646–650.
10. Findley LJ, Gresty MA, Halmagyi GM. Tremor, the cogwheel phenomenon and clonus in Parkinson's disease. J Neurol Neurosurg Psychiatry 1981; 44:534–546.
11. Brooks DJ, Playford ED, Ibanez V, Sawle GV, Thompson PD, Findley LJ et al. Isolated tremor and disruption of the nigrostriatal dopaminergic system: an ^{18}F-dopa PET study. Neurology 1992; 42(8):1554–1560.
12. Rajput AH, Rozdilsky B, Ang L, Rajput A. Significance of parkinsonian manifestations in essential tremor. Can J Neurol Sci 1993; 20:114–117.
13. Cleeves L, Findley LJ, Koller W. Lack of association between essential tremor and Parkinson's disease. Ann Neurol 1988; 24(1):23–26.
14. Louis ED, Levy G, Mejia-Santana H, Cote L, Andrews H, Harris J et al. Risk of action tremor in relatives of tremor-dominant and postural instability gait disorder PD. Neurology 2003; 61(7):931–936.
15. Timmer J, Lauk M, Deuschl G. Quantitative analysis of tremor time series. Electroencephalogr Clin Neurophysiol 1996; 101(5):461–468.
16. Hefter H, Homberg V, Reiners K, Freund HJ. Stability of frequency during long-term recordings of hand tremor. Electroencephalogr Clin Neurophysiol 1987; 67(5):439–446.
17. Spieker S, Boose A, Jentgens C, Dichgans J. Long-term tremor recordings in parkinsonian and essential tremor. J Neural Transm Suppl 1995; 46:339–349.
18. Boose A, Spieker S, Jentgens C, Dichgans J. Wrist tremor: investigation of agonist–antagonist interaction by means of long-term EMG recording and cross-spectral analysis. Electroencephalogr Clin Neurophysiol 1996; 101(4):355–363.
19. Otsuka M, Ichiya Y, Kuwabara Y, Hosokawa S, Sasaki M, Yoshida T et al. Differences in the reduced ^{18}F-Dopa uptakes of the caudate and the putamen in Parkinson's disease: Correlations with the three main symptoms. J Neurol Sci 1996; 136(1–2):169–173.
20. Vingerhoets FJG, Schulzer M, Caine DB, Snow BJ. Which clinical sign of Parkinson's disease best reflects the nigrostriatal lesion? Ann Neurol 1997; 41(1):58–64.
21. Eidelberg D, Moeller JR, Ishikawa T, Dhawan V, Spetsieris P, Chaly T et al. Assessment of disease severity in parkinsonism with fluorine-18-fluorodeoxyglucose and PET. J Nucl Med 1995; 36(3):378–383.
22. Antonini A, Moeller JR, Nakamura T, Spetsieris P, Dhawan V, Eidelberg D. The metabolic anatomy of tremor in Parkinson's disease. Neurology 1998; 51(3):803–810.
23. Louis ED, Tang MX, Cote L, Alfaro B, Mejia H, Marder K. Progression of parkinsonian signs in Parkinson disease. Arch Neurol 1999; 56(3):334–337.
24. Lozza C, Marie RM, Baron JC. The metabolic substrates of bradykinesia and tremor in uncomplicated Parkinson's disease. Neuroimage 2002; 17(2):688–699.
25. Fearnley JM, Lees AJ. Ageing and Parkinson's disease: substantia nigra regional selectivity. Brain 1991; 114:2283–2301.

26. Damier P, Hirsch EC, Agid Y, Graybiel AM. The substantia nigra of the human brain. II. Patterns of loss of dopamine-containing neurons in Parkinson's disease. Brain 1999; 122(Pt 8):1437–1448.

27. Paulus W, Jellinger K. The neuropathologic basis of different clinical subgroups of Parkinson's disease. J Neuropathol Exp Neurol 1991; 50(6):743–755.

28. Jellinger KA. Post mortem studies in Parkinson's disease—is it possible to detect brain areas for specific symptoms? J Neural Trans 1999; 1–29.

29. Magistretti PJ, Pellerin L, Rothman DL, Shulman RG. Energy on demand. Science 1999; 283(5401):496–497.

30. Martin WR, Beckman JH, Calne DB, Adam MJ, Harrop R, Rogers JG et al. Cerebral glucose metabolism in Parkinson's disease. Can J Neurol Sci 1984; 11(suppl 1):169–173.

31. Rougemont D, Baron JC, Collard P, Bustany P, Comar D, Agid Y. Local cerebral glucose utilisation in treated and untreated patients with Parkinson's disease. J Neurol Neurosurg Psychiatry 1984; 47(8):824–830.

32. Baron JC. Consequences des lesions des noyaux gris centraux sur lactivite metabolique cerebrale: Implications cliniques. Rev Neurol 1994; 150:599–604.

33. Eidelberg D, Moeller JR, Dhawan V, Sidtis JJ, Ginos JZ, Strother SC et al. The metabolic anatomy of Parkinson's disease: complementary [18F]fluorodeoxyglucose and [18F]fluorodopa positron emission tomographic studies. Mov Disord 1990; 5(3):203–213.

34. Doder M, Rabiner EA, Turjanski N, Lees AJ, Brooks DJ. Tremor in Parkinson's disease and serotonergic dysfunction—An ^{11}C-WAY 100635 PET study. Neurology 2003; 60(4):601–605.

35. Deuschl G, Krack P, Lauk M, Timmer J. Clinical neurophysiology of tremor. J Clin Neurophysiol 1996; 13(2):110–121.

36. Homberg V, Hefter H, Reiners K, Freund HJ. Differential effects of changes in mechanical limb properties on physiological and pathological tremor. J Neurol Neurosurg Psychiatry 1987; 50(5):568–579.

37. Rack PM, Ross HF. The role of reflexes in the resting tremor of Parkinson's disease. Brain 1986; 109(Pt 1):115–141.

38. Hufschmidt HJ. Proprioceptive origin of parkinsonian tremor. Nature 1963; 200:367–368.

39. Lee RG, Stein RB. Resetting of tremor by mechanical perturbations: a comparison of essential tremor and parkinsonian tremor. Ann Neurol 1981; 10(6):523–531.

40. Britton TC, Thompson PD, Day BL, Rothwell JC, Findley LJ, Marsden CD. Modulation of postural tremors at the wrist by supramaximal electrical median nerve shocks in essential tremor, Parkinson's disease and normal subjects mimicking tremor. J Neurol Neurosurg Psychiatry 1993; 56(10):1085–1089.

41. Britton TC, Thompson PD, Day BL, Rothwell JC, Findley LJ, Marsden CD. Modulation of postural wrist tremors by magnetic stimulation of the motor cortex in patients with Parkinson's disease or essential tremor and in normal subjects mimicking tremor. Ann Neurol 1993; 33:473–479.

42. Pascual-Leone A, Valls-Sole J, Toro C, Wassermann EM, Hallett M. Resetting of essential tremor and postural tremor in Parkinson's disease with transcranial magnetic stimulation. Muscle Nerve 1994; 17(7):800–807.

43. Pollock LJDL. Muscle tone in parkinsonian states. Arch Neurol Psychiatry 1930; 23:303–319.

44. Walsh EG. Muscles, masses and motion. The physiology of normality, hypotonicity, spasticity and rigidity. New York: Mac Keith Press, 1992.
45. Das K, Benzil DL, Rovit RL, Murali R, Couldwell WT. Irving S. Cooper (1922–1985): a pioneer in functional neurosurgery. J Neurosurg 1998; 89(5):865–873.
46. Cooper IS. Neurosurgical alleviation of intention tremor of multiple sclerosis and cerebellar disease. N Engl J Med 1960; 263:441–444.
47. Hassler R, Riechert T, Mundinger F, Umbach W, Ganglberger JA. Physiological observations in stereotaxic operations in extrapyramidal motor disturbances. Brain 1960; 83:337–350.
48. Benabid AL, Pollack P, Gervason C, Hoffman D, Gao DM, Hommel M et al. Long-term suppression of tremor by chronic stimulation of the ventral intermediate thalamic nucleus. Lancet 1991; 337:403–406.
49. Krack P, Pollak P, Limousin P, Benazzouz A, Benabid AL. Stimulation of sub-thalamic nucleus alleviates tremor in Parkinson's disease. Lancet 1997; 350(9092):1675.
50. Kumar R, Lozano AM, Kim YJ, Hutchison WD, Sime E, Halket E et al. Double-blind evaluation of subthalamic nucleus deep brain stimulation in advanced Parkinson's disease. Neurology 1998; 51(3):850–855.
51. Volkmann J, Sturm V, Weiss P, Kappler J, Voges J, Koulousakis A et al. Bilateral high-frequency stimulation of the internal globus pallidus in advanced Parkinson's disease. Ann Neurol 1998; 44:953–961.
52. Pahwa R, Wilkinson S, Smith D, Lyons K, Miyawaki E, Koller WC. High-frequency stimulation of the globus pallidus for the treatment of Parkinson's disease. Neurology 1997; 49(1):249–253.
53. Duffau H, Tzourio N, Caparros-Lefebvre D, Parker F, Mazoyer B. Tremor and voluntary repetitive movement in Parkinson's disease: comparison before and after L-dopa with positron emission tomography. Exp Brain Res 1996; 107(3):453–462.
54. Inase M, Tanji J. Thalamic distribution of projection neurons to the primary motor cortex relative to afferent terminal fields from the globus pallidus in the macaque monkey. J Comp Neurol 1995; 353(3):415–426.
55. Parker F, Tzourio N, Blond S, Petit H, Mazoyer B. Evidence for a common network of brain structures involved in parkinsonian tremor and voluntary repetitive movement. Brain Res 1992; 584(1–2):11–17.
56. Deiber M-P, Pollak P, Passingham R, Landais P, Gervason C, Cinotti L et al. Thalamic stimulation and suppression of parkinsonian tremor. Evidence of a cerebel-lar deactivation using positron emission tomography. Brain 1993; 116:267–279.
57. Deuschl G, Wilms H, Krack P, Würker M, Heiss WD. Function of the cerebellum in Parkinsonian rest tremor and Holmes' tremor. Ann Neurol 1999; 46(1):126–128.
58. Llinas R, Yarom Y. Electrophysiology of mammalian inferior olivary neurones in vitro. Different types of voltage-dependent ionic conductances. J Physiol 1981; 315:549–567.
59. Jahnsen H, Llinas R. Electrophysiological properties of guinea-pig thalamic neurones: an *in vitro* study. J Physiol 1984; 349:205–226.
60. Pare D, Curro'Dossi R, Steriade M. Neuronal basis of the parkinsonian resting tremor: a hypothesis and its implications for treatment. Neuroscience 1990; 35(2):217–226.

61. Hutchison WD, Lozano AM, Tasker RR, Lang AE, Dostrovsky JO. Identification and characterization of neurons with tremor-frequency activity in human globus pallidus. Exp Brain Res 1997; 113(3):557–563.

62. Lemstra AW, Verhagen ML, Lee JI, Dougherty PM, Lenz FA. Tremor-frequency (3–6 Hz) activity in the sensorimotor arm representation of the internal segment of the globus pallidus in patients with Parkinson's disease. Neurosci Lett 1999; 267(2):129–132.

63. Hutchison WD, Benko R, Dostrovsky JO, Lang AE, Lozano AM. Coherent relation of rest tremor and pallidal tremor cells in Parkinson's disease patients. Mov Disord 1998; 13(suppl 2):3218.

64. Bergman H, Wichmann T, Karmon B, DeLong MR. The primate subthalamic nucleus. II. Neuronal activity in the MPTP model of parkinsonism. J Neurophysiol 1994; 72:507–520.

65. Raz A, Vaadia E, Bergman H. Firing patterns and correlations of spontaneous discharge of pallidal neurons in the normal and the tremulous 1-methyl-4-phenyl-1,2,3,6-tetrahydropyridine vervet model of parkinsonism. J Neurosci 2000; 20(22):8559–8571.

66. Lenz FA, Tasker RR, Kwan HC, Schnider S, Kwong R, Murayama Y et al. Single unit analysis of the human ventral thalamic nuclear group: correlation of thalamic "tremor cells" with the 3–6 Hz component of parkinsonian tremor. J Neurosci 1988; 8(3):754–764.

67. Steriade M, Deschenes M. The thalamus as a neuronal oscillator. Brain Res 1984; 320(1):1–63.

68. Zirh TA, Lenz FA, Reich SG, Dougherty PM. Patterns of bursting occurring in thalamic cells during parkinsonian tremor. Neuroscience 1998; 83(1):107–121.

69. Lozano AM, Lang AE, Hutchison WD. Pallidotomy for tremor. Mov Disord 1998; 13:107–110.

70. Samuel M, Caputo E, Brooks DJ, Schrag A, Scaravilli T, Branston NM et al. A study of medial pallidotomy for Parkinson's disease: clinical outcome, MRI location and complications. Brain 1998; 121(1):59–75.

71. Hutchison WD, Allan RJ, Opitz H, Levy R, Dostrovsky JO, Lang AE et al. Neurophysiological identification of the subthalamic nucleus in surgery for Parkinson's disease. Ann Neurol 1998; 44(4):622–628.

72. Lozano AM, Hutchison WD, Tasker RR, Lang AE, Junn F, Dostrovsky JO. Microelectrode recordings define the ventral posteromedial pallidotomy target. Stereotact Funct Neurosurg 1998; 71(4):153–163.

73. Taha JM, Favre J, Baumann TK, Burchiel KJ. Tremor control after pallidotomy in patients with Parkinson's disease: Correlation with microrecording findings. J Neurosurg 1997; 86(4):642–647.

74. Filion M, Tremblay L. Abnormal spontaneous activity of globus pallidus neurons in monkeys with MPTP-induced parkinsonism. Brain Res 1991; 547:142–151.

75. Hutchison WD, Levy R, Dostrovsky JO, Lozano AM, Lang AE. Effects of apomorphine on globus pallidus neurons in parkinsonian patients. Ann Neurol 1997; 42(5):767–775.

76. Lozano AM, Lang AE, Levy R, Hutchison W, Dostrovsky J. Neuronal recordings in Parkinson's disease patients with dyskinesias induced by apomorphine. Ann Neurol 2000; 47(4):S141–S146.

77. Merello M, Lees AJ, Balej J, Cammarota A, Leiguarda R. GPi firing rate modification during beginning-of-dose motor deterioration following acute administration of apomorphine. Mov Disord 1999; 14(3):481–483.
78. Limousin P, Krack P, Pollak P, Benazzouz A, Ardouin C, Hoffmann D et al. Electrical stimulation of the subthalamic nucleus in advanced Parkinson's disease. N Engl J Med 1998; 339(16):1105–1111.
79. Moro E, Scerrati M, Romito LM, Roselli R, Tonali P, Albanese A. Chronic subthalamic nucleus stimulation reduces medication requirements in Parkinson's disease. Neurology 1999; 53(1):85–90.
80. Kleiner-Fisman G, Fisman DN, Sime E, Saint-Cyr JA, Lozano AM, Lang AE. Long-term follow up of bilateral deep brain stimulation of the subthalamic nucleus in patients with advanced Parkinson disease. J Neurosurg 2003; 99(3):489–495.
81. Rodriguez MC, Guridi OJ, Alvarez L, Mewes K, Macias R, Vitek J et al. The subthalamic nucleus and tremor in Parkinson's disease. Mov Disord 1998; 13:111–118.
82. Levy R, Hutchison WD, Lozano AM, Dostrovsky JO. High-frequency synchronization of neuronal activity in the subthalamic nucleus of parkinsonian patients with limb tremor. J Neurosci 2000; 20(20):7766–7775.
83. Levy R, Ashby P, Hutchison WD, Lang AE, Lozano AM, Dostrovsky JO. Dependence of subthalamic nucleus oscillations on movement and dopamine in Parkinson's disease. Brain 2002; 125(6):1196–1209.
84. Wichmann T, Bergman H, DeLong MR. The primate subthalamic nucleus. III. Changes in motor behavior and neuronal activity in the internal pallidum induced by subthalamic inactivation in the MPTP model of parkinsonism. J Neurophysiol 1994; 72:521–530.
85. Patel NK, Heywood P, O'Sullivan K, McCarter R, Love S, Gill SS. Unilateral subthalamotomy in the treatment of Parkinson's disease. Brain 2003; 126(5):1136–1145.
86. Su PC, Tseng HM, Liu HM, Yen RF, Liou HH. Treatment of advanced Parkinson's disease by subthalamotomy: one-year results. Mov Disord 2003; 18(5):531–538.
87. Plenz D, Kital ST. A basal ganglia pacemaker formed by the subthalamic nucleus and external globus pallidus. Nature 1999; 400(6745):677–682.
88. Middleton FA, Strick PL. Basal ganglia and cerebellar loops: motor and cognitive circuits. Brain Res Rev 2000; 31(2–3):236–250.
89. Strick PL. How do the basal ganglia and cerebellum gain access to the cortical motor areas? Behav Brain Res 1985; 18(2):107–123.
90. Timmermann L, Gross J, Dirks M, Volkmann J, Freund HJ, Schnitzler A. The cerebral oscillatory network of parkinsonian resting tremor. Brain 2003; 126(1):199–212.
91. Raethjen J, Lindemann M, Schmaljohann H, Wenzelburger R, Pfister G, Deuschl G. Multiple oscillators are causing parkinsonian and essential tremor. Mov Disord 2000; 15(1):84–94.
92. Benabid AL, Benazzouz A, Hoffmann D, Limousin P, Krack P, Pollak P. Long-term electrical inhibition of deep brain targets in movement disorders. Mov Disord 1998; 13:119–125.
93. Halliday GM, Blumbergs PC, Cotton RG, Blessing WW, Geffen LB. Loss of brainstem serotonin- and substance P-containing neurons in Parkinson's disease. Brain Res 1990; 510(1):104–107.

94. Braak H, Braak E, Yilmazer D, Schultz C, De Vos RAI, Jansen ENH. Nigral and extranigral pathology in Parkinson's disease. J Neural Transm Park Dis Dement Sect 1995; 46:15–31.
95. Braak H, Del Tredici K, Rüb U, De Vos RAI, Steur ENHJ, Braak E. Staging of brain pathology related to sporadic Parkinson's disease. Neurobiol Aging 2003; 24(2):197–211.
96. Wilms H, Sievers J, Deuschl G. Animal models of tremor. Mov Disord 1999; 14(4):557–571.
97. Ohye C, Shibazaki T, Hirai T, Wada H, Kawashima Y, Hirato M et al. A special role of the parvocellular red nucleus in lesion-induced spontaneous tremor in monkeys. Behav Brain Res 1988; 28(1–2):241–243.
98. Nini A, Feingold A, Slovin H, Bergman H. Neurons in the globus pallidus do not show correlated activity in the normal monkey, but phase-locked oscillations appear in the MPTP model of parkinsonism. J Neurophysiol 1995; 74:1800–1805.
99. Bergman H, Raz A, Feingold A, Nini A, Nelken I, Hansel D et al. Physiology of MPTP tremor. Mov Disord 1998; 13:29–34.
100. Perez-Otano I, Oset C, Luquin MR, Herrero MT, Obeso JA, Del Rio J. MPTP-induced parkinsonism in primates: pattern of striatal dopamine loss following acute and chronic administration. Neurosci Lett 1994; 175(1–2):121–125.
101. Pifl C, Schingnitz G, Hornykiewicz O. The neurotoxin MPTP does not reproduce in the rhesus monkey the interregional pattern of striatal dopamine loss typical of human idiopathic Parkinson's disease. Neurosci Lett 1988; 92(2):228–233.
102. Elsworth JD, Deutch AY, Redmond DE Jr, Taylor JR, Sladek JR Jr, Roth RH. Symptomatic and asymptomatic 1-methyl-4-phenyl-1,2,3,6-tetrahydropyridine-treated primates: biochemical changes in striatal regions. Neuroscience 1989; 33(2):323–331.
103. Parent A, Lavoie B. The heterogeneity of the mesostriatal dopaminergic system as revealed in normal and parkinsonian monkeys. Adv Neurol 1993; 60:25–33.
104. Hantraye P, Varastet M, Peschanski M, Riche D, Cesaro P, Willer JC, Maziere M. Stable parkinsonian syndrome and uneven loss of striatal dopamine fibres following chronic MPTP administration in baboons. Neuroscience 1993; 53:169–178.
105. Schneider JS, Yuwiler A, Markham CH. Selective loss of subpopulations of ventral mesencephalic dopaminergic neurons in the monkey following exposure to MPTP. Brain Res 1987; 411(1):144–150.
106. Ballard PA, Tetrud JW, Langston JW. Permanent human parkinsonism due to 1-methyl-4-phenyl-1,2,3,6-tetrahydropyridine (MPTP): seven cases. Neurology 1985; 35(7):949–956.
107. Tetrud JW, Langston JW. MPTP-induced parkinsonism as a model for Parkinson's disease. Acta Neurol Scand Suppl 1989; 126:35–40.
108. Tetrud JA, Langston JW. MPTP-Induced Parkinsonism and Tremor. In: Findley LJ, Koller W, eds. Handbook of Tremor. [22], 319–332. 1995. New York: Marcel Dekker, Inc. Neurological Disease and Therapy. Koller W.
109. Boraud T, Bezard E, Bioulac B, Gross CE. Ratio of inhibited-to-activated pallidal neurons decreases dramatically during passive limb movement in the MPTP-treated monkey. J Neurophys 2000; 83(3):1760–1763.
110. Ordenstein L. Sur la paralysie et la sclerose en plague generalise. Paris: Martinet, 1867.

111. Duvoisin RC. Cholinergic–anticholinergic antagonism in parkinsonism. Arch Neurol 1967; 17(2):124–136.

112. Cholinesterases and anticholinesterase agents. New York, Springer, Berlin Heidelberg, 1963.

113. Parkes JD, Baxter RC, Marsden CD, Rees JE. Comparative trial of benzhexol, amantadine, and levodopa in the treatment of Parkinson's disease. J Neurol Neurosurg Psychiatry 1974; 37(4):422–426.

114. Strang RR. Kemadrin in the treatment of parkinsonism: a double blind and one-year follow-up study. Curr Med Drugs 1965; 28:27–32.

115. Burke RE. The relative selectivity of anticholinergic drugs for the M1 and M2 muscarinic receptor subtypes. Mov Disord 1986; 1(2):135–144.

116. Farnebo LO, Fuxe K, Hamberger B, Ljungdahl H. Effect of some antiparkinsonian drugs on catecholamine neurons. J Pharm Pharmacol 1970; 22(10):733–737.

117. Obeso JA, Matsumura M. Anticholinergics and amantadine. In: Koller W, ed. Handbook of Parkinson's Disease. New York: Marcel-Dekker, 1987:309–316.

118. Koller WC. Pharmacologic treatment of parkinsonian tremor. Arch Neurol 1986; 43(2):126–127.

119. Friedman JH, Koller WC, Lannon MC, Busenbark K, Swanson-Hyland E, Smith D. Benztropine versus clozapine for the treatment of tremor in Parkinson's disease. Neurology 1997; 48(4):1077–1081.

120. Fermaglich J, O'Doherty DS. Effect of gastric motility on levodopa. Dis Nerv Syst 1972; 33(9):624–625.

121. Yahr MD, Clough CG, Bergmann KJ. Cholinergic and dopaminergic mechanisms in Parkinson's disease after long term levodopa administration. Lancet 1982; 2(8300):709–710.

122. Fahn S, David E. Orofacio-lingual dyskinesia due to anticholinergic medication. Trans Am Neurol Assoc 2003; 97:277–279.

123. Birket-Smith E. Abnormal involuntary movements in relation to anticholinergics and levodopa therapy. Acta Neurol Scand 1975; 52(2):158–160.

124. Sivertsen B, Dupont E, Mikkelsen B, Mogensen P, Rasmussen C, Boesen F et al. Selegiline and levodopa in early or moderately advanced Parkinson's disease: a double-blind controlled short- and long-term study. Acta Neurol Scand Suppl 1989; 126:147–152.

125. Elble RJ. Tremor and dopamine agonists. Neurology 2002; 58(4):S57–S62.

126. Navan P, Findley LJ, Jeffs JAR, Pearce RKB, Bain PG. Double-blind, single-dose, cross-over study of the effects of pramipexole, pergolide, and placebo on rest tremor and UPDRS part III in Parkinson's disease. Mov Disord 2003; 18(2):176–180.

127. Korczyn AD, Brooks DJ, Brunt ER, Poewe WH, Rascol O, Stocchi F. Ropinirole versus bromocriptine in the treatment of early Parkinson's disease: a 6-month interim report of a 3-year study. Mov Disord 1998; 13(1):46–51.

128. Kunig G, Pogarell O, Moller JC, Delf M, Oertel WH. Pramipexole, a nonergot dopamine agonist, is effective against rest tremor in intermediate to advanced Parkinson's disease. Clin Neuropharmacol 1999; 22(5):301–305.

129. Moller JC, Oertel WH. Pramipexole in the treatment of advanced Parkinson's disease. Eur J Neurol 2000; 7(suppl 1):21–25.

130. Jansen EN. Clozapine in the treatment of tremor in Parkinson's disease. Acta Neurol Scand 1994; 89(4):262–265.

131. Friedman JH, Lannon MC. Clozapine-responsive tremor in Parkinson's disease. Mov Disord 1990; 5(3):225–229.
132. Pakkenberg H, Pakkenberg B. Clozapine in the treatment of tremor. Acta Neurol Scand 1986; 73(3):295–297.
133. Bonuccelli U, Ceravolo R, Salvetti S, D'Avino C, Del Dotto P, Rossi G et al. Clozapine in Parkinson's disease tremor—Effects of acute and chronic administration. Neurology 1997; 49(6):1587–1590.
134. Koller WC, Herbster G. Adjuvant therapy of parkinsonian tremor. Arch Neurol 1987; 44(9):921–923.
135. Olson WL, Gruenthal M, Mueller ME, Olson WH. Gabapentin for Parkinsonism: a double-blind, placebo-controlled, crossover trial. Am J Med 1997; 102(1):60–66.
136. Pact V, Giduz T. Mirtazapine treats resting tremor, essential tremor, and levodopa-induced dyskinesias. Neurology 1999; 53(5):1154.
137. Gordon PH, Pullman SL, Louis ED, Frucht SJ, Fahn S. Mirtazapine in Parkinsonian tremor. Parkinsonism Relat Disord 2002; 9(2):125–126.
138. Jankovic J, Cardoso F, Grossman RG, Hamilton WJ. Outcome after stereotactic thalamotomy for Parkinsonian, essential, and other types of tremor. Neurosurgery 1995; 37:680–686.
139. Diederich N, Goetz CG, Stebbins GT, Klawans HL, Nittner K, Koulosakis A et al. Blinded evaluation confirms long-term asymmetric effect of unilateral thalamotomy or subthalamotomy on tremor in Parkinson's disease. Neurology 1992; 42(7):1311–1314.
140. Laitinen LV, Bergenheim AT, Hariz MI. Leksell's posteroventral pallidotomy in the treatment of Parkinson's disease. J Neurosurg 1992; 76(1):53–61.
141. Fine J, Duff J, Chen R, Chir B, Hutchison W, Lozano AM et al. Long-term follow-up of unilateral pallidotomy in advanced Parkinson's disease. N Engl J Med 2000; 342(23):1708–1714.
142. De Brie RMA, De Haan RJ, Nijssen PCG, Rutgers AWF, Beute GN, Bosch DA et al. Unilateral pallidotomy in Parkinson's disease: a randomized, single-blind, multicentre trail. Lancet 1999; 354:1665–1669.
143. Baron MS, Vitek JL, Bakay RA, Green J, Kaneoke Y, Hashimoto T et al. Treatment of advanced Parkinson's disease by posterior GPi pallidotomy: 1-year results of a pilot study. Ann Neurol 1996; 40(3):355–366.
144. Trepanier LL, Saint-Cyr JA, Lozano AM, Lang AE. Neuropsychological consequences of posteroventral pallidotomy for the treatment of Parkinson's disease. Neurology 1998; 51(1):207–215.
145. Scott R, Gregory R, Hines N, Carroll C, Hyman N, Papanasstasiou V et al. Neuropsychological, neurological and functional outcome following pallidotomy for Parkinson's disease—A consecutive series of eight simultaneous bilateral and twelve unilateral procedures. Brain 1998; 121(4):659–675.
146. Obeso JA, Guridi J, Rodriguez-Oroz MC, Agid Y, Bejjani P, Bonnet AM et al. Deep-brain stimulation of the subthalamic nucleus or the pars interna of the globus pallidus in Parkinson's disease. N Engl J Med 2001; 345(13):956–963.
147. Lozano AM, Dostrovsky J, Chen R, Ashby P. Deep brain stimulation for Parkinson's disease: disrupting the disruption. Lancet Neurol 2002; 1(4):225–231.
148. Koller W, Pahwa R, Busenbark K, Hubble J, Wilkinson S, Lang A et al. High-frequency unilateral thalamic stimulation in the treatment of essential and parkinsonian tremor. Ann Neurol 1997; 42(3):292–299.

149. Limousin P, Speelman JD, Gielen F, Janssens M. Multicentre European study of thalamic stimulation in parkinsonian and essential tremor. J Neurol Neurosurg Psychiatry 1999; 66(3):289–296.

150. Hariz GM, Bergenheim AT, Hariz MI, Lindberg M. Assessment of ability/disability in patients treated with chronic thalamic stimulation for tremor. Mov Disord 1998; 13(1):78–83.

151. Krack P, Pollak P, Limousin P, Hoffmann D, Xie J, Benazzouz A et al. Subthalamic nucleus or internal pallidal stimulation in young onset Parkinson's disease. Brain 1998; 121(3):451–457.

152. Ghika J, Villemure JG, Fankhauser H, Favre J, Assal G, Ghika-Schmid F. Efficiency and safety of bilateral contemporaneous pallidal stimulation (deep brain stimulation) in levodopa-responsive patients with Parkinson's disease with severe motor fluctuations: a 2-year follow-up review. J Neurosurg 1998; 89(5):713–718.

153. Visser-Vandewalle V, van der LC, Temel Y, Nieman F, Celik H, Beuls E. Long-term motor effect of unilateral pallidal stimulation in 26 patients with advanced Parkinson disease. J Neurosurg 2003; 99(4):701–707.

154. Durif F, Lemaire JJ, Debilly B, Dordain G. Long-term follow-up of globus pallidus chronic stimulation in advanced Parkinson's disease. Mov Disord 2002; 17(4):803–807.

155. Vingerhoets G, Van Der Linden C, Lannoo E, Vandewalle V, Caemaert J, Wolters M et al. Cognitive outcome after unilateral pallidal stimulation in Parkinson's disease. J Neurol Neurosurg Psychiatry 1999; 66(3):297–304.

156. Krack P, Batir A, Van Blercom N, Chabardes S, Fraix V, Ardouin C et al. Five-year follow-up of bilateral stimulation of the subthalamic nucleus in advanced Parkinson's disease. NEJM 2003; 349(20):1925–1934.

157. Deuschl G, Lauk M, Timmer J. Tremor classification and tremor time series analysis. Chaos 1995; 5(1):48–51.

158. Hellwig B, Häussler S, Lauk M, Guschlbauer B, Köster B, Kristeva-Feige R et al. Tremor-correlated cortical activity detected by electroencephalography. Clin Neurophysiol 2000; 111(5):806–809.

159. Volkmann J, Joliot M, Mogilner A, Ioannides AA, Lado F, Fazzini E et al. Central motor loop oscillations in parkinsonian resting tremor revealed by magnetoencephalography. Neurology 1996; 46(5):1359–1370.

14

Dystonic Tremor

Joseph Jankovic and Nicte I. Mejia

Baylor College of Medicine, Houston, Texas, USA

I. INTRODUCTION

Dystonia is a neurological syndrome characterized by involuntary, sustained, patterned and often repetitive muscle contractions of opposing muscles, causing twisting movements, abnormal postures, or both (1). While in some patients with dystonia the abnormal posture may be sustained, in others the dystonic movement is repetitive, thus resembling tremor. The term dystonic tremor was introduced during the 1980s, when movement disorder specialists recognized that tremor was a common finding in patients with dystonia (2). Although this movement disorder has had numerous proposed definitions (2–5) and its pathophysiological basis is still not fully understood, an effort has been made to separate this condition from other tremor syndromes and classify it as a distinct type of tremor (6).

II. DEFINITION AND CLINICAL CHARACTERISTICS OF DYSTONIC TREMOR

The Scientific Committee of the Movement Disorder Society on the Consensus Statement on Tremor defined dystonic tremor based on clinical criteria as an action, either postural or kinetic, tremor occurring in a body part or extremity, which is affected by dystonia (6). This definition highlights the importance of underlying dystonia in this form of tremor. Dystonic tremor may occur in the setting of any primary or secondary dystonia, consequently the epidemiology of dystonic tremor is the epidemiology of dystonia, neither of which has been extensively studied. In one study of a North England population the prevalence of generalized dystonia was estimated to be 1.42 per 100,000 and 12.9 per 100,000 for focal dystonia (7). Much higher prevalence of primary dystonia, 732 per 100,000 was reported in a population over age 50 years studied at Bruneck, South Tyrol, in northern Italy (8).

Dystonic tremor is an action tremor occurring in a body part or extremity which is affected by dystonia. This type of tremor is usually localized, presenting with irregular amplitude and variable frequency (3–7 Hz, with a peak at 5 Hz) (2). Dystonic tremor, an actual component of the dystonia, is most obvious when the patient voluntarily attempts to move in the direction opposite to the force of the dystonia. Thus, if the patient has torticollis to the right but attempts to maintain a primary position, then lateral oscillation of the head (dystonic tremor) might be seen as the patient attempts to look straight ahead. However, when the patient stops resisting the dystonic pulling of the neck, the dystonic tremor ceases (this position is referred to as "the null point"). This type of tremor may be exacerbated by muscular contractions and tends to decrease in amplitude with the employment of sensory tricks. An example of a sensory trick ("geste antagonistique") is touching the chin or neck in an attempt to stop the dystonia (2). Although antagonistic gestures are not included in the current criteria used to define dystonic tremor, it is useful to take their existence into consideration when differentiating this condition from other types of tremor. Dystonic tremor may resemble myoclonus if accompanied by jerk-like movements; 15 of 45 (33%) patients with idiopathic dystonia and tremor that were studied clinically and with electromyography (EMG) had EMG features consistent with myoclonus (9).

III. DIAGNOSIS AND PATHOPHYSIOLOGY

The diagnosis of dystonic tremor is based on the clinical history and physical findings. Criteria have been postulated for the diagnosis of this condition, providing a sub-classification into possible, probable, and definite dystonic tremor. Family history should be taken into consideration when evaluating patients with tremor and dystonia; tremor may be an isolated finding in patients with dystonic relatives (usually referred to as dystonia gene-associated tremor) (10). Electromyographic recordings of patients with dystonic tremor have shown that bursts of muscle contraction occur in an un-synchronized activity of agonist and antagonist muscles, with variable amplitude (3–12 Hz) and duration (50–300 ms) (10). Although some studies disagree on the utility of EMG criteria for distinguishing dystonic tremor from other types of tremor such as enhanced physiological tremor or essential tremor (11), other studies (12) suggest that this technology may be useful in differentiating dystonic tremor from conditions such as essential tremor, and also help differentiate conditions in which tremor and dystonia are present.

There is currently a limited understanding of the pathophysiology of dystonic tremor (13,14). One of the reasons for this paucity of knowledge is that there is considerable uncertainty about the relationship between dystonia, dystonic tremor and essential tremor (15). This uncertainty is particularly true with head and hand tremor. Head oscillation associated with cervical dystonia can be divided into two broad categories: essential-type tremor or dystonic tremor. Although the two types of tremor can usually be identified clinically, the differentiation may be aided by the use of EMG (16). The essential-type tremor is usually more regular and has a higher (>7 Hz, with peaks at 9 and 11 Hz) frequency than the dystonic tremor (3–7 Hz, with a peak at 5 Hz). Also, patients with coexistent essential-type tremor continue to have the oscillation of the head regardless of the direction of the force of the dystonia; in contrast dystonic tremor ceases when the patient stops resisting the dystonic pulling ("null point"). Using this clinical differentiation, head tremor, identified in 60% of all patients with cervical dystonia, was categorized as "dystonic" in 38%, "essential" in 30%, and a combination "dystonic-essential" in 8% (4). Deuschl et al. (17) provided support for this clinical differentiation by employing EMG polygraphic recordings to study patients with cervical dystonia. In all patients with low-frequency tremor, thought to be dystonic in origin, the EMG tremor activity ceased when the patients used "geste antagonistique"; this phenomenon was not observed in patients with essential tremor. A study of 45 patients with arm tremor and cervical dystonia (12) noted that cervical dystonia patients with dystonic arm tremor had significantly more severe tremor than cervical dystonia patients with essential arm tremor.

Due to the variable character of dystonic tremor, another important differential diagnosis is psychogenic tremor. Clinical clues to the diagnosis of psychogenic tremor, such as easy distractibility while performing concentration tasks and entrainment to a new frequency or rate, are useful to differentiate psychogenic from organic causes of tremor. A recent study evaluating the use of a coherence entrainment test (CET) to differentiate psychogenic, dystonic and other organic tremors (18) found this test to have a 100% concordance with the clinical diagnosis when comparing clinically certain cases and controls ($n = 23$), suggesting that the use of a CET is a powerful way to identify dystonic tremor.

IV. MANAGEMENT

The understanding of the differences between essential tremor and dystonic tremor is not merely academic, since it may determine which treatment modalities should be employed (19). Treatment of patients with dystonic tremor is usually based on the available treatments for dystonia (20). Oral medications such as benzodiazepines (e.g., clonazepam, lorazepam, diazepam) and anticholinergic drugs (e.g., trihexyphenidyl, benztropine) are usually the initial treatment used to relieve the underlying dystonia, but the response to therapy is usually limited by its relative lack of efficacy and adverse effects. Therefore, chemodenervation with botulinum toxin (BTX) has become the first-line treatment for dystonia (21). BTX acts at the neuromuscular junction by binding to presynaptic cholinergic nerve terminals and interfering with acetylcholine release, relieving the abnormal muscle contractions or spasms, and thus improving dystonic tremor. The efficacy of BTX has been demonstrated in various studies; for example, 92% of 303 patients with medically intractable cervical dystonia had a significant improvement in function and control of head-neck movement after BTX (22). Although BTX is usually well tolerated, some of the side effects that might occur are usually related to focal weakness; for example, dysphagia was the most common complication encountered in 14% of 659 patients treated with BTX (22). Most complications of BTX therapy resolve spontaneously, usually within 2 weeks (23). Finally, surgical options such as pallidotomy, and deep brain stimulation of the ventrointermediate (VIM) nucleus of the thalamus or globus pallidus interna are also available to treat dystonic tremor in carefully selected patients, and have proven to aid in decreasing its frequency and intensity (14,24,25).

V. CONCLUSION

There is still much to learn about the pathophysiology of dystonic tremor. Advancement in the understanding of the basis of this disease will help structure a more comprehensive definition of dystonic tremor, and provide tools for the development of new management strategies.

REFERENCES

1. Jankovic J, Fahn S. Dystonic disorders. In: Jankovic J, Tolosa E, eds. Parkinson's Disease and Movement Disorders, 4th ed. Philadelphia, PA: Lippincott Williams and Wilkins, 2002:331–357.
2. Deuschl G. Dystonic tremor. Rev Neurol (Paris) 2003; 159:900–905.
3. Couch JR. Dystonia and tremor in spasmodic torticollis. Adv Neurol 1976; 14:245–258.
4. Jankovic J, Leder S, Warner D, Schwartz K. Cervical dystonia: clinical findings and associated movement disorders. Neurology 1991; 41:1088–1091.

5. Rosenbaum F, Jankovic J. Focal task-specific tremor and dystonia: categorization of occupational movement disorders. Neurology 1988; 38:522–527.
6. Deuschl G, Bain P, Brin M, Scientific-Committee. Consensus statement of the Movement Disorder Society on Tremor. Mov Disord 1998; 13:2–23.
7. Duffey P, Butler AG, Hawthorne MR, Barnes H. The epidemiology of primary dystonia in the North England. In: Fahn S, Marsden CD, DeLong DR, eds. Dystonia 3, Adv Neurol. Vol. 78. Philadelphia: Lippincott-Raven, 1998:121–125.
8. Muller J, Kiechl S, Wenning GK et al. The prevalence of primary dystonia in the general community. Neurology 2002; 59:941–943.
9. Jedynak CP, Bonnet AM, Agid Y. Tremor and idiopathic dystonia. Mov Disord 1991; 3:230–236.
10. Lucking CH, Hellwig B. Uncommon tremors. In: Mark Hallett, ed. Movement Disorders: Handbook of Clinical Neurophysiology. Elsevier, 2003:397–415.
11. Chan J, Brin MF, Fahn S. Idiopathic cervical dystonia: clinical characteristics. Mov Disord 1991; 6:119–126.
12. Munchau A, Schrag A, Chuang C, Mac Kinnon CD, Bhatia KP, Quinn NP, Rothwell JC. Arm tremor in cervical dystonia differs from essential tremor and can be classified by onset age and spread of symptoms. Brain 2001; 124:1765–1776.
13. Deuschl G, Raethjen J, Lindemann M, Krack P. The pathophysiology of tremor. Muscle Nerve 2001; 24:716–735.
14. Deuschl G, Bergman H. Pathophysiology of nonparkinsonian tremors. Mov Disord 2002; 17:S41–S48.
15. Jankovic J. Essential tremor: A heterogenous disorder. Mov Disord 2002; 17:638–644.
16. Deuschl G, Krack P, Lauk M, Timmer J. Clinical electrophysiology of tremor. J Clin Neurophysiol 1996; 13:110–122.
17. Deuschl G, Heinen F, Kleedorfer B et al. Clinical and polymyographic investigation of spasmodic torticollis. J Neurol 1992; 239:9–15.
18. McAuley J, Rothwell J. Identification of psychogenic, dystonic, and other organic tremors by a coherence entrainment test. Mov Disord 2004; 19:253–267.
19. Rivest J, Marsden CD. Trunk and head tremor as isolated manifestations of dystonia. Mov Disord 1990; 5:60–65.
20. Cooper G, Rodnitzky R. The many forms of tremor. Postgraduate Medicine 2000; 108:57–58, 61–64, 70.
21. Jankovic J. Botulinum toxin in clinical practice. J Neurol Neurosurg Psychiatry 2004; 75:951–957.
22. Jankovic J, Schwartz K. Botulinum toxin treatment of tremors. Neurology 1991; 41:1185–1188.
23. Jankovic J. Treatment of cervical dystonia with botulinum toxin. Mov Disord 2004; 19(suppl 8):S109–S115.
24. Ondo WG, Desaloms M, Krauss JK, Jankovic J, Grossman RG. Pallidotomy and thalamotomy for dystonia. In: Krauss JK, Jankovic J, Grossman RG, eds. Surgery for Parkinson's Disease and Movement Disorders. Philadelphia: Lippincott Williams and Wilkins, 2001:299–306.
25. Brin MF, Germano I, Danisi F, Weisz D, Olanow CW. Deep brain stimulation in the treatment of dystonia. In: Krauss JK, Jankovic J, Grossman RG, eds. Surgery for Parkinson's Disease and Movement Disorders. Philadelphia: Lippincott Williams and Wilkins, 2001:307–315.

15

Cerebellar Tremor

Lauren C. Seeberger

Colorado Neurological Institute Movement Disorders Center, Englewood, Colorado, USA

Robert A. Hauser

University of South Florida and Tampa General Healthcare, Tampa, Florida, USA

I. DEFINITION

Cerebellar tremor is a proximal 3–5 Hz action tremor in one or both extremities ipsilateral to a lesion of the deep cerebellar nuclei or the outflow tracts of these nuclei in the superior cerebellar peduncle. Action tremor occurs during voluntary contraction of skeletal muscles and is categorized as postural or kinetic. Postural tremor refers to oscillation of a body part while it is maintained against gravity, such as holding the arms out. Kinetic tremor refers to oscillation during guided voluntary movement and may be evident on finger-to-nose testing, or during activities such as eating or drinking. Kinetic tremors are further divided into simple kinetic or intention tremors. Simple kinetic tremor occurs during directed voluntary movements. Intention tremor is characterized by increasing amplitude of oscillation during pursuit of a target. The terms intention tremor and cerebellar tremor are often used interchangeably.

Cerebellar tremor amplitude increases as the limb is visually guided to a target. It can be elicited by finger-to-nose or heel-knee-shin testing. The tremor is usually perpendicular to the direction of movement and variable in amplitude. There may also be a postural tremor component when the limb is maintained in an outstretched position. Cerebellar tremor can be unilateral or bilateral and may involve one or both extremities on a side. A clinical diagnosis of cerebellar tremor is made only when there is predominant intention tremor of low frequency (usually <5 Hz) without a rest tremor (1).

Cerebellar tremor should be differentiated from the incoordinated ataxic limb movements that also occur with cerebellar dysfunction. Limb ataxia is a general term that refers to gross irregular decomposition of limb movements. Poor performance in smooth, fluid, rapid alternating movements is called dysdiadochokinesis and dyssynergia is a loss of coordination leading to breakdown of "en mass" movements into individual parts. Dysmetria is the inability to properly execute targeted movements and may result in hypometria (undershooting target) or hypermetria (overshooting target). In contrast to these abnormalities of movement, the dominant feature of tremor is the rhythmic nature of the oscillation.

II. ANATOMY OF THE CEREBELLUM

The cerebellum is comprised of two hemispheres joined by a midline vermis. It lies in the posterior fossa dorsal to the fourth ventricle and is connected to the brainstem by the superior, middle, and inferior cerebellar peduncles. These paired structures contain afferent and efferent tracts to and from the cerebellum. Transversely, the cerebellum is divided into three lobes: the anterior lobe responsible for coordination of gait and posture, the posterior lobe for guiding movements and modulating tone of the ipsilateral limbs, and the flocculonodular lobe which has extensive connections to the vestibular system for maintenance of orientation in space. There are three layers in the cortex of the cerebellum: the outer molecular layer, the Purkinje layer, and the inner granular layer. The Purkinje cells are the sole efferents from the cerebellar cortex and their processes connect extensively in the deep nuclei of the ipsilateral hemisphere. Arising from these nuclei (dentate, emboliform, globose and fastigial) are major pathways out of the cerebellum through the superior and inferior peduncles. Those that are most important for control of movement arise in the ipsilateral dentate nucleus and travel through the ipsilateral superior peduncle to synapse in the contralateral red nucleus or thalamus.

There are three well-described neuronal loops from the cerebellum: the dentato-rubro-thalamo-cortico-ponto-cerebellar loop, the dentato-rubro-olivo-cerebellar loop, and the fastigio-vestibulo-cerebellar loop (2). The Purkinje cell efferent projections have inhibitory effects on the deep cerebellar nuclei mediated by the transmitter gamma-aminobutyric acid (GABA) (3). The cerebellar nuclei exert excitatory effects on their targets, mediated by glutamate. The principle afferent loops back to the Purkinje cells are also excitatory. There is a somatotopic arrangement of neurons in the cerebellar hemispheres, although not as precise as that seen in the cerebrum.

III. PATHOPHYSIOLOGY OF CEREBELLAR TREMOR

There are three theories about how the normal cerebellum guides and controls movement (4). The first is that the cerebellum acts through a feedback system. This system uses constant feedback to the cerebellum from peripheral receptors; visual, vestibular, and somatosensory, to adjust ongoing movement and posture. A lesion study in cats supports the role of cerebellar outflow neurons in correcting ongoing movement initiated by the motor cortex (5).

The second theory is that the cerebellum uses feedforward control. According to this theory, the cerebellum generates planned motor sequences that are sent to the motor cortex in anticipation of movement. This enables movements to be accomplished more quickly, especially learned movements. Evidence shows that there is activation of the dentate nucleus that precedes intended movement (4).

Lastly, the efferent copy concept stipulates that the motor cortex provides the cerebellum with a "copy" of the motor plan that is being sent to effector muscles prior to movement. The cerebellum then provides short loop corrections back to the motor cortex even before movement is completed. It stands to reason that the development of pathologic tremor involves dysfunction of one or more of these control systems allowing oscillation to occur. These systems are dynamic and depending on the situation, one may prevail over the others. The most important cerebellar pathways for movement control involve the cerebello-dentato-rubro-thalamic circuit. Cerebellar tremor is caused by a lesion of these deep lateral cerebellar nuclei or their outflow pathways in the superior cerebellar peduncle (6), up to but not beyond the red nucleus (7). Lesions proximal to the decussation result in ipsilateral tremor and those distal to the decussation result in contralateral tremor (8). Injury to the cerebellar cortex itself does not initiate tremor (9,10).

There are three types of oscillatory mechanisms that may explain generation of tremor: (1) mechanical oscillation of the joints and their muscles, (2) reflex oscillation through afferent muscle spindle pathways to the central nervous system, and (3) central oscillation by groups of neurons within the central nervous system. It is likely that cerebellar tremor results from a combination of these oscillatory mechanisms brought about by dysfunction of cerebellar-based motor control.

Mechanical oscillation. Mechanical forces can decrease but do not eliminate cerebellar tremor, indicating some susceptibility of the tremor to mechanical forces. Animal studies have shown a change in cerebellar tremor characteristics depending on the mechanical state of the limb (11,12). Specifically, tremor frequency and amplitude can be altered by changing mechanical load (resistance and mass), as well as by changing the position of the limb. However, the tremor is less affected by these mechanical changes than changes in the reflex pathway.

Reflex oscillation. There are feedback loops between the cerebellum and muscle spindle afferents. Cerebellar ablation causes depression of both flexor and extensor muscle spindle afferents (13). Evidence that this afferent system has an important role in cerebellar tremor comes from both monkey and human studies (12,14). In monkeys with a cerebellar lesion, tremor can be induced by increasing muscle tone through posture holding or active movement, or with drugs that cause hypertonicity (15). In nine patients with cerebellar tremor and poorly legible handwriting, blood pressure cuff inflation that induced ischemia sufficient to temporarily block peripheral input reduced tremor in some and markedly improved their handwriting (14). These studies indicate that peripheral input may contribute to cerebellar tremor. Increased gain in the system coupled with reflex conduction delay may set up oscillations in muscles (16). Nonetheless, the genesis of cerebellar tremor cannot come only from muscle afferents as kinetic tremor has been experimentally produced by cerebellar ablations in deafferented animals (13,17).

Some studies implicate a change in timing in antagonist muscle firing which sets up oscillations through long loop reflex pathways to the motor cortex. In the disease state, the cerebellum is not able to effectively use feedforward control to fine-tune movement so it must rely on proprioceptive feedback which causes delays in firing that result in oscillating contractions of muscles (6,18). Abnormal firing patterns in these unstable long loop pathways, from peripheral input to cerebellum to motor cortex, are considered to be the primary cause of tremor in cerebellar disease.

Independent oscillators. There are two regions of the central nervous system (CNS) shown to have a predisposition to oscillation, the inferior olive and the thalamic relay nuclei (16). There is no evidence currently that independent central oscillation alone causes cerebellar tremor but the cerebellum is intimately linked to these two regions. Evidence that the cerebellum itself has an important role in the generation of tremor comes from positron emission tomography (PET) imaging studies showing hyperactivity of the cerebellum in other types of tremor (19,20). Dash noted that tremor began prior to any movement related feedback of sensation thereby suggesting a central component to generation of tremor (14). Recently, repetitive transcranial magnetic stimulation of the motor cortex areas of the forearm muscles was shown to cause terminal tremor in healthy subjects (21). The stimulation led to an inability to effectively terminate movement and oscillations began.

In summary, dysfunction of central control over movement finely tuned by the cerebellum through feedback, feedforward, and efferent copy mechanisms causes oscillation that is based on abnormal central processing and response to peripheral proprioceptive and mechanical input.

IV. ETIOLOGY OF CEREBELLAR TREMOR

There are many causes of cerebellar tremor. The most common causes are multiple sclerosis (MS), trauma, and degenerative diseases. Rarely do any of these disorders present with tremor as an isolated feature. A variety of other signs of cerebellar dysfunction are usually present depending on the areas of the cerebellum or outflow tracts that are affected. As a general rule, degenerative or toxic cerebellar dysfunction causes bilateral tremor whereas focal disease processes, such as a mass, infarction, or plaque, cause unilateral tremor. The appearance of the tremor itself does not distinguish the various etiologies. Cerebellar tremor is never a sign of normal aging.

Tremor and other cerebellar signs are often seen in MS, especially with disease progression. A study of 100 randomly selected MS patients referred to a tertiary center revealed that 37% had tremor, with 27% having some disability as a result, and 10% describing themselves as "incapacitated" by the tremor (22). In the majority of patients, tremor started in the arms, and the most common appearance was a mixed action tremor (postural and kinetic). In this population, kinetic tremor was most likely to cause disability (22).

Cerebellar tremor can be a late consequence of head injury. Brain stem cerebellar syndrome is a fairly common sequelae of brain trauma (23) and has been shown pathologically to be caused by direct injury to the cerebellum with a reduction of Purkinje cells and neurons of the dentate nucleus as well as shear injury of brain stem cerebellar connections (24). In one study, tremor emerged between two weeks and six months after severe closed head injury in 19% of survivors (25). In 58% of those, tremor resolved in less than one year. In another study, tremor emerged up to 18 months after head injury (25). Infarctions in the superior cerebellar peduncle or lateral cerebellar hemisphere can also cause delayed onset cerebellar tremor (26).

Cerebellar degenerative diseases may be inherited or spontaneous and genetic testing is available for the most commonly inherited spinocerebellar ataxias (Table 15.1). There has been a recent description of a rat model of hereditary Purkinje cell loss manifesting ataxia and a 3–5 Hz whole body tremor (27).

Toxic causes of cerebellar tremor include chronic alcoholism, lithium, heavy metal intoxication, and some medications (28), including anticonvulsants, antidepressants and neuroleptics. The tremor caused by lithium may be permanent because of gliosis and neuronal loss in the cerebellar cortex and dentate nuclei (6). Other causes of cerebellar tremor include neoplasm, paraneoplastic

Table 15.1 Causes of Cerebellar Tremor

	Genetic test available
Trauma	
Closed head injury	
Hypoxia	
Stroke	
Cerebellar neoplasm	
Hyperthermia	
Inherited	
Spinocerebellar ataxias	
SCA-12, SCA-16, SCA-19	SCA1-SCA 17
FXTAS	Fragile X DNA Test
Diseases	
Multiple sclerosis	
OPCA/MSA	
Wilson's disease	
Paraneoplastic syndrome	Hu, Yo, CV2, MaTa,
Creutzfeldt-Jacob disease	Ri, CAR, LEMS
Guillain-Barre syndrome	
Endocrinopathy	
hyperthyroid	
hypoparathyroid	
hypoglycemia (insulinoma)	
Infectious	
Rubella	
H. *influenzae*	
Rabies	
Varicella infection or vaccination	
Drug effects	
ETOH	
Lithium	
Heavy metal	
Anticonvulsants	
Antidepressants	
Neuroleptics	
Chemotherapeutic agents	

Note: ETOH, ethanol; FTXAS, Fragile X associated tremor and ataxia; OPCA, olivopontocerebellar atrophy; MSA, multiple system atrophy.

syndromes, Wilson's disease and other inherited metabolic diseases, endocrinopathies, and infections (29).

Patient history, neurological examination, and ancillary evaluations usually lead the clinician to a working diagnosis. Magnetic resonance imaging (MRI) of the brain is recommended in any case of new onset cerebellar tremor. It is helpful to assess the cerebellum for degeneration, infarction, white matter disease, plaques, traumatic injury, or tumor. In olivopontocerebellar atrophy (OPCA), the MRI characteristically demonstrates atrophy of the pons, cerebellum and middle cerebellar peduncles, as well as T2 weighted hyperintensity of the transverse pontine fibers, cerebellar white matter, and middle cerebellar peduncles (30). If an adult patient has a rapidly progressive course of ataxia with no known family history, consider testing for paraneoplastic syndromes and if accompanied by cognitive changes consider Creutzfeldt-Jakob disease. Electrophysiologic studies of tremor frequency may be helpful in the diagnosis of cerebellar tremor as few types of tremor have such low frequency (31).

A tremor syndrome was described by Hagerman et al. (32) named Fragile X associated tremor and ataxia (FXTAS). The patient is typically a middle-aged man [usually >50 years old (33)] who develops dementia, intention tremor, ataxia, parkinsonism and autonomic dysfunction. There may be a family history of mental retardation. Genetic testing for the CGG trinucleotide repeat in the fragile X mental retardation 1 gene (FMR1) shows an abnormally increased number of repeats (55–200 repeats), although not in the range that causes full-blown Fragile X syndrome (>200 repeats). FXTAS is an inclusion disease, like many of the other inherited forms of cerebellar degeneration, with eosinophilic intranuclear inclusions found in neurons and astrocytes throughout the brain (33). MRI of the brain may demonstrate hyperintensity in the middle cerebellar peduncles and the white matter near the dentate nucleus (34).

V. TREATMENT OF CEREBELLAR TREMOR

Symptomatic treatments focus on altering neurotransmitter activity, primarily serotonin and GABA. There are little data to support any particular pharmacologic approach and cerebellar tremor remains difficult to treat. Open label studies and case reports have suggested several medications that may have some benefit including propranolol, primidone, glutethimide, carbamazepine, isoniazid, clonazepam, buspirone, and topiramate (35–43). However, there have been few randomized double-blind trials (42,44–49).

Many of the medications tried for cerebellar tremor have been used to treat essential tremor. Braham et al. (50), found beneficial effects on ataxia and intention tremor in two brothers with familial ataxia treated with propranolol 120 mg/day, yet, in a crossover treatment trial of six patients, propranolol was not found to benefit cerebellar tremor (47). Two patients with MS-related tremor given primidone, at varying doses, showed tremor reduction and improved hand control (42). A short-term trial of glutethimide, a schedule II sedative hypnotic, in eight individuals with cerebellar tremor resulted in functional improvement and quantitative reduction in tremor with 50% choosing to remain on treatment (40).

In a 10 patient single-blind study, carbamazepine significantly reduced cerebellar tremor amplitude and clinical tremor scores at 15 (400 mg/day) and 30 days (600 mg/day). Improvement correlated with mean carbamazepine plasma levels (37). Seven of the 10 patients chose to stay on long-term treatment and attempts to lower the carbamazepine dose were associated with worsening of tremor. An open-label study of three patients with cerebellar tremor following stroke noted marked efficacy of carbamazepine at 600 mg/day (serum levels between 5.8 and 9.6 μg/mL) with return of tremor severity upon cessation of the agent (36). It has been postulated that the mechanism by which carbamazepine ameliorates cerebellar tremor is through reduction of repetitive neuronal firing in the ventral intermediate (VIM) nucleus of the thalamus (35).

Evidence as to whether isoniazid can reduce cerebellar tremor has been mixed. Limited improvement from isoniazid up to 1000 mg/day was reported by Duquette et al. (51) in 13 MS patients with ten patients showing slight improvement on one or more assessments. However, other trials with isoniazid reported better success with doses up to 1200 mg/day (39,46,52). Sabra et al., described improvement in four patients with MS-related tremor at doses of isoniazid between 800 and 1200 mg/day (52). This was followed by a placebo-controlled, double-blind trial in six MS patients titrated to isoniazid 1200 mg/day with four reporting global improvement and demonstrating tremor reduction on blinded videotape analysis (46). The effect of the medication was best at higher doses. In a double-blind, crossover trial of isoniazid (mean daily dose 935 mg) for action tremor in MS patients, 75% had only minimal improvement based on separate ratings by three neurologists, but two-thirds of those wished to continue therapy after the trial (49). Koller (47) conducted a double-blind crossover trial in six patients using isoniazid, propranolol, and intravenous ethyl alcohol, and found that none improved tremor severity. However, tremor reduction may be under-recognized by clinical assessments. In one study of isoniazid for cerebellar tremor, no benefit was identified using objective clinical assessments but four of five patients noted symptomatic improvement. In these patients, polarized light goniometry revealed a two to three fold reduction in tremor (39). Isoniazid inhibits γ-aminobutyric acid-aminotransferase, the first step in the enzymatic breakdown of GABA, and therefore increases GABA concentration. GABA is the major inhibitory neurotransmitter of the efferent pathways of the cerebellum and cerebral spinal fluid (CSF) levels of GABA are known to be reduced in some degenerative cerebellar ataxias (53). Isoniazid has many adverse effects including the potential for hepatic toxicity and liver function testing should be monitored regularly.

Other treatments to enhance GABA have been tried. Weiss et al. (54), reported marked improvement in upper extremity cerebellar tremor in one case after an intrathecal baclofen pump was placed for bilateral lower extremity spasticity. In addition, benzodiazepines have been reported to improve some cases of cerebellar tremor (35,55) and these medications facilitate GABAergic transmission at Purkinje neurons (56). In a study by Sechi et al. (43), the GABA agonist, topiramate was employed in doses up to 200 mg/day (average 122 mg/day) in nine patients with seven taking it as monotherapy and two in combination with carbamazepine. The patients [5 with MS, 2 with inherited degenerative disease, 1 with paraneoplastic syndrome, and 1 cerebrovascular accident (CVA)] were tested using an antigravity maneuver, goal-directed movements, and a free-hand writing task. There were significant reductions in both postural and intention tremor in the treated group but three of nine patients terminated early due to side effects. These results suggest that a placebo-controlled trial of topiramate using a slower titration in an effort to lessen side effects is warranted (43).

Buspirone hydrochloride, a serotonin agonist, has been evaluated in one open-label and one double-blind trial for cerebellar ataxia (41,44). The open label trial of buspirone 60 mg/day found significant overall benefit in ataxia in the mild-moderate group, particularly for those with lower extremity dysfunction (41). The mild-moderate group also rated themselves improved overall. Similarly, a double-blind study of buspirone (44) for cerebellar ataxia demonstrated improvement in kinetic scores. Neither of these studies specifically evaluated tremor. The therapeutic mechanism of action of buspirone in this setting is unknown, but may be related to serotonergic activity in the cerebellar cortex, independent of any anxiolytic or anti-depressant effect (41,44).

The intravenous and oral forms of ondansetron, a 5-HT 3 receptor antagonist, have been studied as possible treatments for cerebellar tremor. A double-blind trial evaluating oral ondansetron, 16 mg/day vs. placebo, in 45 patients with various cerebellar disorders showed no significant improvement in upper extremity tremor (45). Likewise, MS patients treated in an open-label study with a single dose of intravenous ondansetron failed to demonstrate improvement of tremor on functional tasks (57). These results do not support the findings of an earlier double-blind trial of intravenous ondansetron in MS and familial cerebellar degeneration in which tremor was improved (48).

VI. NONPHARMACOLOGIC INTERVENTIONS

Because medical intervention for cerebellar tremor is of limited benefit, therefore, non-pharmacologic approaches have been explored. Attempts at decreasing tremor amplitude and power have focused primarily on mechanical forces to quell the shaking limb. One method is to apply weights to the limb (58,59); another is to use tremor damping devices. Aisen and colleagues (60) demonstrated by use of orthoses that viscous damping loads lessen proximal tremor power and improve performance of tracking and other tasks. The biggest damping loads were less effective than smaller loads, indicating that too much damping leads to worsening of motor performance. Because damping by viscous loads improves both tremor and performance, it may provide a more effective treatment than traditional mass loading. In clinical practice, the response to weighting the limb is variable. Several authors have proposed that when feasible, a patient might be able to decrease tremor by working a task from memory rather than visual guidance (61,62).

VII. SURGICAL INTERVENTIONS

A wide variety of tremor types improve after VIM nucleus thalamotomy, reflecting this area's role as a common pathway for rhythmic activity in the brain (25). The VIM is the major receptor zone for output from the lateral cerebellar nuclei and is the target for thalamotomy. Narabayashi (63) described rhythmic, large-spiked burst discharges in the VIM synchronous with contralateral body tremor and proposed that lesions of this nucleus would disrupt the tremor circuit propagated by central and peripheral mechanisms. He considered intention tremor to be one of the movements most successfully improved by thalamotomy.

Thalamotomy has been used to treat cerebellar tremor arising from various causes, including trauma, MS, and stroke (64–66). In a series of seven mostly pediatric trauma-induced cases of intention tremor, Marks (64) reported improvement in tremor and function in six of seven patients who underwent thalamotomy. However, there were no specific measures of function or tremor assessment reported and two of the seven experienced transient hemiparesis following surgery. Similarly, in eight head trauma patients with mixed tremor undergoing thalamotomy, Andrew et al. (25), described marked improvement in all eight due to resolution of postural tremor and reduction of kinetic tremor but temporary worsening of dysarthria, ataxia, and weakness. There were no measures of tremor or function used to quantify these results. Post-traumatic movements can spontaneously improve within the first year after injury and patients should generally not be referred for surgery within this time (25,64).

A larger study of thalamotomy for cerebellar tremor of various etiologies (22 essential tremor, 46 MS, 11 post-traumatic, 9 post stroke, and 7 idiopathic) found that most patients experienced improvement in several domains including tremor severity, motor dexterity, and ability to drink from a cup without spilling (66). MS patients had a significant number of post operative complications (44 events in 53 surgeries including persistent cognitive dysfunction, hemiparesis, dysarthria, gait ataxia, arm ataxia, and numbness) and worsening of MS was observed in 8.7% despite perioperative steroid treatment. The majority of MS patients were evaluated for one year or less with more than half exhibiting recurrence of some tremor within the first year after surgery. Of the 25 patients who underwent thalamotomy for cerebellar tremor, the best improvement was for poststroke tremor. Another study of thalamotomy for MS cerebellar tremor (65) demonstrated overall rates of sustained improvement in arm tremor of about 70% (67). In this study (65), relapse of MS was observed in three of 24 patients (12.5%) given no perioperative steroid or adrenocorticotropic hormone (ACTH) treatment. Although most patients expressed satisfaction with their result some patients were not satisfied, usually due to lack of sustained benefit and high expectations for continued improvement. In addition, there was a lack of correlation of any clinical parameter (impairment of arm function due to severity of tremor, duration of MS, age or gender) to success of the procedure (65). Patient selection is therefore difficult. The risks of lack of sustained improvement in tremor and possible relapse of MS symptoms must be explained to potential surgical candidates along with possible benefits. It has been reported recently that frequency analysis of a wrist tracking task may predict those patients who are most likely to benefit from thalamotomy (68).

Bilateral thalamotomy is usually avoided because of the high risk of dysarthria and dysphagia (69).

Deep brain stimulation (DBS) of the VIM nucleus has now been used to treat cerebellar tremor (70–76). DBS does not improve the associated signs of dyssynergia and dysmetria which may be the most disabling aspects of the cerebellar dysfunction. Therefore, candidates for DBS must be carefully selected and reasonable expectations for outcomes set. The advantages of DBS include no permanent lesion, the potential for bilateral placement in patients with bilateral tremor, and adjustability of stimulation settings if tremor control wanes. In a study by Geny et al. (71), 69.2% of 13 patients with MS tremor undergoing DBS had reduction in tremor amplitude (mostly proximal), although none had complete resolution of tremor. Patients reported fatigue during activities of daily living to be improved along with tremor improvement. There were few postsurgical complications which differ from the reports of thalamotomy. The authors report good tremor amplitude reduction over time (mean of 13 months) with frequent stimulation parameter adjustments and also some recovery of functional use in the arms in most patients (71). In two studies of DBS for different tremor types, including some individuals with MS tremor, dysarthria was reported in $\sim$30% of those having bilateral DBS or a unilateral DBS placed contralateral to a thalamotomy lesion (77,78). Change in stimulation parameters was reported to help the dysarthria but resulted in less tremor control. A long term (mean of 32 months) study of DBS in nine medically refractory MS patients demonstrated a reduction of tremor in all, though improvement was greatest initially (72). Average Bain-Finchley tremor scale scores were 5.4 before surgery, 1.7 at six months, and 2.1 at last follow-up. Extended Disability Status Scale (EDSS) scores worsened over time and were on average, 6.7 before surgery, 6.8 at six months, and 7.8 at long-term follow-up. Thus, improvement in tremor scores persisted despite the fact that disability scores worsened. This is consistent with continued benefit for tremor despite progression of the underlying disease. Only one patient had a decline on neuropsychological testing and MRI did not reveal new plaques related to the electrodes in any subject. Within one month of surgery, one-third had exacerbations of MS symptoms, requiring steroid therapy (72). However, one-third, had long term restitution of their ability to feed themselves and maintain independent personal hygiene when stimulated. DBS for MS tremor is safe and effective. In addition, some patients may have sustained benefit but the progressive nature of MS makes it difficult to assess functional outcomes from surgery over time (72). This finding is likely to hold true for any neurodegenerative cause of cerebellar tremor. Better outcome tools are required to truly determine functional outcome, disability, and quality of life following DBS (75,79). These concerns should be addressed in future trials of surgical treatment for cerebellar tremor. Although there are limitations in functional improvement as currently measured, the resistance to medical treatment and debilitating aspects of this tremor along with the low morbidity and mortality rate of DBS make the surgery an acceptable option for those appropriately selected patients with moderately to severely disabling cerebellar tremor.

REFERENCES

1. Dueschl G, Bain P, Brin M, Committee AHS. Consensus statement of the movement disorder society on tremor. Mov Disord 1998; 13(suppl 3):2–23.
2. Daube JR, Reagan TJ, Sandok BA, Westmoreland BF. Medical neurosciences: an approach to anatomy, pathology, and physiology by systems and levels. 2nd ed. Boston: Little, Brown and Company, 1986.
3. Schulman JA. Chemical neuroanatomy of the cerebellar cortex. In: Emson PC, ed. Chemical Neuroanatomy. New York: Raven Press, 1983:209–228.
4. Johnson DS, Montgomery EB. Pathophysiology of cerebellar disorders. In: Watts RL, Koller WC, eds. Movement Disorders: Neurologic Principles and Practice. New York: McGraw-Hill, 1997:587–610.
5. Li Volsi G, Pacitti C, Perciavalle V, Sapienza S, Urbano A. Interpositus nucleus influences on pyramidal tract neurons in the cat. Neuroscience 1982; 7(8):1929–1936.
6. Elble RJ. Central mechanisms of tremor. J Clin Neurophysiol 1996; 13(2):133–144.
7. Cooper IS. A cerebellar mechanism in resting tremor. Neurology 1966; 16(10):1003–1015.
8. Carrea RM, Mettler FA. Function of the primate brachium conjunctivum and related structures. J Comp Neurol 1955; 102(1):151–322.
9. Cole JD. Hemispheric lesions and tremor. In: Findley LJ, Koller WC, eds. Handbook of Tremor Disorders. New York: Marcel Dekker, 1995:429–441.
10. Soriano V. Contribution of John F. Fulton to the study of cerebellar function. Int J Neurol 1970; 7(2):108–112.
11. Vilis T, Hore J. Effects of changes in mechanical state of limb on cerebellar intention tremor. J Neurophysiol 1977; 40(5):1214–1224.
12. Flament D, Vilis T, Hore J. Dependence of cerebellar tremor on proprioceptive but not visual feedback. Exp Neurol 1984; 84(2):314–325.
13. Gilman S. The nature of cerebellar dyssynergia. Mod Trends Neurol 1970; 5:60–79.
14. Dash BM. Role of peripheral inputs in cerebellar tremor. Mov Disord 1995; 10(5):622–629.
15. Gemba H, Sasaki K, Yoneda Y, Hashimoto S, Mizuno N. Tremor in the monkey with a cerebellar lesion. Exp Neurol 1980; 69(1):173–182.
16. Rothwell JC. Physiology and anatomy of possible oscillators in the central nervous system. Mov Disord 1998; 13(suppl 3):24–28.
17. Gilman S, Carr D, Hollenberg J. Kinematic effects of deafferentation and cerebellar ablation. Brain 1976; 99:311–330.
18. Elble RJ. Animal models of action tremor. Mov Disord 1998; 13(suppl 3):35–39.
19. Jenkins IH, Frackowiak RS. Functional studies of the human cerebellum with positron emission tomography. Rev Neurol (Paris) 1993; 149(11):647–653.
20. Boecker H, Brooks DJ. Functional imaging of tremor. Mov Disord 1998; 13(suppl 3):64–72.
21. Topka H, Mescheriakov S, Boose A, Kuntz R, Hertrich I, Seydel L, Dichgans J, Rothwell J. A cerebellar-like terminal and postural tremor induced in normal man by transcranial magnetic stimulation. Brain 1999; 122(pt 8):1551–1562.
22. Alusi SH, Worthington J, Glickman S, Bain PG. A study of tremor in multiple sclerosis. Brain 2001; 124(pt 4):720–730.
23. Roberts AH. Long-term prognosis of severe accidental head injury. Proc R Soc Med 1976; 69(2):137–141.

24. Marks PV. Post-traumatic cerebellar syndrome: a clinico-pathological study. J Neurol Neurosurg Psychiatry 1990; 53:448.
25. Andrew J, Fowler CJ, Harrison MJG. Tremor after head injury and its treatment by stereotaxic surgery. J Neurol Neurosurg Psychiatry 1982; 45:815–819.
26. Lin JJ, Chang DC. Delayed onset of hand tremor related to cerebellar hemorrhage. Mov Disord 1999; 14(1):189–191.
27. Clark BR, LaRegina M, Tolbert DL. X-linked transmission of the shaker mutation in rats with hereditary Purkinje cell degeneration and ataxia. Brain Res 2000; 858(2):264–273.
28. Lang AE, Weiner WJ, eds. Drug-Induced Movement Disorders. Mount Kisco: Futura Publishing Company, Inc., 1992.
29. Gilman S. Clinical features and treatment of cerebellar disorders. In: Watts RL, Koller WC, eds. Movement Disorders: Neurologic Principles and Practice. New York: McGraw-Hill, 1997:576–585.
30. Savoiardo M, Strada L, Girotti F, Zimmerman RA, Grisoli M, Testa D, Petrillo R. Olivopontocerebellar atrophy: MR diagnosis and relationship to multisystem atrophy. Radiology 1990; 174(3 pt 1):693–696.
31. Dueschl G, Krack P, Lauk M, Timmer J. Clinical neurophysiology of tremor. J Clin Neurophysiol 1996; 13(2):110–121.
32. Hagerman RJ, Leehey M, Heinrichs W, Tassone F, Wilson R, Hills J, Grigsby J, Gage B, Hagerman PJ. Intention tremor, parkinsonism, and generalized brain atrophy in male carriers of fragile X. Neurology 2001; 57(1):127–130.
33. Hagerman PJ. Fragile X-associated tremor/ataxia syndrome. Ment Retard Dev Disabil Res Rev 2004; 10(1):25–30.
34. Brunberg JA, Jacquemont S, Hagerman RJ, Berry-Kravis EM, Grigsby J, Leehey MA, Tassone F, Brown WT, Greco CM, Hagerman PJ. Fragile X premutation carriers: characteristic MR imaging findings of adult male patients with progressive cerebellar and cognitive dysfunction. AJNR Am J Neuroradiol 2002; 23(10):1757–1766.
35. Sandyk R. Successful treatment of cerebellar tremor with clonazepam. Clin Pharm 1985; 4(6):615, 618.
36. Sechi GP, Pirisi A, Agnetti V, Piredda M, Zuddas M, Tanca S, Piras ML, Aiello I, Deserra F, Rosati G. Efficacy of carbamazepine on cerebellar tremors in patients with superior cerebellar artery syndrome. J Neurol 1989; 236(8):461–463.
37. Sechi GP, Zuddas M, Piredda M, Agnetti V, Sau G, Piras ML, Tanca S, Rosati G. Treatment of cerebellar tremors with carbamazepine: A controlled trial with long-term follow-up. Neurology 1989; 39:1113–1115.
38. Jabbari B, Scherokman B, Gunderson CH, Rosenberg ML, Miller J. Treatment of movement disorders with trihexyphenidyl. Mov Disord 1989; 4(3):202–212.
39. Francis DA, Grundy D, Heron JR. The response to isoniazid of action tremor in multiple sclerosis and its assessment using polarised light goniometry. J Neurol Neurosurg Psychiatry 1986; 49(1):87–89.
40. Aisen ML, Holzer M, Rosen M, Dietz M, McDowell F. Glutethimide treatment of disabling action tremor in patients with multiple sclerosis and traumatic brain injury. Arch Neurol 1991; 48(5):513–515.
41. Lou J-S, Goldfarb L, McShane L, Gatev P, Hallett M. Use of buspirone for treatment of cerebellar ataxia. Arch Neurol 1995; 52:982–988.
42. Henkin Y, Herishanu YO. Primidone as a treatment for cerebellar tremor in multiple sclerosis-two case reports. Isr J Med Sci 1989; 25(12):720–721.

43. Sechi GP, Agnetti V, Sulas FMI, Sau G, Corda D, Pitzolu MG, Rosati G. Effects of topiramate in patients with cerebellar tremor. Progress in Neuro-Psychopharmacology & Biological Psychiatry 2003; 27:1023–1027.
44. Trouillas P, Xie J, Adeleine P, Michel D, Vighetto A, Honnorat J, Dumas R, Nighoghossian N, Laurent B. Buspirone, a 5-hydroxytryptamine 1A agonist, is active in cerebellar ataxia. Arch Neurol 1997; 54:749–752.
45. Bier JC, Dethy S, Hildebrand J, Jacquy J, Manto M, Martin JJ, Seeldrayers P. Effects of the oral form of ondansetron on cerebellar dysfunction. A multi-center double-blind study. J Neurol 2003; 250(6):693–697.
46. Hallett M, Lindsey JW, Adelstein BD, Riley PO. Controlled trial of isoniazid therapy for severe postural cerebellar tremor in multiple sclerosis. Neurology 1985; 35(9):1374–1377.
47. Koller WC. Pharmacologic trials in the treatment of cerebellar tremor. Archives of Neurology 1984; 41:280–281.
48. Rice GP, Lesaux J, Vandervoort P, Macewan L, Ebers GC. Ondansetron, a 5-HT3 antagonist, improves cerebellar tremor. J Neurol Neurosurg Psychiatry 1997; 62(3):282–284.
49. Bozek CB, Kastrukoff LF, Wright JM, Perry TL, Larsen TA. A controlled trial of isoniazid therapy for action tremor in multiple sclerosis. J Neurol 1987; 243:36–39.
50. Braham J, Sadeh M, Turgman J, Sarova-Pinchas I. Beneficial effect of propranolol in familial ataxia. Ann Neurol 1979; 5(2):207.
51. Duquette P, Pleines J, du Souich P. Isoniazid for tremor in multiple sclerosis: a controlled trial. Neurology 1985; 35(12):1772–1775.
52. Sabra AF, Hallett M, Sudarsky L, Mullally W. Treatment of action tremor in multiple sclerosis with isoniazid. Neurology 1982; 32(8):912–913.
53. Wasielewski PG, Burns JM, Koller WC. Pharmacologic treatment of tremor. Mov Disord 1998; 13(suppl 3):90–100.
54. Weiss N, North RB, Ohara S, Lenz FA. Attenuation of cerebellar tremor with implantation of an intrathecal baclofen pump: the role of gamma-aminobutyric acidergic pathways. Case report. J Neurosurg 2003; 99(4):768–771.
55. Trelles L, Trelles JO, Castro C, Altamirano J, Benzaquen M. Successful treatment of two cases of intention tremor with clonazepam. Ann Neurol 1984; 16(5):621.
56. Costa E, Guidotti A, Mao CC. Evidence for involvement of GABA in the action of benzodiazepines: studies on rat cerebellum. Adv Biochem Psychopharmacol 1975; 14:113–130.
57. Gbadamosi J, Buhmann C, Moench A, Heesen C. Failure of ondansetron in treating cerebellar tremor in MS patients—an open-label pilot study. Acta Neurol Scand 2001; 104(5):308–311.
58. Hewer RL, Cooper R, Morgan MH. An investigation into the value of treating intention tremor by weighting the affected limb. Brain 1972; 95(3):579–590.
59. Morgan MH, Hewer RL, Cooper R. Application of an objective method of assessing intention tremor—a further study on the use of weights to reduce intention tremor. J Neurol Neurosurg Psychiatry 1975; 38(3):259–264.
60. Aisen ML, Arnold A, Baiges I, Maxwell S, Rosen M. The effect of mechanical damping loads on disabling action tremor. Neurology 1993; 43:1346–1350.
61. Sanes JN, LeWitt PA, Mauritz KH. Visual and mechanical control of postural and kinetic tremor in cerebellar system disorders. J Neurol Neurosurg Psychiatry 1988; 51(7):934–943.

62. Mitoma H. Intention tremor exaggerated by visually guided movement. Eur Neurol 1996; 36:177–178.
63. Narabayashi H. Analysis of intention tremor. Clin Neurol Neurosurg 1992; 94(suppl):S130–132.
64. Marks PV. Stereotactic surgery for post-traumatic cerebellar syndrome: an analysis of seven cases. Stereotact Funct Neurosurg 1993; 60(4):157–167.
65. Critchley GR, Richardson PL. Vim thalamotomy for the relief of the intention tremor of multiple sclerosis. Br J Neurosurg 1998; 12(6):559–562.
66. Shahzadi S, Tasker RR, Lozano A. Thalamotomy for essential and cerebellar tremor. Stereotact Funct Neurosurg 1995; 65:11–17.
67. Haddow LJ, Mumford M, Whittle IR. Stereotactic treatment of tremor due to Multiple Sclerosis. Neurosurg Q 1997; 7(1):23–34.
68. Liu X, Aziz TZ, Miall RC, Rowe J, Alusi SH, Bain PG, Stein JF. Frequency analysis of involuntary movements during wrist tracking: a way to identify ms patients with tremor who benefit from thalamotomy. Stereotact Funct Neurosurg 2000; 74(2):53–62.
69. Selby G. Stereotactic surgery for the relief of Parkinson's disease. 2. An analysis of the results in a series of 303 patients (413 operations). J Neurol Sci 1967; 5(2):343–375.
70. Hooper J, Taylor R, Pentland B, Whittle IR. A prospective study of thalamic deep brain stimulation for the treatment of movement disorders in multiple sclerosis. Br J Neurosurg 2002; 16(2):102–109.
71. Geny C, Nguyen JP, Pollin B, Feve A, Ricolfi F, Cesaro P, Degos JD. Improvement of severe postural cerebellar tremor in multiple sclerosis by chronic thalamic stimulation. Mov Disord 1996; 11(5):489–494.
72. Schulder M, Sernas TJ, Karimi R. Thalamic stimulation in patients with multiple sclerosis: long-term follow-up. Stereotact Funct Neurosurg 2003; 80:48–55.
73. Benabid AL, Benazzous A, Hoffmann D, Limousin P, Krack P, Pollak P. Long-term electrical inhibition of deep brain targets in movement disorders. Mov Disord 1998; 13(suppl 3):119–125.
74. Lozano AM. VIM thalamic stimulation for tremor. Arch Med Res 2000; 31(3):266–269.
75. Berk C, Carr J, Sinden M, Martzke J, Honey C. Thalamic deep brain stimulation for the treatment of tremor due to multiple sclerosis: a prospective study of tremor and quality of life. J Neurosurg 2002; 97:815–820.
76. Montgomery EB Jr, Baker KB, Kinkel RP, Barnett G. Chronic thalamic stimulation for the tremor of multiple sclerosis. Neurology 1999; 53(3):625–628.
77. Siegfried J, Lippitz B. Chronic electrical stimulation of the VL-VPL complex and of the pallidum in the treatment of movement disorders: personal experience since 1982. Stereotact Funct Neurosurg 1994; 62(1–4):71–75.
78. Taha JM, Janszen MA, Favre J. Thalamic deep brain stimulation for the treatment of head, voice, and bilateral limb tremor. J Neurosurg 1999; 91(1):68–72.
79. Matsumoto J, Morrow D, Kaufman K, Davis D, Ahlskog JE, Walker A, Sneve D, Noseworthy J, Rodriguez M. Surgical therapy for tremor in multiple sclerosis. Neurology 2001; 57:1876–1882.

16

Holmes Tremor

Arif Dalvi

University of Chicago, Chicago, Illinois, USA

I. INTRODUCTION

In 1904 Gordon Holmes, then a resident medical officer at the National Hospital in London, published a series of nine cases with the common theme of an unusual tremor (1). The tremor was noted to have a static and dynamic component. The static component in most cases consisted of a regular and coarse tremor with a frequency of 3–5 Hz, that was difficult to control with volition, and increased with attempts at inhibition. The dynamic component consisted of an irregular intention-type tremor similar to that seen in multiple sclerosis. Associated findings included diplopia, ptosis, oculomotor palsies, hemiparesis, hemianopsia, emotional lability, and parkinsonian symptoms such as mask-like facial appearance, shuffling gait, rigidity, and bradykinesia. The presence of these findings varied from case to case. A vascular etiology or tumor were the probable causes in these early case reports.

A key anatomical observation in this series was the sparing of the corticospinal tracts. In one of the cases the tremor became less intense as the patient developed worsening hemiplegia with involvement of the corticospinal tracts. Holmes argued that the red nucleus was involved in the pathophysiology of the tremor based on the following considerations: the symptomatology or pathological findings were localizable to the superior cerebellar peduncle or the red nucleus; the tremor was similar to one created by lesioning the superior cerebellar peduncle in apes; and in a case report where such a tremor was seen, autopsy findings showed an isolated degeneration of the rubrospinal tract.

The term "rubral tremor" gained acceptance although Holmes himself did not use this term. The red nucleus was proposed as the primary anatomic substrate. Subsequent evidence both from case reports and animal studies indicated that the involvement of the red nucleus was not a sine qua non for this tremor. However other midbrain structures were implicated and hence the term "midbrain tremor" was coined. More recently the Consensus Statement of the Movement Disorders Society recommended the term Holmes tremor (2).

The consensus statement attempted to settle the debate on the name of this tremor. Other terms used include rubral tremor, midbrain tremor, thalamic tremor, myorhythmia, and Benedikt's syndrome. Names that included topographic descriptions were avoided given the awareness that the tremor can occur due to lesions outside the classic locations such as the red nucleus and the thalamus. The acceptance of the term Holmes tremor also credits Gordon Holmes' early description of the tremor. The consensus statement emphasizes that the dopaminergic system and the cerebellothalamic system play a role in the pathophysiology of this tremor. Thalamic tremor is considered a subtype of Holmes tremor. The preferred usage in such a case is the labeling of the clinical syndrome as Holmes tremor, and the etiology as a tremor following a midbrain/thalamic lesion.

II. CLINICAL FEATURES

The Consensus Statement uses the following criteria to define Holmes tremor (2):

1. Rest and intention tremor. In many patients postural tremor is also present. The tremor rhythm is often not as rhythmic as other tremors.
2. Slow frequency, usually <4.5 Hz.
3. If the time when the lesion occurred can be identified (e.g., as in a cerebrovascular accident), a variable delay (usually 4 weeks to 2 years) between the lesion and the first occurrence of the tremor is typical.

The key features of the tremor are the presence of a rest tremor, an exacerbation by sustained posture, and a further amplification with movement. The tremor is usually accompanied by other neurological signs. Two specific syndromes have been described in conjunction with the tremor. Claude syndrome is a combination of Holmes tremor, ataxia, and ipsilateral third nerve palsy. The addition of contralateral corticospinal tract findings defines Benedikt syndrome (3).

III. ETIOLOGY

Stroke and trauma to the midbrain are the most common causes of Holmes tremor, however, structural lesions in the vicinity of the midbrain can also cause Holmes tremor.

A. Stroke

Cerebrovascular disease was the most common etiology in Holmes' original series. Holmes tremor secondary to bilateral thalamic infarction has also been reported. Tan et al. (4) reported two children with a combined resting-postural-kinetic tremor caused by bithalamic infarction. Generalized seizures and diffuse spike-wave discharges predominantly over the left frontal area were seen on electroencephalography (EEG) in one patient, leading to the initial diagnosis of epilepsia partialis continua. However, clinical observation and video-EEG monitoring of the movements did not show an EEG correlate, favoring a diagnosis of rubral tremor. In both patients magnetic resonance imaging (MRI) revealed ischemic lesions in thalami bilaterally but failed to reveal any mesencephalic lesions. Holmes tremor has been reported following acute subarachnoid hemorrhage due to the rupture of a subthalamic arteriovenous malformation (5) and with mesencephalic infarction occurring as a complication of decompression surgery for trigeminal neuralgia (6).

B. Trauma

Samie et al. (7) reported three patients with post-traumatic midbrain tremors with radiographic and pathological confirmation of the localization. All three cases occurred in the setting of a head injury following a motor vehicle accident. In all cases the tremor had a delayed onset with the interval ranging from six to 18 months. In two of the cases, addition of a neuroleptic medication played a role in the development of the tremor. Both these patients had some reduction in tremor with benztropine. The third patient had remarkable reduction in tremor with levodopa. A delay in development of tremor is one of the hallmarks of this clinical entity. While four weeks to two years is typical, the tremor was reported in one case to develop 23 years after the initial insult (8).

C. Infection

The earliest description of such a tremor was by Benedikt who described a syndrome consisting of a contralateral tremor and an ipsilateral oculomotor nerve palsy (9). The lesion was localized to the midbrain tegmentum and affected the red nucleus and the oculomotor nerve. The patient was also noted to have left hemiparesis in addition to left-sided tremor. Autopsy revealed multiple brain tuberculomas including one in the right cerebral peduncle along with destruction of the oculomotor nerve. Any appropriately localized infectious lesion of midbrain structures can produce the tremor. A number of case reports implicate toxoplasmosis as a causative factor for Holmes tremor (10–12). This may occur in the setting of an human immunodeficiency virus (HIV) positive patient (13). In such cases concomitant infection with tuberculosis may contribute. Tieve et al. (14) described a case of neuroparacoccidioidomycosis that presented with a midbrain mass lesion associated with Holmes tremor.

D. Neoplasms

Midbrain tumors can cause Holmes tremor. These include midbrain angioma (15) and germinoma (16). Holmes tremor may also present as part of a paraneoplastic syndrome (17,18). Radiation therapy of tumors in this region may result in Holmes tremor (19). Surgical resections in the vicinity of the midbrain may also result in Holmes tremor. Pahwa et al. (20) reported Holmes tremor following surgical resection of a midbrain cavernous hemangioma. The tremor occurred approximately three months after partial resection and was intractable to medical treatment. The patient had a marked improvement after thalamic stimulation. Samadani et al. (21) also reported a patient with Holmes tremor related to a cavernous angioma that worsened after surgical resection and was improved with deep brain stimulation of the thalamus.

E. Neuroleptic Medications and Toxins

Friedman (22) reported Holmes tremor induced by fluphenazine that improved with benztropine and bromocriptine. The patient had an old, post-traumatic cerebellar lesion with ataxia and a mild postural tremor. However, after fluphenazine injections he developed a marked worsening of the tremor and a resting component. Lorazepam and benztropine alone did not help. However combination therapy with benztropine and bromocriptine improved the tremor. One of the patients in the series of post-traumatic tremor reported by Samie et al. (7) also developed tremor six months after a head injury and ten days following administration of haloperidol. The tremor had some response to benztropine. Substance abuse with toluene has also caused Holmes tremor (23). Imaging in this case revealed lesions in the basal ganglia, thalamus and red nucleus. The tremor persisted despite discontinuation of toluene. It was medically intractable but responded to thalamotomy.

F. Demyelination

While postural tremors are common in multiple sclerosis, a study evaluating tremor in 100 patients with multiple sclerosis did not reveal any patients with Holmes tremor (24).

IV. PATHOPHYSIOLOGY

Holmes tremor has features in common with parkinsonian and cerebellar tremor. Midbrain lesions involving the cerebellorubrothalamic pathways or other subcortical lesions are implicated in the pathophysiology (25). Both the dopaminergic nigrostriatal system and the cerebellothalamic system are involved according to autopsy and positron emission tomography (PET) data. Lesions along the fiber tracts of these systems can also result in Holmes tremor (26).

A case report by Deuschl et al. (27) illustrates the role of the cerebellum in parkinsonian rest tremor and Holmes tremor. They described a patient who developed Parkinson's disease 17 years after resection of his right cerebellum because of a Lindau tumor. He had a classic parkinsonian 4.3 Hz resting tremor on the left side but a 3.1 Hz resting, postural, and intention tremor on the right side compatible with Holmes tremor. This case suggests that both functional deficits, cerebellar and nigrostriatal, come together to produce Holmes tremor. The cerebellum could modulate the tremor frequency of parkinsonian rest tremor and may prevent the rest tremor from transforming into a postural and goal-directed tremor.

Tremor following lesions of the ventromedial tegmentum in primates resembles Holmes tremor (28) and responds to levodopa or anticholinergic medications. Isolated substantia nigra lesions are insufficient in inducing tremor in the animal model. Additional lesions in the cerebellothalamic fibers and the parvocellular division of the red nucleus are required (29).

V. TREATMENT

The treatment of Holmes tremor includes management of the underlying etiology and symptomatic control of tremor. Treatment of structural lesions may help alleviate the tremor. Heran et al. (30) reported improvement in Holmes tremor following drainage of neuroepithelial cysts. Treatment of infectious causes is indicated. However, resolution of underlying lesions may not correlate with cessation of the tremor. Koppel and Daras (11) reported a case of Holmes tremor due to a toxoplasma abscess with persistent tremor despite resolution of the lesion on imaging.

A review of the pathophysiology (26,31) would indicate that treatment modalities should affect the nigrostriatal component and cerebellar outflow systems. Early reports (32,33) indicated that levodopa could suppress the tremor. More recent reports support this observation of successful treatment with levodopa alone (34,35) or in combination with other agents such as isoniazid (12), anticholinergics (7), or carbamazepine (36). In a report of Holmes tremor following a midbrain hemorrhage the resting tremor component responded to levodopa, while the kinetic component improved with the addition of carbamazepine (36). This response to levodopa is not universal and other agents have been tried. Treatment with benzodiazepines, in particular clonazepam has been reported to be helpful in post-traumatic Holmes tremor (37). Botulinum toxin injections may be considered in patients with Holmes tremor unresponsive to oral medications (38). However, achieving functional improvement with botulinum toxin in tremor disorders is difficult due to the possibility of hand weakness which is a dose-dependent side effect. The postural component of the tremor is more responsive than the resting or intention components (39).

Surgery is an option in patients with severe Holmes tremor intractable to medical modalities who do not have significant comorbid illnesses or cognitive deficits (40). Both ventralis intermedius (VIM) thalamotomy (16,23) and posteroventral pallidotomy (41) have been reported to be effective. However, deep brain stimulation is currently the preferred modality due to its lower risk of complications (40). Thalamic stimulation of the VIM nucleus has been effective in Holmes tremor occurring after resection of midbrain angiomas (20,21), or pontine hemorrhages (42). Romanelli et al. (43) reported a case where the addition of the subthalamic nucleus as a secondary target was required to control resting tremor that persisted after the postural and kinetic components had responded to VIM stimulation. Pallidal stimulation has also been tried but only with partial success (6).

REFERENCES

1. Holmes G. On certain tremors in organic cerebral lesions. Brain 1904; 27:327–375.
2. Deuschl G, Bain P, Brin M. Consensus statement of the Movement Disorder Society on Tremor. Ad Hoc Scientific Committee. Mov Disord 1998; 13(suppl 3):2–23.
3. Bogousslavsky J, Maeder P, Regli F, Meuli R. Pure midbrain infarction: clinical syndromes, MRI, and etiologic patterns. Neurology 1994; 44(11):2032–2040.
4. Tan H, Turanli G, Ay H, Saatci I. Rubral tremor after thalamic infarction in childhood. Pediatr Neurol 2001; 25(5):409–412.
5. Defer GL, Remy P, Malapert D, Ricolfi F, Samson Y, Degos JD. Rest tremor and extrapyramidal symptoms after midbrain haemorrhage: clinical and 18F-dopa PET evaluation. J Neurol Neurosurg Psychiatry 1994; 57(8):987–989.
6. Fernandez HH, Friedman JH, Centofanti JV. Benedikt's syndrome with delayed-onset rubral tremor and hemidystonia: a complication of tic douloureux surgery. Mov Disord 1999; 14(4):695–697.
7. Samie MR, Selhorst JB, Koller WC. Post-traumatic midbrain tremors. Neurology 1990; 40(1):62–66.
8. Krack P, Deuschl G, Kaps M, Warnke P, Schneider S, Traupe H. Delayed onset of "rubral tremor" 23 years after brainstem trauma. Mov Disord 1994; 9(2):240–242.

9. Benedikt M. The Classical Brain Stem Syndromes. Springfield, IL: Charles C Thomas, 1991.

10. Daras M, Koppel BS, Samkoff L, Marc J. Brainstem toxoplasmosis in patients with acquired immunodeficiency syndrome. J Neuroimaging 1994; 4(2):85–90.

11. Koppel BS, Daras M. "Rubral" tremor due to midbrain Toxoplasma abscess. Mov Disord 1990; 5(3):254–256.

12. Pezzini A, Zavarise P, Palvarini L, Viale P, Oladeji O, Padovani A. Holmes' tremor following midbrain Toxoplasma abscess: clinical features and treatment of a case. Parkinsonism Relat Disord 2002; 8(3):177–180.

13. Mattos JP, Rosso AL, Correa RB, Novis SA. Movement disorders in 28 HIV-infected patients. Arq Neuropsiquiatr 2002; 60(3-A):525–530.

14. Teive HA, Zanatta A, Germiniani FM, Almeida SM, Werneck LC. Holmes' tremor and neuroparacoccidioidomycosis: a case report. Mov Disord 2002; 17(6):1392–1394.

15. Leung GK, Fan YW, Ho SL. Rubral tremor associated with cavernous angioma of the midbrain. Mov Disord 1999; 14(1):191–193.

16. Kim MC, Son BC, Miyagi Y, Kang JK. Vim thalamotomy for Holmes' tremor secondary to midbrain tumour. J Neurol Neurosurg Psychiatry 2002; 73(4):453–455.

17. Golbe LI, Miller DC, Duvoisin RC. Paraneoplastic degeneration of the substantia nigra with dystonia and parkinsonism. Mov Disord 1989; 4(2):147–152.

18. Simonetti F, Pergami P, Aktipi KM, Giardini G, Ceroni M, Lattuada P et al. Paraneoplastic "rubral" tremor: a case report. Mov Disord 1998; 13(3):612–614.

19. Pomeranz S, Shalit M, Sherman Y. "Rubral" tremor following radiation of a pineal region vascular hamartoma. Acta Neurochir (Wien) 1990; 103(1–2):79–81.

20. Pahwa R, Lyons KE, Kempf L, Wilkinson SB, Koller WC. Thalamic stimulation for midbrain tremor after partial hemangioma resection. Mov Disord 2002; 17(2):404–407.

21. Samadani U, Umemura A, Jaggi JL, Colcher A, Zager EL, Baltuch GH. Thalamic deep brain stimulation for disabling tremor after excision of a midbrain cavernous angioma. Case report. J Neurosurg 2003; 98(4):888–890.

22. Friedman JH. "Rubral" tremor induced by a neuroleptic drug. Mov Disord 1992; 7(3):281–282.

23. Miyagi Y, Shima F, Ishido K, Yasutake T, Kamikaseda K. Tremor induced by toluene misuse successfully treated by a Vim thalamotomy. J Neurol Neurosurg Psychiatry 1999; 66(6):794–796.

24. Alusi SH, Worthington J, Glickman S, Bain PG. A study of tremor in multiple sclerosis. Brain 2001; 124(Pt 4):720–730.

25. McAuley JH, Marsden CD. Physiological and pathological tremors and rhythmic central motor control. Brain 2000; 123(Pt 8):1545–1567.

26. Deuschl G, Bergman H. Pathophysiology of nonparkinsonian tremors. Mov Disord 2002; 17(suppl 3):S41–S48.

27. Deuschl G, Wilms H, Krack P, Wurker M, Heiss WD. Function of the cerebellum in Parkinsonian rest tremor and Holmes' tremor. Ann Neurol 1999; 46(1):126–128.

28. Wilms H, Sievers J, Deuschl G. Animal models of tremor. Mov Disord 1999; 14(4):557–571.

29. Ohye C, Shibazaki T, Hirai T, Wada H, Kawashima Y, Hirato M et al. A special role of the parvocellular red nucleus in lesion-induced spontaneous tremor in monkeys. Behav Brain Res 1988; 28(1–2):241–243.

30. Heran NS, Berk C, Constantoyannis C, Honey CR. Neuroepithelial cysts presenting with movement disorders: two cases. Can J Neurol Sci 2003; 30(4):393–396.
31. Vidailhet M, Jedynak CP, Pollak P, Agid Y. Pathology of symptomatic tremors. Mov Disord 1998; 13(suppl 3):49–54.
32. Findley LJ, Gresty MA. Suppression of "rubral" tremor with levodopa. Br Med J 1980; 281(6247):1043.
33. Berkovic SF, Bladin PF. Rubral tremor: clinical features and treatment of three cases. Clin Exp Neurol 1984; 20:119–128.
34. Vidailhet M, Dupel C, Lehericy S, Remy P, Dormont D, Serdaru M et al. Dopaminergic dysfunction in midbrain dystonia: anatomoclinical study using 3-dimensional magnetic resonance imaging and fluorodopa F 18 positron emission tomography. Arch Neurol 1999; 56(8):982–989.
35. Velez M, Cosentino C, Torres L. Levodopa-responsive rubral (Holmes') tremor. Mov Disord 2002; 17(4):741–742.
36. Harmon RL, Long DF, Shirtz J. Treatment of post-traumatic midbrain resting-kinetic tremor with combined levodopa/carbidopa and carbamazepine. Brain Inj 1991; 5(2):213–218.
37. Jacob PC, Pratap Chand R. Posttraumatic rubral tremor responsive to clonazepam. Mov Disord 1998; 13(6):977–978.
38. Jankovic J, Schwartz K. Botulinum toxin treatment of tremors. Neurology 1991; 41(8):1185–1188.
39. Henderson JM, Ghika JA, Van Melle G, Haller E, Einstein R. Botulinum toxin A in non-dystonic tremors. Eur Neurol 1996; 36(1):29–35.
40. Deuschl G, Bain P. Deep brain stimulation for tremor: patient selection and evaluation. Mov Disord 2002; 17(suppl 3):S102–S111.
41. Miyagi Y, Shima F, Ishido K, Moriguchi M, Kamikaseda K. Posteroventral pallidotomy for midbrain tremor after a pontine hemorrhage. Case report. J Neurosurg 1999; 91(5):885–888.
42. Shepherd GM, Tauboll E, Bakke SJ, Nyberg-Hansen R. Midbrain tremor and hypertrophic olivary degeneration after pontine hemorrhage. Mov Disord 1997; 12(3):432–437.
43. Romanelli P, Bronte-Stewart H, Courtney T, Heit G. Possible necessity for deep brain stimulation of both the ventralis intermedius and subthalamic nuclei to resolve Holmes tremor. Case report. J Neurosurg 2003; 99(3):566–571.

17

Orthostatic Tremor

Michele Tinazzi

*Institute of Neurology, London, UK and Neurology Unit,
Azienda Ospedaliera di Verona, Verona, Italy*

Willibald Gerschlager

*Institute of Neurology, London, UK and
Krankenhaus der Barmherzigen Brüder, Vienna, Austria*

Kailash P. Bhatia

*Institute of Neurology and National Hospital for Neurology
and Neurosurgery, London, UK*

I. INTRODUCTION

Orthostatic tremor, first described by Heilman in 1984, is a rare condition characterized by unsteadiness when standing that is relieved when sitting or walking, and is accompanied by a rapid 13–18 Hz tremor of the legs (1). Orthostatic tremor was initially classified as a variant of essential tremor (2,3), because of the presence of a postural arm tremor resembling essential tremor in some cases. According to the Consensus Statement of the Movement Disorder Society on tremor (4), orthostatic tremor is defined as a subjective feeling of unsteadiness during stance that is usually relieved during sitting or lying, associated with visible and occasionally palpable fine amplitude rippling of the leg muscles when standing, and accompanied by a rapid 13–18 Hz tremor of the legs. Currently, orthostatic tremor is considered a distinct tremor disorder that it is thought to arise from a central generator in the cerebellum or brainstem.

However, little is known about the demographic features, natural history, progression and response to treatment of orthostatic tremor. It is also unclear how commonly arm tremor and other features are associated with orthostatic tremor, and whether there are different subgroups of orthostatic tremor. One reason for this lack of information could be the relative rarity of this disorder, since most reports have described only a few cases, without detailed clinical analysis and follow up. A series of 30 patients (5) and a review of 41 cases with a clinical and electrophysiological diagnosis of orthostatic tremor (6) have been reported.

In this review we will describe different aspects of orthostatic tremor, including classification, demographic variables, medical history, clinical and neurophysiological features, pathophysiology and treatment.

II. ETIOLOGY AND CLASSIFICATION

Orthostatic tremor is generally considered to be an idiopathic disorder as brain imaging and other investigations are usually normal. Only rarely, orthostatic tremor has been described in patients with pontine lesions (7), aquaeduct stenosis or with a relapsing polyradiculoneuropathy (8), cerebellar degeneration (9,10) or following head trauma (11,12). Although not all these patients had typical orthostatic tremor (some displayed a lower frequency than the typical 14–18 Hz bursts) these reports could be considered forms of symptomatic orthostatic tremor.

In a review of 41 orthostatic tremor patients, 31 (over 75%) could be classified as idiopathic based on their clinical features and normal investigations including brain imaging (6). These patients were classified as having "primary orthostatic tremor." This group of patients was further divided into two subgroups: those with additional postural arm tremor ($n = 24$), and those without postural arm tremor or "pure orthostatic tremor" ($n = 7$). McManis and Sharbrough (5) had also reported that 9 out of 30 orthostatic tremor patients had a postural tremor on routine clinical examination although a 13–18 Hz arm tremor was present in 27 of them when the arms were involved in weight-bearing tasks.

Additional neurological features were evident in 10 out of 41 orthostatic tremor patients (25%) defined as "orthostatic tremor plus" (6). Six of these 10 had parkinsonism: four of these had typical Parkinson's disease (PD). One had vascular and one had drug-induced parkinsonism. This is consistent with rare reports of patients in whom orthostatic tremor was associated with PD (13,14). Among the remaining four patients, two had restless legs syndrome (RLS) and one had tardive dyskinesia and one orofacial dyskinesias of uncertain etiology. One patient with PD and the patient with vascular parkinsonism also had RLS.

III. EPIDEMIOLOGY

As there are no epidemiological data, the incidence and prevalence of orthostatic tremor are unknown. However, orthostatic tremor is considered to be a rare disorder and so far, mostly case reports or studies in small groups of patients have been described.

A. Demographical Variables: Age, Sex and Onset Age

Orthostatic tremor appears to be a disorder of middle-aged or elderly people with a mean age of onset ~55 years and with a female predominance (~65%) (5,6). In the series of patients of Gerschlager et al. (6) the mean onset age was significantly earlier in women (50.4 ± 14.2) vs. men (60.0 ± 13.1) and the mean disease duration was significantly longer in women (mean ± SD: 12.4 ± 8.4 years) as compared with men (6.1 ± 4.4 years). Orthostatic tremor seemed to be underdiagnosed as on an average, it took 5.7 years (SD: 4.3) from the initial symptoms until a diagnosis of orthostatic tremor was made (6). In many patients ($n = 10$) the orthostatic tremor symptoms were initially mistaken for PD, RLS or considered psychogenic.

B. Family History

A family history of orthostatic tremor appears to be an uncommon feature. In the series of McManis and Sharbrough (5) of the 24 patients in whom family history was known, eight had a family history of movement disorders (4 had family members with typical upper limb essential tremor and in 2 others essential tremor was likely by history, one patient was said to have a similarly affected parent, and 1 had a parent with PD). Gerschlager et al. (6) reported that of the 36 patients in whom family history was detailed, eight had a family history of movement disorders. Among the 20 (of 24) in whom family history was available in the "orthostatic tremor with postural arm tremor" group, two patients reported similar symptoms of leg tremor in a sibling (sisters in both cases). Three patients had first-degree relatives with postural arm tremor. One patient reported that her aunt had the same problems when standing still, another had a first degree relative with postural arm tremor, and one had an uncle with probable PD.

IV. CLINICAL AND NEUROPHYSIOLOGICAL FEATURES

Orthostatic tremor is typically characterized by: (1) a subjective feeling of unsteadiness during stance but only in severe cases during gait (usually without any disturbance during sitting or lying); (2) sparse clinical findings that are mostly limited to a visible and sometimes only palpable fine-amplitude rippling of the leg (quadriceps or gastrocnemius) muscles when standing; and (3) electromyographic (EMG) recordings (e.g., from the quadriceps muscle) that show a typical 13–18 Hz pattern. The diagnosis of orthostatic tremor is based upon clinical presentation and EMG findings according to the Consensus Statement of the Movement Disorder Society (4).

Tremor may still be less conspicuous than the dramatic compensatory maneuvers adopted by the patient in an effort to minimize the symptoms of unsteadiness when standing. Patients may stand in a slightly stooped posture with a widened stance, with their legs stiffly extended and claw at the floor with their toes or shuffle their feet in an attempt to steady themselves. Finally, they may reach to grasp at nearby secure objects for further support. Both the leg tremor and the sensation of unsteadiness appear a few seconds after standing still, and are relieved by walking, sitting down, or leaning against a support (12,15–22). The condition under which this tremor occurs is in the stance phase of the gait (16). Tremor is more pronounced in the leg and trunk (cervical, thoracic and lumbar paraspinal) muscles, but can also be detected in upper limb muscles during certain postural maneuvers. Arm tremor is rarely accompanied by complaints of shaking and varies in frequency depending on arm posture.

Physiological studies have revealed that the 16 Hz tremor occurs not only in the antigravity muscles but also in forearm flexor muscles of the leg, the trunk and arm muscles (15,16,18–20). In addition to the muscles innervated by the spinal cord, the cranial nerves are also involved (23), indicating that all motor nuclei have this unique pattern with the possible exception of the extraocular muscles, which have not been tested. The activity of the muscles in orthostatic tremor is highly coherent in all muscles tested (15,16,18,20,22). Muscles from both sides of the body and from the upper limbs, lower limbs, and cranial nerves are all coherent. This is a unique finding among tremors assessed with coherence analysis (22). McAuley et al. (22), using frequency domain analysis of postural muscle EMG signals, have assessed the tremor frequency and the time relation between bursts of activity in different muscles during execution of different postural tasks in orthostatic tremor patients. The authors found a link between the 16 Hz range EMG oscillations between different muscles which is characterized by a complex pattern of phase lags between these muscles that does not simply reflect the different motor conduction times from a single central oscillator down the descending pathways to different muscles.

The pattern varied between subjects and on performing different postural tasks, but was constant if a subject repeatedly performed the same task. They concluded that the complex pattern of timing could represent the unmasking of normal processes that become peripherally manifest as a result of the abnormally strong 16 Hz central oscillation. Such timing relations could reflect the passage of motor commands through complex central nervous system (CNS) neural networks that are relatively fixed while performing a certain task but vary for different tasks. Alternatively, they may represent a more active process where the postural motor system controls linkage between muscles through a phase-dependent code.

An important feature is that the tremor cannot be reset by a peripheral nerve stimulus, unlike some examples of essential tremor (16,24). These features all confirm a unique and central oscillator underlying this tremor. This oscillator must be strong enough to dominate normal corticospinal and bulbospinal activity, because single-unit recordings have shown that individual units are activated only at 16 Hz or at lower harmonics (e.g., 8, 4, 2 Hz, etc.) of the 16 Hz pattern (19). Thus, the motor neurons receive such a strong excitatory potential at the time of each tremor burst that additional excitatory potentials in the pauses between the tremor bursts are not able to increase the membrane potential to firing threshold. This firing pattern excluded a purely spinal mechanism of orthostatic tremor (19).

A. Relationship between Orthostatic Tremor and Postural Arm Tremor

Orthostatic tremor was initially classified as a variant of essential tremor (2,3,25) because of the presence of a postural arm tremor resembling essential tremor in some cases. In the series reported by Gerschlager et al. (6), 24 out of 31 patients with primary orthostatic tremor had additional postural arm tremor. McManis and Sharbrough (5) reported that 9 out of 30 orthostatic tremor patients had a postural tremor on routine clinical examination although a 13–18 Hz arm tremor was present in 27 of them when the arms were involved in weight-bearing tasks. These reports indicate that postural upper limb tremor is a frequent finding in primary orthostatic tremor patients. Whether it represents essential tremor or another form of tremor, perhaps even part of the syndrome of orthostatic tremor, has long been a matter of debate.

In essential tremor, leg tremor has been reported to occur in 15–30% of patients (26) but it is unusual for patients to describe a profound sensation of unsteadiness when standing. However, patients with essential tremor may complain of leg tremor when standing still (25,26). On clinical examination, essential tremor of the legs appears as an action tremor on standing and it is also evident during the activation of the leg muscles in any posture, irrespective of whether the patient is seated or walking. Essential tremor has a frequency of ~6–8 Hz, which occasionally can be reset by a peripheral stimulus, unlike orthostatic tremor.

In the study of Gerschlager et al. (6), age, onset age or duration of orthostatic tremor symptoms did not differ between the "pure orthostatic tremor" and "orthostatic tremor with postural arm tremor" groups. However, eight patients with "orthostatic tremor with postural arm tremor" had benefit from alcohol and five had a family history of a movement disorder, usually tremor, although it must be pointed out that these cases only constituted a small minority (8/24 alcohol benefit, 5/24 positive family history). In contrast, none of the patients with "pure orthostatic tremor" had a family history of a movement disorder and none had benefit from alcohol. Response to alcohol was not reported in the study of McManis and Sharbrough (5). Also, in a meta-analysis of 25 orthostatic tremor patients. Britton et al. (16) pointed out that the majority of their patients, had a postural arm tremor but only one had a modest benefit from alcohol.

It has been suggested that the postural 6–8 Hz arm tremor in orthostatic tremor patients might be a subharmonic of the high-frequency orthostatic tremor spreading throughout the body (22). The high frequency of the tremor and high coherence of tremor activity between the involved muscle groups, including the corresponding muscles on both sides of the body in orthostatic tremor, have led some authors to suggest that orthostatic tremor and essential tremor are probably different entities (5,8,16,22). Unfortunately in the large series of patients reported by Gerschlager et al. (6), electrophysiological assessment of the arm tremor was not carried out and the presence of arm tremor in this large number of patients became clear only during the retrospective analysis of the clinical details of the case notes. Thus, at present it remains uncertain whether the postural arm tremor in these orthostatic tremor patients is the same as essential tremor, whether orthostatic tremor leg tremor in these cases is part of essential tremor, or whether the postural arm tremor is part of orthostatic tremor (22). Further studies, including the discovery of genes for "classic" essential tremor may clarify this issue.

From the pharmacological point of view, orthostatic tremor and essential tremor appear to respond to different medications. Alcohol or β-adrenergic blocker responsiveness is not a feature of orthostatic tremor, yet both these drugs may produce dramatic improvement in essential tremor. Only clonazepam and primidone have been reported to improve orthostatic tremor.

All these findings suggest that, although there may be some overlap between orthostatic tremor and essential tremor, the presence of many clinical and neurophysiological differences between these two tremors, lead to the conclusion that they may represent distinct tremor syndromes.

It has also been speculated whether the presence of essential tremor, which is thought to be due to cerebellar dysfunction (27), could increase the susceptibility to develop orthostatic tremor by the double lesion model (6) discussed subsequently.

B. Relationship between Orthostatic Tremor, Parkinsonism and Other Movement Disorders

Orthostatic tremor can be associated with idiopathic PD (13,14). Two reports have suggested that dopaminergic drugs are of benefit in some patients with orthostatic tremor (13,28). Other cases of orthostatic tremor and associated idiopathic PD, one of whom had additional RLS/periodic limb movements in sleep, has been recently reported by Gerschlager et al. (6). Furthermore, orthostatic tremor was associated, in one patient each, with other forms of parkinsonism such as vascular parkinsonism (plus RLS), and drug-induced parkinsonism (6). Another patient had tardive dyskinesia while being treated with the dopamine blocking agent trifluoperazine. Gerschlager et al. (6) suggested that the association of parkinsonism and orthostatic tremor may be more than just chance and could suggest the pathophysiological mechanisms of orthostatic tremor. Gerschlager et al. (6) also pointed out the association of orthostatic tremor with RLS in four patients, two of whom, also had parkinsonism.

V. PATHOPHYSIOLOGY

Given the clinical features associated with orthostatic tremor there has been speculation about the pathophysiological mechanisms (6). Orthostatic tremor is considered to be caused by a central oscillator since high frequency tremor bursts are time locked in arm, leg, truncal and even facial muscles and peripheral stimulation does not reset the tremor (15,16,18,22,23). Some reports have suggested that the central generator may be located in the posterior fossa, because orthostatic tremor has been associated with lesions in the cerebellum and pons, but not with lesions in the cerebral hemispheres (7,9,10). A functional imaging study demonstrated that orthostatic tremor is associated with increased bilateral cerebellar activity (29). Moreover, it was reported that orthostatic tremor could be reset by electrical stimulation over the posterior fossa (16,24). The authors speculated that pontocerebellar fibers, which project to brainstem centers involved in postural control, may have been affected by the electrical stimulation. Since inhibition of voluntary EMG produced by stimulation over tendons, which has been attributed to effects from Golgi tendon organs (GTO), was not modulated in synchrony with the tremor, the authors concluded that the tremor is not expressed through GTO interneurons. Whatever the generator of orthostatic tremor, it is likely that it does not project directly to the motor neurons, but instead through fast conducting fibers, presumably the reticulospinal tract (24). These findings are of particular interest if considered with the possibility that orthostatic tremor may be associated with other movement disorders, such as parkinsonian syndromes and RLS.

Parkinsonian syndromes and also RLS are considered to be caused by dopaminergic deficiency or dysfunction (30–33). Also, electrophysiological abnormalities suggesting brainstem involvement occur in both PD and RLS (31,34–38). It has been hypothesized that brainstem abnormalities could result in disinhibition of reticulospinal excitatory responses and may cause an abnormal recruitment of spinal motor neurons. Thus it is possible that an abnormally active, but possibly structurally intact, oscillator in the posterior fossa is the cause of primary orthostatic tremor, whereas orthostatic tremor with other neurological signs may be the result of dysfunction of modulatory control of a higher motor center (the basal ganglia and/or brainstem) (6). These authors have suggested that subtle subclinical abnormalities of dopamine transmission at the level of the basal ganglia preceding the manifestation of PD, parkinsonian syndromes or RLS, could result in reticulospinal disinhibition and, consequently, deficient control of the oscillator leading to abnormal rhythmic activity manifesting as orthostatic tremor. Conceivably, this would happen only in susceptible individuals with pre-existing, yet subclinical, abnormalities of this oscillator. In other words, in these individuals orthostatic tremor would only develop if such a subtle oscillator dysfunction was coupled with another insult, for example, at the level of the basal ganglia or in the cerebellum as in essential tremor. In fact, a recent study found dopaminergic dysfunction, as evidenced by reduced dopamine transporter on single photon emission tomography (SPECT), in patients with orthostatic tremor alone (without any features of parkinsonism) (39). Similar "double lesion" models have been put forward in blepharospasm and cervical dystonia (40,41).

A. Clinical Course

Orthostatic tremor is generally considered a life-long condition once the movement disorder has started. However, the only available long-term follow-up study is that described by Gerschlager et al. (6). In this study, although no rating scales were used, in most orthostatic tremor patients (31 out of 41) the symptom severity was relatively unchanged over the years. However, in six cases the symptom severity (namely the amount of time they could stand still) subjectively got worse over the years.

Progression of symptoms has also been noted occasionally in the literature (3,8,13,14,16,42,43). All these observations suggest that only in a minority, orthostatic tremor may spread from the legs to the trunk and arms, and some patients can become symptomatic even when seated. However, a thorough prospective study using clinical and electrophysiological methods in a large cohort of patients is required to clarify this issue. One can conclude that orthostatic tremor symptoms can progress in some patients but in the large majority the condition remains static after initial onset.

VI. THERAPY

There is no generally accepted therapy for orthostatic tremor. Because this condition is very rare, and there are no prospective or controlled studies; only case reports or open studies in small groups of patients have been published. In general, clonazepam has been considered the first line treatment for orthostatic tremor and the improvement has been described as sustained (1–3,5,12,42–45). However, other investigators did not find a lasting response (16,21). In the study of Gerschlager et al. (6), only three out of 18 patients had a sustained benefit from clonazepam. In the same study, good and lasting improvement to primidone was observed in three out of seven patients while another four patients had some improvement only in the first few months of treatment. Others have also described this response pattern (3,5,18,46,47).

Similarly levodopa has been said to be beneficial. A good response was reported with 250 mg of levodopa three times daily over an eight week assessment period in five out of eight patients (13). Another patient taking clonazepam, described by Sander et al. (12), was said to show further improvement after the addition of 300 mg of sustained release levodopa twice daily (16). However, although levodopa may have some modulatory potential on the severity of orthostatic tremor, only two out of 15 patients described by Gerschlager et al. (6), both with typical PD experienced any long-lasting benefit (>2 years) on levodopa. Some patients may have a good response to valproic acid (5). Other drugs including propranolol, phenytoin, carbamazepine, lioresal, and acetazolamide seem to be ineffective.

REFERENCES

1. Heilman KM. Orthostatic tremor. Arch Neurol 1984; 41:880–881.
2. Papa SM, Gershanik OS. Orthostatic tremor: an essential tremor variant? Mov Disord 1988; 3:97–108.
3. FitzGerald PM, Jankovic J. Orthostatic tremor: an association with essential tremor. Mov Disord 1991; 6:60–64.
4. Deuschl G, Bain P, Brin M, and an Ad Hoc Scientific Committee. Consensus statement of the movement disorder society on tremor. Mov Disord 1998; 13:2–23.
5. McManis PG, Sharbrough FW. Orthostatic tremor: clinical and electrophysiologic characteristics. Muscle Nerve 1993; 16:1254–1260.
6. Gerschlager W, Münchau A, Katzenschlager R, Brown P, Rothwell JC, Quinn N, Lees AJ, Bhatia KP. Natural history and syndromic associations of orthostatic tremor: a review of 41 patients. Mov Disord 2004; 19(7):788–795.
7. Benito-Leon J, Rodriguez J, Orti-Pareja M, Ayuso-Peralta L, Jimenez-Jimenez FJ, Molina JA. Symptomatic orthostatic tremor in pontine lesions. Neurology 1997; 49:1439–1441.
8. Gabellini AS, Martinelli P, Gulli MR, Ambrosetto G, Ciucci G, Lugaresi E. Orthostatic tremor: essential and symptomatic cases. Acta Neurol Scand 1990; 81:113–117.
9. Setta F, Jaquy J, Hildebrand J, Manto MU. Orthostatic tremor associated with cerebellar ataxia. J Neurol 1998; 245:299–302.
10. Manto MU, Setta F, Legros B, Jaquy J, Godeaux E. Resetting of orthostatic tremor associated with cerebellar cortical atrophy by transcranial magnetic stimulation. Arch Neurol 1999; 56:1497–1500.
11. Sanitate SS, Meerschaert JR. Orthostatic tremor: delayed onset following head trauma. Arch Phys Med Rehabil 1993; 74:886–889.
12. Sander HW, Masdeu JC, Tavoulareas G, Walters A, Zimmermann T, Chokroverty S. Orthostatic tremor: an electrophysiological analysis. Mov Disord 1998; 13:735–738.
13. Wills AJ, Brusa L, Wang HC, Brown P, Marsden CD. Levodopa may improve orthostatic tremor: case report and trial of treatment. J Neurol Neurosurg Psychiatry 1999; 66:681–684.

14. Apartis E, Tison F, Arne P, Jedynak CP, Vidailhet M. Fast orthostatic tremor in Parkinson's disease mimicking primary orthostatic tremor. Mov Disord 2001; 16:1133–1136.
15. Thompson PD, Rothwell JC, Day BL, Berardelli A, Dick JP, Kachi T, Marsden CD. The physiology of orthostatic tremor. Arch Neurol 1986; 43:584–587.
16. Britton TC, Thompson PD, van der Kamp W, Rothwell JC, Day BL, Findley LJ, Marsden CD. Primary orthostatic tremor: further observations in six cases. J Neurol 1992; 239:209–217.
17. Britton TC, Thompson PD. Primary orthostatic tremor. BMJ 1995; 310:143–144.
18. Deuschl G, Lücking CH, Quintern J. Orthostatic tremor: clinical aspects, pathophysiology and therapy. EEG EMGZ. Elektroenzephalogr Elektromyogr Verwand Geb 1987; 18:13–19.
19. Deuschl G, Raethjen J, Lindemann M, Krack P. The pathophysiology of tremor. Muscle and Nerve 2001; 24:716–735.
20. Boroojerdi B, Ferbert A, Foltys H, Kosinski CM, Noth J, Schwarz M. Evidence for a non-orthostatic origin of orthostatic tremor. J Neurol Neurosurg Psychiatry 1999; 66:284–288.
21. Uncini A, Onofrj M, Basciani M, Cutarella R, Gambi D. Orthostatic tremor: report of two cases and an electrophysiological study. Acta Neurol Scand 1989; 79:119–122.
22. McAuley JH, Britton TC, Rothwell JC, Findley LJ, Marsden CD. The timing of primary orthostatic tremor bursts has a task-specific plasticity. Brain 2000; 123:254–266.
23. Koster B, Lauk M, Timmer J, Poersch M, Guschlbauer B, Deuschl G, Lucking CH. Involvement of cranial muscles and high intermuscular coherence in orthostatic tremor. Ann Neurol 1999; 45:384–388.
24. Wu YR, Ashby P, Lang AE. Orthostatic tremor arises from an oscillator in the posterior fossa. Mov Disord 2001; 16:272–279.
25. Wee AS, Subramony SH, Currier RD. "Orthostatic tremor" in familial-essential tremor. Neurology 1986; 36:1241–1245.
26. Cleeves L, Cowan J, Findley LG. Orthostatic tremor: diagnostic entity or variant of essential tremor. J Neurol Neurosurg Psychiatry 1987; 52:130–131.
27. Britton TC, Thompson PD, Day BL, Rothwell JC, Findley LJ, Marsden CD. Rapid wrist movements in patients with essential tremor. The critical role of the second agonist burst. Brain 1994; 117:39–47.
28. Finkel MF. Pramipexole is a possible effective treatment for primary orthostatic tremor (shaky leg syndrome). Arch Neurol 2000; 57:1519–1520.
29. Wills AJ, Thompson PD, Findley LJ, Brooks DJ. A positron emisson tomography study of primary orthostatic tremor. Neurology 1996; 46:747–752.
30. Gershanik OS. Drug-induced movement disorders. Curr Opin Neurol Neurosurg 1993; 6:369–376.
31. Bucher SF, Seelos KC, Oertel WH, Reiser M, Trenkwalder C. Cerebral generators involved in the pathogenesis of the restless legs syndrome. Ann Neurol 1997; 41:639–645.
32. Turjanski N, Lees AJ, Brooks DJ. Striatal dopaminergic function in restless legs syndrome: ^{18}F-dopa and ^{11}C-raclopride PET studies. Neurology 1999; 52:932–973.
33. Sethi KD. Movement disorders induced by dopamine blocking agents. Semin Neurol 2001; 21:59–68.
34. Wechsler LR, Stakes JW, Shahani BT, Busis NA. Periodic leg movements of sleep (nocturnal myoclonus): an electrophysiological study. Ann Neurol 1986; 19:168–173.

35. Delwaide PJ, Pepin JL, Maertens de Noordhout A. The audiospinal reaction in parkinsonian patients reflects functional changes in reticular nuclei. Ann Neurol 1993; 33:63–69.
36. Briellmann RS, Rosler KM, Hess CW. Blink reflex excitability is abnormal in patients with periodic leg movements in sleep. Mov Disord 1996; 11:710–714.
37. Lozza A, Pepin JL, Rapisarda G, Moglia A, Delwaide PJ. Functional changes of brain-stem reflexes in Parkinson's disease. Conditioning of the blink reflex R2 component by paired and index finger stimulation. J Neural Transm 1997; 104:679–687.
38. Bara-Jimenez W, Aksu M, Graham B, Sato S, Hallett M. Periodic limb movements in sleep. State dependent excitability of the spinal flexor reflex. Neurology 2000; 54:1609–1616.
39. Katzenschlager R, Costa D, Gerschlager W, Sullivan JO, Zijlmans J, Gacinov S, Pirker W, Wills A, Bhatia K, Lees AJ, Brown P. Dopamine transporter imaging with ^{123}I-FP-CIT-SPECT demonstrates dopaminergic deficit in orthostatic tremor. Ann Neurol 2003; 53:489–496.
40. Schicatano EJ, Basso MA, Evinger C. Animal model explains the origins of the cranial dystonia benign essential blepharospasm. J Neurophysiol 1997; 77:2842–2846.
41. Munchau A, Corna S, Gresty MA, Bhatia KP, Palmer JD, Dressler D, Quinn NP, Rothwell JC, Bronstein AM. Abnormal interaction between vestibular and voluntary head control in patients with spasmodic torticollis. Brain 2001; 124:47–59.
42. Gates PC. Orthostatic tremor (shaky legs syndrome). Clin Exp Neurol 1993; 30:66–71.
43. Poersch M. Orthostatic tremor: combined treatment with primidone and clonazepam [letter]. Mov Disord 1994; 9:467.
44. Vieregge P, Kompf D. Orthostatischer Tremor. Aktuel Neurol 1990; 17:69–72.
45. Brunotte P, Poburski R. Orthostatischer Tremor. Aktuel Neurol 1991; 17:36.
46. Zwan van der A, Verwey JC, van Gijn J. Relief of orthostatic tremor by primidone. Neurology 1988; 38:1332.
47. Willeit J, Deisenhammer F, Ransmayr G, Gerstenbrand F. Orthostatischer Tremor. Dtsch Med Wochenschr 1991; 116:1509–1512.

18

Task-Specific Tremor

Natividad P. Stover and Ray L. Watts

*University of Alabama at Birmingham,
Birmingham, Alabama, USA*

I. DEFINITION AND HISTORICAL BACKGROUND

Task-specific tremor is a kinetic tremor that appears or becomes exacerbated during highly skilled learned motor activities (1). This type of tremor is frequently denominated occupational tremor or focal tremor related to a particular action. The tremor usually occurs only when performing a specific repetitive task unique to each individual, but at times it may appear while performing similar movements and/or different activities that involve the same group of muscles.

The tremor may be evident as soon as the patient initiates the specific activity or it may have a latency period of a few seconds to a few minutes after beginning the performance of the task.

Primary writing tremor is the most frequent example of task-specific tremor. It was first described by Rothwell et al. (2) in 1979 in a 20 year old patient who complained of jerking of the right forearm manifested mainly during the act of writing. Active pronation of his forearm produced several beats of pronation/supination tremor. Many other cases of tremor resembling this first description have been reported.

Other task-specific tremors have been described in the hand only while swinging a golf club (3), only during bowing a violin (4), and only when holding a glass or a cup of a certain weight and size at a certain distance (5). Soland et al. (6) described nine cases of focal tremor induced by different tasks: when gripping an object in the palm of the left hand, without postural tremor and being able to write normally with this hand, head tremor in a horn player, tremor of the upper extremity while golfing, tremor of the index finger after soft tissue injury and removal of a plaster cast in a dental student with difficulty holding his dental instruments but without problem with handwriting or with other tasks, tremor in the hand when drinking from a saucer but not from a cup, hand tremor while throwing darts, head tremor when shooting, hand tremor while holding an ophthalmoscope in a specific position, and arm tremor in a bricklayer while using a trowel. Many other cases of isolated focal tremor when performing a specific activity have been reported in the voice (7,8), tongue (9), chin (10), jaw (11), and smile (12). Other examples include focal task-specific tremors and dystonias in musicians, athletes, tailors, cobblers, florists, fencers, turners, tinmen (5,13), telegraphists and typists (14) and in nurses while handling a syringe.

II. EPIDEMIOLOGY AND MEDICAL HISTORY

There are no prospective epidemiologic studies of this condition and the cases are usually not frequent in movement disorder clinics. Most of the cases of task-specific tremor are young to middle age adults and the condition is associated with a repetitive task that the patient usually performs on a daily basis. Bain et al. (15) reported a mean age of onset of 50.1 years and Klawans et al. (16) reported six patients with primary writing tremor with ages of eight to 54. Five patients described by Elble et al. (17) had an age range from 44 to 61 years. Kachi et al. (3) reported nine patients aged 21 to 61 with a mean age of 44 years and Ravits et al. (18) reported five patients aged 12 to 76 with a mean age of 47 years. Some cases had a family history of a similar disorder (19), but most of the cases were sporadic. There is an overwhelming predominance of males in the reported cases, but females are affected as well.

Specific data from the medical history are required, including the onset of the tremor, specific tasks that provoke the tremor, history of associated trauma, either focal or head trauma before the symptoms appeared, past neurological disease, family history of neurologic disorders, especially tremor and dystonia, sequence of spread including symmetry and laterality, alcohol sensitivity, medications, drug abuse, toxic exposures as well as associated signs of bradykinesia and akinesia, muscle tone changes, postural abnormalities and associated symptoms.

III. MANIFESTATIONS OF TASK-SPECIFIC TREMOR AND ASSOCIATED CONDITIONS

It is unknown whether task-specific tremor represents a type of essential tremor, a variant of dystonia, or a third distinct pathophysiologic entity. Another possibility is that all these symptoms may represent different manifestations of abnormal motor control in the spectrum of the same disease, since many times the clinical picture overlaps.

Task-specific tremor is seen most commonly in the hands, and specifically the right hand is the most affected area in the majority of the cases described, but the tongue, palate, wrists or fingers may be involved. Localization of the tremor in one hand is the standard but bilateral hand involvement has been described when the patient tried to write with the nonaffected hand (16,20). The tremor frequency is usually in the range of 4–10 Hz, and most of the cases have a frequency of 5–7 Hz.

The coexistence of tremor and dystonia is particularly evident in patients with task-specific movement disorders. Although position and task sensitivity provide few clues to the underlying etiology of tremor, its presence should raise the possibility of an underlying dystonia. Some authors defend the position that isolated focal, position specific, and task-specific tremor is probably a form of dystonia (6,17–19,21).

The presence of dystonia may not be evident on examination, and electromyographic (EMG) recording may be necessary to record the abnormal coactivation of antagonist muscles (6), a typical sign of dystonic movements. In other cases the subtle dystonic posturing of the affected limb may be overshadowed by the severity of the tremor. Many occupational dystonias often have an associated tremor and this is particularly evident in patients with writer's cramp, musician's cramp, or focal dystonias in which it is common to see an associated tremor. In this regard, it is postulated that these task-specific tremors may represent a type of focal dystonia. The dystonic posturing may have a latency period after writing several lines of a text and the tremor may be the only manifestation at the beginning of the task (22). Several studies have described patients with a combination of focal tremor and dystonia in the same limb (6). Marsden and Harrison (23) described eight patients in whom writer's cramp was the presenting symptom in a review of 42 patients with idiopathic torsion dystonia. This may represent a *forme fruste* of generalized dystonia in some cases.

Several authors have argued that task-specific tremor is a variant of essential tremor because it shares some of its electrophysiologic and clinical characteristics and responds to medications frequently used for essential tremor as well as alcohol (3,15,24–26). The typical picture in writing tremor consists of a rhythmic pronation/supination of the hand when attempting to write, the same pattern that is seen in essential tremor. Biary and Koller (9) described 20 patients with tongue tremor when the tongue was protruded associated with ET. In this study, dystonia, myoclonus, and tremor of other body parts were present in some patients. They concluded that this may represent a postural tremor of the tongue. The action or postural tremor of essential tremor may be considered a multi-task tremor and task-specific tremor may represent a subtype of typical essential tremor. Postural tremor is frequently seen in both conditions. One difference between task-specific tremor and essential tremor is the lack of family history in the former, a common characteristic of essential tremor. Another difference is that task-specific tremor is usually unilateral and has the tendency to remain focal. On the other hand, a family study of hereditary essential tremor in 20 patients and 141 relatives performed by Bain et al. (27) showed no cases of task-specific tremor or isolated head, tongue, voice, jaw, trunk or leg tremors.

Trauma is another condition that has been associated in this spectrum of symptoms. Four patients with primary writing tremor in the study of Bain et al. (15) had a history of preceding trauma to the dominant hand, one with a fracture of the metacarpal bones and a residual bony deformity, one with a mallet deformity of the ring finger and two with a history of carpal tunnel syndrome. The role of trauma in precipitating movement disorders is another element to suggest a link between focal task-specific tremor and dystonia. Peripheral trauma is a well documented trigger of focal dystonia (28–30). The trauma may not be the etiology of the disorder but may facilitate the manifestation of the symptoms in patients with a genetic predisposition.

The first case described of primary writing tremor had a history of meningitis at the age of nine with full recovery after treatment with antibiotics, and a latency of three years until he developed the tremor while writing. One of the patients described by Soland et al. (6) in his series of focal task-specific tremors, had a history of head trauma with a sequelae of dysarthria as a result of the insult. Past medical history of perinatal hypoxia has also been described in two patients with primary writing tremor (16).

Finally, tremor on handwriting or performing other tasks may occur as part of a more widespread and extensive neurological disorder such as Parkinson's disease, parkinsonism, essential tremor, or dystonia, and a complete neurological examination to determine associated signs and symptoms is warranted before designating the disorder as an isolated primary task-specific tremor. Although isolated tremor can occur in Parkinson's disease, it usually affects the arm and/or the leg, does not have task-specificity, and is frequently associated with other symptoms like bradykinesia and rigidity (31–34).

Cohen et al. (19) studied seven members of a family who had different types of movement disorders: two had essential tremor, two (twins) had typical writer's cramp, a form of focal dystonia, one had both essential tremor and writer's cramp, one had primary writing tremor and one had uncharacterized tremor. The high incidence of tremor and focal dystonia in this family suggests a genetic transmission. The appearance of subclinical tremor in one of the monozygotic twins with writer's cramp suggests that tremor and dystonia can be manifestations of the same genetic defect.

A. Primary Writing Tremor

Writing tremor has been extensively studied clinically after the initial description by Rothwell et al. (3,16,18,19,25,35–39). Two forms of primary writing tremor have been described: (1) type specific tremor characterized by tremor appearing during writing only, (2) tremor that occurs when the hand adopts a writing position, known as position specific or position sensitive tremor (15). Some patients with writing tremor also have dystonic posturing, and some patients with writer's cramp have tremor. Careful clinical and electrophysiological examination of the patient with writing tremor described by Rothwell et al., showed short bursts of rhythmic oscillations, synchronicity in all muscles, and at times myoclonic jerks of 4–6 Hz in the hand and the arm. The pronator teres muscle fired at a higher frequency that the rest of the muscles. The tremor frequency and the fact that the symptoms in this patient improved with alcohol, at least temporarily, are two characteristics seen in patients with essential tremor. Deep tendon reflexes, coordination exam, electroencephalogram (EEG), nerve conduction studies and somatosensory evoked potentials were within normal limits, and he did not have family history of neurologic disorders. Stretch-reflex amplitudes and latencies were normal in the cases studied. Some series of patients described patterns of abnormal coactivation of muscles in the arm and shoulder in the EMG studies which represented an association with writer's cramp. Nearly half of the patients with writer's cramp exhibited a superimposed tremor. Many patients develop incapacitating tremor while writing or drawing and they may be forced to change many activities and their occupation.

B. Task-Specific Jaw Tremor

Miles et al. (11) described a patient with a prominent highly specific 5–6 Hz jaw tremor that began only when the patient drank from a cup or a glass, when the teeth were together or when moving the jaw voluntarily to the right, but the tremor did not occur when eating. Neurologic exam and magnetic resonance imaging (MRI) of the brain were normal. This tremor was restricted to the mandible and confined to the digastric muscle. The jaw opening muscles did not contain muscle spindles, they did not have involvement of the antagonist masseter and there was not a reciprocal inhibitory reflex as was found in the limbs. EMG recording demonstrated high amplitude, rhythmical bursting activity in the digastric muscle at ~6 Hz and the EMG activity of the left and right masseters was minimal. The same pattern of tremor was found when the patient placed the front teeth edge to edge. The etiology of the tremor was hypothesized to be from a central oscillator that drives the masticatory muscles at a frequency of 5 Hz without increased muscle spindle excitability. Whether this is a pure task-specific tremor or it is related to a focal dystonia is unclear.

C. Tremor of the Smile

Jacome et al. (12) observed isolated bilateral idiopathic 5–6 Hz tremor of the face induced only by spontaneous or volitional contraction of the risori muscles in a 27-year-old woman with a nine year history of perioral tremor. In this case, the father had a similar tremor and the neurological examination and brain MRI were normal. Unilateral muscle contraction of the risorius induced ipsilateral tremor only. EEG showed no myoclonic jerks and EMG studies were normal. This tremor was considered a focal task-specific tremor or an action tremor that may represent a form of familial essential tremor.

D. Voice Tremor

Isolated voice tremor is present if vocalization is tremulous but no other parts of the body show tremor (8). This is an involuntary rhythmic oscillation in the pitch and loudness of vocal sounds, mainly vowels, resulting in tremulous and quivering speech and voice arrest at times (7). Tremor occurs when patients pronounce long words or sounds (40). The tremor frequency varies from 3–8 Hz. Voice tremor is present in 20% of patients with essential tremor (21,27,41–43). This tremor must be differentiated from spasmodic dysphonia that is related to dystonia of the laryngeal muscles. Video examination of the vocal cords is usually helpful in differentiating these conditions. Abductor dysphonia produces a whispering, low volume speech pattern, usually without tremor, and adductor dysphonia produces a hoarse strained voice, arising from hyperadduction of the true and false vocal cords (44–48). Voice tremor does occur in other conditions such as Parkinson's disease, cerebellar disease or amyotrophic lateral sclerosis, together with other manifestations.

E. Tongue Tremor

Biary and Koller (9) described three patients with isolated tongue tremor at a frequency of 4–6 Hz when the tongue was protruded. In this study, one patient had tongue tremor and writing tremor, one had tongue tremor and spasmodic torticollis, and one had tremor in the tongue, hands, head, and lips. The rest of the 20 patients in this study had tongue and hand tremor. The frequency of the tongue tremor was the same as the hand tremor in individual patients.

IV. PATHOPHYSIOLOGY OF TASK-SPECIFIC TREMOR

It is unclear why the tremor associated with task-specific movement disorders occurs only during such a limited range of possible movements. It may be that the activation of different muscles by a determined oscillator could depend on the command signal used to select different tasks. Several surveys failed to identify clearly involved risk factors. One of the strongest points in support of a common pathogenetic mechanism in the different task-specific and non task-specific movement disorders is their occurrence in different members of the same family.

Rothwell et al., in one patient with writing tremor, were able to abolish the tremor by partial motor point anesthesia of the pronator teres muscle and he concluded that the tremor was originated by an abnormal response to muscle spindle discharge and increased excitability of the involved muscles. Rondot et al. (49) also noted that motor point anesthesia of a critical or oscillator muscle may abolish postural tremor in essential tremor and tremor associated with cerebellar disease. They argued that such tremor was generated by proprioceptive input from the critical muscle. There is, however, a growing body of evidence supporting the notion that central oscillators are important in the generation of physiological and pathological tremors. Intracellular recordings have demonstrated that neurons in the inferior olive and other brain stem and subcortical nuclei have spontaneous oscillatory activity (50–53).

The relationship between task-specific tremor and other movement disorders is not clearly defined. Central etiology is most likely the best explanation in patients with focal task-specific tremor or dystonia and even though the symptoms may exist in isolation they frequently overlap. The task-specific jaw tremor reported by Miles et al. (11) suggests that the tremor originates from a central oscillator that drives the masticatory muscles, since the jaw opening muscles are not involved in a reciprocal inhibitory reflex with the masseters.

Recent investigations of musicians and other patients with focal dystonias support the idea that these patients have a central disorder of motor control since the representation in the primary sensory cortex of the part of the body that is affected is markedly disordered in dystonic patients and in primate models of dystonia. In patients with primary writing tremor there is no evidence for excessive overflow in the rhythmic EMG activity and forearm reciprocal inhibition is normal in most of the patients. Cortical activation patterns and somatosensory cortical representation are also abnormal in patients with focal dystonia during the performance of motor tasks with significant increases in the size of the receptive fields. This is especially evident in cases of tremor or dystonia after trauma. There is an ongoing debate regarding whether the use or overuse of a group of muscles involved in a specific task plays a role in the genesis of the abnormal movement.

The concept that a focal movement disorder may occur as part of a more widespread motor disturbance has been proposed in several series of patients. Rosenbaum and Jankovic (5) performed a study of 28 patients with focal task-specific disorders: one group had focal tremor alone, another group had dystonia alone and a third group had a combination of tremor and dystonia. The coexistence of focal tremor and focal dystonia in the same limb in 10 patients of this study suggests a link between these focal disorders.

V. DISABILITY AND TREATMENT

The fact that the tremor usually affects a specific task that the patient performs frequently can be quite disabling and compromise employment. One of the strongest factors that relates the task-specific tremor to essential tremor or dystonia is that this tremor responds to medications that are beneficial for these conditions. Also, task-specific tremor may be temporarily relieved by the use of alcohol, a hallmark of many cases of essential tremor (Refs. 3,15,24,26).

Case reports describe improvement with the use of beta blockers and primidone, as well as with anticholinergic medications and benzodiazepines (Ref. 15). The best result with beta blockers has been reported with propanolol, but other medications in this category may also be effective (Refs. 7,24). The strategy to start treatment with one or another depends on associated factors or concomitant medical problems. If alcohol intake has a beneficial effect on the symptoms, starting with medications that are effective for essential tremor are the first recommended step. Treatment with amantadine, levodopa or dopamine agonists has not been reported to be effective (Ref. 5).

Anticholinergic medications are the next group of medications that have been associated with control of the symptoms in task-specific tremor but a close vigilance of the patients is warranted as side effects are a frequent occurrence (Ref. 27). A combination of medications is another option in patients resistant to monotherapy.

Botulinum toxin is also an option in some cases, but tremor reduction is often accompanied by weakness. The study of the muscles that may have a major contribution in the abnormal movements may be the best way to choose the muscles to be targeted with botulinum toxin treatment (54–57).

Deep brain stimulation of the ventralis intermedius (VIM) nucleus of the thalamus or thalamotomy has reduced primary writing tremor in several open label studies (58–61).

REFERENCES

1. Deuschl G, Bain P, Brin M. Consensus statement of the Movement Disorder Society on tremor. Ad Hoc Scientific Committee. Mov Disord 1998; 13(3):2–23.
2. Rothwell JC, Traub MM, Marsden CD. Primary writing tremor. J Neurol Neurosurg Psychiatry 1979; 42:1106–1114.
3. Kachi T, Rothwell JC, Cowan JMA, Marsden CD. Writing tremor: its relationship to benign essential tremor. J Neurol Neurosurg Psychiatry 1995; 48:545–550.
4. Cleeves L, Findley LJ, Marsden CD. Odd tremors. In: Marsden CD, Fahn S, eds. Movement Disorders 3. Oxford: Butterworth-Heinemann, 1994:434–458.
5. Rosenbaum F, Jankovic J. Focal task-specific tremor and dystonia: categorization of occupational movement disorders. Neurology 1988; 38(4):522–527.
6. Soland VL, Bhatia KP, Volonte MA, Marsden CD. Focal task-specific tremors. Mov Disord 1996; 11(6):665–670.

7. Koller WC, Graner D, Mlcoch A. Essential voice tremor: treatment with propanolol. Neurology 1985; 35:106–108.
8. Hachinski VC, Thomsen IV, Buch NH. The nature of primary vocal tremor. Can J Neurol Sci 1975; 2:195–197.
9. Biary N, Koller WC. Essential tongue tremor. Mov Disord 1987; 2:25–29.
10. Fahn S. Atypical, rare and unclassified tremors. In: Findley LJ, Capildeo R, eds. Movement Disordes: Tremor. London: Macmillan, 1984:85–93.
11. Miles TS, Findley LJ, Rothwell JC. Electrophysiological observations on an unusual, task-specific jaw tremor. J Neurol Neurosurg Psychiatry 1997; 63(2):251–254.
12. Jacome DE, Yanez GF. Tremors of the smile. J Neurol Neurosurg Psychiatry 1987; 50:489–490.
13. Sheedy MP, Marsden CD. Writer's cramp, a focal dystonia. Brain 1982; 105:461–480.
14. Marsden CD. The focal dystonias. Clin Neuropharmacol 1986; 9(2):49–60.
15. Bain PG, Findley LJ, Britton TC, Rothwell JC, Gresty MA, Thompson PD, Marsden CD. Primary writing tremor. Brain 1995; 118:1461–1472.
16. Klawans HL, Glantz R, Tanner CM, Goetz CG. Primary writing tremor: a selective action tremor. Neurology 1982; 32:203–206.
17. Elble RJ, Moody C, Higgins C. Primary writing tremor. A form of focal dystonia? Mov Disord 1990; 5:118–126.
18. Ravits J, Hallet M, Baker M, Wilkins D. Primary writing tremor and myoclonic writer's cramp. Neurology 1985; 35(9):1387–1391.
19. Cohen LG, Hallett M, Sudarsky L. A single family with writer's cramp, essential tremor, and primary writing tremor. Mov Disord 1987; 2:109–116.
20. Jimenez-Jimenez FJ, Cabrera-Valdivia F, Orti-Pareja M, Gasalla T, Tallon-Barranco A, Zurdo M. Bilateral primary writing tremor. Eur J Neurol 1998; 5(6): 613–614.
21. Elble RJ. Diagnostic criteria for essential tremor and differential diagnosis. Neurology 2000; 54(4):2–6.
22. Koller WC, Glatt S, Biary N, Rubino FA. Essential tremor variants: effect of treatment. Clin Neuropharmacol 1987; 10:342–350.
23. Marsden CD, Harrison MJG. Idiopathic torsion dystonia (dystonia musculorum deformans): a review of forty-two patients. Brain 1974; 97:797–810.
24. Koller WC, Martyn B. Writing tremor: its relationship to essential tremor. J Neurol Neurosurg Psychiatry 1986; 49:220.
25. Martinelli P, Gabellini AS, Gulli MR, Lugaresi E. different clinical features of essential tremor: a 200-patient study. Acta Neurol Scand 1987; 75:106–111.
26. Koller WC, Biary N. Effect of alcohol on tremors: comparison with propanolol. Neurology 1984; 34:221–222.
27. Bain PG, Findley LJ, Thompson PD, Gresty MA, Rothwell JC, Harding AE, Marsden CD. A study of hereditary essential tremor. Brain 1994; 117:805–824.
28. Lee MS, Rinne JO, Ceballos-Baumann A, Thompson PD, Marsden CD. Dystonia after head trauma. Neurology 1994; 44:1374–1378.
29. Frucht SJ, Fahn S, Ford B. Focal task-specific dystonia induced by peripheral trauma. Mov Disord 2000; 15(2):348–350.
30. Frucht SJ, Fahn S, Greene PE, O'Brien C, Gelb M, Truong DD, Welsh J, Factor S, Ford B. The natural history of embouchure dystonia. Mov Disord 2001; 16(5):899–906.

31. Morrison S, Newell KM. Limb stiffness and postural tremor in the arm. Motor Control 2000; 4(3):293–315.
32. Ackermann H, Konczak J, Hertrich I. The temporal control of repetitive articulatory movements in Parkinson's disease. Brain and Language 1997; 56(2):312–319.
33. Watts RL, Mandir AS, Ahn KJ, Juncos JL, Zakers GO, Freeman A. Electrophysiologic analysis of early Parkinson's disease. Neurology 1991; 41(2):44–48; discussion 48–49.
34. Brooks DJ, Playford ED, Ibanez V, Sawle GV, Thompson PD, Findley LJ, Marsden CD. Isolated tremor and disruption of the nigrostriatal dopaminergic system: an 18F-dopa PET study. Neurology 1992; 42:1554–1560.
35. Anonymous. Writing tremor and writing dystonia. Mov Disord 1990; 5:354–355.
36. Nicaretta DH, Pereira JS, Pimentel NL. Writing tremor: report of a case. Arq Neuropsiquiatr 1994; 52:87–89.
37. Kim JS, Lee Mc. Writing tremor after discrete cortical infarction. Stroke 1994; 25:2280–2282.
38. Wills AJ, Jenkins IH, Thompson PD, Findley LJ, Brooks DJ. A positrom emission tomography study of cerebral activation with essential tremor and writing tremor. Arch Neurol 1995; 52(3):299–305.
39. Bain PG, Mally J, Gresty M, Findley LJ. Assessing the impact of essential tremor on upper limb function. J Neurol 1993; 241(1):54–61.
40. Brown JR, Simpson J. Organic voice tremor. Neurology 1963;13:520–525.
41. Lou JS, Jankovic J. Essential tremor: clinical correlates in 350 patients. Neurology 1991; 47:234–238.
42. Findley LJ, Gresty MA. Head, facial, and voice tremor. Adv Neurol 1988; 49:239–253.
43. Massey EW, Paulson GW. Essential vocal tremor: clinical characteristics and response to therapy. South Med J 1985; 78:316–317.
44. Aminoff MJ, Dedo HH, Izdebski K. Clinical aspects of spasmodic dysphonia. J Neuro Neurosurg Psychiatry 1978; 41:361–365.
45. Aronson AE, Brown JR, Litin EM, Pearson JS. Spastic dysphonia. II: Comparison with essential (voice) tremor and other neurologic and psychogenic dysphonias. J Speech Hear Disord 1968; 33:219–231.
46. Blitzer A, Brin MF, Stewart C, Aviv J, Fahn S. Abductor laryngeal dystonia: a series treated with botulinum toxin. Laryngoscope 1992; 102:163–167.
47. Pool KD, Freeman FJ, Finitzo T, Hayashi MM, Chapman SB, Devous MD, Close LG Sr, Kondraske GV, Mendelsohn D, Schaefer SD. Heterogeneity in spasmodic dysphonia. Neurologic and voice findings. Arch Neurol 1991; 48:305–309.
48. Hillel AD. The study of laryngeal muscle activity in normal human subjects and in patients with laryngeal dystonia using multiple fine-wire electromyography. Laryngoscope 2001; 111(97):1–47.
49. Rondot MD, Korn H, Scherrer J. Suppression of an entire limb tremor by anesthetizing a selective muscular group. Arch Neurol 1968; 19:421–429.
50. Lamarre Y. Animal models of physiological, essential and parkinsonian-like tremors. In: Findley LJ, Capildeo R, eds. Movement Disorders: Tremor. New York: Oxford University Press, 1984:183–194.
51. Llinas RR. The intrinsic electrophysiological properties of mammalian neurons: insights into central nervous system functions. Science 1988; 242:1654–1664.
52. Kepler TB, Marder E, Abbott LF. The effect of electrical coupling on the frequency of model neuronal oscillators. Science 1990; 248:83–85.

53. Schnitzler A, Gross J, Timmermann L. Synchronised oscillations of the human sensorimotor cortex. Acta Neurobiol Exp (Wars) 2000; 60(2):271–287.
54. Jankovic J. Treatment of tremors with botulinum toxin. In: Jankovic J, ed. Neurological Disease and Therapy. Therapy with Botulinum Toxin. Vol. 25. New York: Marcel Dekker, 1994:493–502.
55. Jankovic J, Schwartz K. Botulinum toxin treatment of tremors. Neurology 1991; 41:1185–1188.
56. Ludlow CL, Sedory SE, Fujita M, Naunton RF. Treatment of voice tremor with botulinum toxin injection. Neurology 1989; 39(1):353.
57. Ludlow CL. Treatment of speech and voice disorders with botulinum toxin. JAMA 1990; 264:2671–2675.
58. Deuschl G, Bain P. Deep brain stimulation for tremor [correction of trauma]: patient selection and evaluation. Mov Disord 2002; 17(3):S102–S111.
59. Ohye C, Miyazaki M, Hirai T, Shibasaki T, Nakajima H, Nageseki Y. Primary writing tremor treated by stereotaxic selective thalamotomy. J Neurol Neurosurg Psychiatry 1982; 45:988–997.
60. Hirai T, Miyazaki M, Nakajima H, Shibasaki T, Ohye C. The correlation between tremor characteristics and the predicted volume of effective lesions in stereotaxic nucleus ventralis intermedius thalamotomy. Brain 1983; 106:1001–1018.
61. Minguez-Castellanos A, Carnero-Pardo C, Gomez-Camello A et al. Primary writing tremor treated by chronic thalamic stimulation. Mov Disord 1999; 14:1030–1033.

19

Neuropathic Tremor

David S. Saperstein and Richard J. Barohn

University of Kansas Medical Center, Kansas City, Kansas, USA

Tremor may be observed in patients with peripheral nerve disorders. The occurrence of tremor in immune-mediated demyelinating and hereditary peripheral neuropathies has been the most extensively documented, and a peripheral neuropathy patient with tremor is most likely to have one of these disorders. Tremor may also occur in certain forms of inherited motor neuron disease, such as spinal muscular atrophy and X-linked bulbospinal atrophy. It remains unknown why some peripheral neuropathy patients develop tremor while other similarly affected patients do not. Genetic factors may play a role in some cases. This chapter will review the most common tremor syndromes associated with peripheral nerve disorders.

I. IMMUNE-MEDIATED POLYNEUROPATHIES

Tremor is mentioned as a feature in some patients with Guillain-Barré syndrome (especially the rare, relapsing form of this disease) (1,2) and chronic inflammatory demyelinating polyneuropathy (CIDP) (3). However, the strongest association and most extensive documentation of tremor has been for patients with demyelinating neuropathy associated with a monoclonal protein, most commonly IgM. In these cases, the monoclonal protein typically represents a monoclonal gammopathy of undetermined significance (MGUS). This entity is described in the literature under a number of different names, such as CIDP-MGUS, IgM neuropathy, and anti-myelin associated glycoprotein (MAG) neuropathy. It is now clear that this peripheral nerve disorder is distinct from CIDP and shows consistent clinical features: male predominance, older age of onset, slow progression, predominantly sensory manifestations, especially sensory ataxia, and poor response to immunomodulating therapies (4,5). Nerve conduction studies show demyelinating features, but a distinct and consistent feature is significantly prolonged motor distal latencies (4,5). In 50–70% of cases the IgM monoclonal protein recognizes MAG (4). It is unclear whether there are clinically relevant differences between IgM demyelinating neuropathy patients with or without MAG reactivity (4). Serum immune fixation electrophoresis is more sensitive than routine protein electrophoresis for detection of a monoclonal protein (6). A small percentage of MAG-positive patients will not have a detectable monoclonal protein (7). Therefore, in patients who have clinical and nerve conduction study features classic for IgM demyelinating neuropathy but who lack a monoclonal protein, a MAG assay can help confirm the diagnosis.

Upper extremity tremor occurs in 40–90% of patients with IgM demyelinating neuropathy (3,8–13). This tremor is postural with a frequency of 3–6 Hz (3,14). There may also be a kinetic component. There is a single report of rest tremor (11). The tremor involves distal muscles, usually at or below the wrist. The presence of tremor is not associated with upper extremity proprioceptive loss, weakness or other clinical exam findings (3,13,14). The occurrence of tremor varies among patients at similar stages of the neuropathy (13), and many patients never develop tremor despite a long disease duration. In one series, tremor appeared a mean of three years after the onset of neuropathy (14). Tremor is rarely the presenting symptom (10,14), and only one reported patient had a family history of tremor (14). There are other important ways in which the tremor that occurs in IgM demyelinating neuropathy contrasts from essential tremor such as male predominance, late age of onset, and poor response to ethanol (14). In addition, the percentage of IgM demyelinating neuropathy patients with tremor is more than 10-fold greater than the expected prevalence of essential tremor (14).

The precise pathophysiology of this tremor remains uncertain. Delayed and/or distorted afferent input has been postulated, but this fails to explain why some, but not other, patients develop tremor (14). Several series found indirect evidence of central nervous system involvement. Leger et al. (12) found three of 12 patients with central conduction latencies. In another series, six of 12 patients had abnormal visual evoked potentials (15). White matter lesions may be seen on brain magnetic resonance imaging (MRI) scans of these patients, but these findings are not clearly abnormal for age (12,16). Bain et al. (14) did not find any clear abnormalities of central conduction using somatosensory evoked potentials and magnetic stimulation. More impressive evidence for central involvement has come from functional imaging. Positron emission tomography (PET) scans show that patients with IgM demyelinating neuropathy and tremor show activation of the cerebellar hemispheres (17,18). This is the same finding seen in patients with essential tremor (17–19).

The tremor in IgM demyelinating neuropathy patients does not respond to immunomodulating therapies (3,13,14). This is not surprising since the neuropathic deficits do not respond well to such therapies either (4). Mixed and modest improvement from tremor-specific therapies, such as propranolol and clonazepam, has been described (3,14). This tremor is often not a significant problem for the patient; however, when tremor is bothersome or interferes with activities, therapies used for essential tremor are a treatment option. Weide et al. (20) described a patient whose tremor and neuropathy improved following treatment with rituximab. Rituximab is a chimeric mouse–human monoclonal antibody directed against the B cell surface membrane protein CD20. Treatment with rituximab prevents B cell production and is used in the treatment of certain B cell lymphomas. Two small, open series have reported improved symptoms and findings in some IgM demyelinating neuropathy patients following rituximab treatment, but tremor is not mentioned (21,22). Experience with rituximab in IgM demyelinating neuropathy is still limited and it remains to be seen what role this agent will play in management. There is a single report of deep brain stimulation (DBS) used to treat tremor in IgM demyelinating neuropathy. Ruzicka et al. (23) described good tremor suppression and functional improvements in a 72-year-old man with a 21 year history of tremor treated with DBS of the ventral intermediate (VIM) thalamic nucleus.

II. HEREDITARY MOTOR AND SENSORY NEUROPATHY

Hereditary motor and sensory neuropathy, also known as Charcot-Marie-Tooth (CMT) disease, is characterized by foot deformities, weakness, and atrophy affecting primarily the anterior compartment muscles in the lower leg. In 1926, Roussy and Lévy (24) described seven patients from a large, multigenerational kindred with an autosomal dominant peripheral neuropathy demonstrating clinical features of CMT, but also prominent tremor and gait unsteadiness. This gave rise to the term "Roussy-Lévy syndrome" (RLS) to describe patients with a CMT phenotype and postural tremor. From the beginning there were suspicions that RLS and CMT represented the same disorder (25). This was supported by nerve biopsies from RLS patients showing a hypertrophic demyelinating neuropathy, suggestive of CMT type 1 (26–28).

Several different genes are responsible for CMT 1. Approximately 70% of the cases of CMT 1 are caused by a duplication of the PMP22 gene on chromosome 17 (CMT 1A) and 20% are caused by mutations in the myelin protein zero

(MPZ) gene on chromosome 1 (CMT 1B). Demyelinating CMT can also be caused by mutations in the connexin 32 gene on the X chromosome (CMT X). Thomas et al. (29) examined the phenotype of 61 patients with CMT 1A. Thirteen percent had a RLS phenotype. This phenotype, however, is genetically heterogeneous. Genetic testing of members of the original family studied by Roussy and Lévy revealed mutations in MPZ (CMT 1B) (30). A RLS phenotype has also been associated with CMT X (31). Among RLS families, some affected members will have a RLS phenotype whereas others (carrying the same mutation) will have a typical CMT phenotype without tremor (29,31,32). In one CMT X family, a women manifested tremor but no clinical features of neuropathy (31). The presence of tremor in some family members but not others raises the question of a second gene defect. In these families tremor is not usually seen in family members without neuropathy, arguing against a co-occurrence of CMT and essential tremor as an explanation for the RLS phenotype. The mechanism for tremor in these patients is not known. Since the tremor resembles that seen in patients with IgM demyelinating neuropathy, it is tempting to speculate a shared pathogenesis. Tremor is not restricted to CMT patients with demyelinating neuropathies and can be observed in axonal CMT (type 2) (25). Overall, tremor can be seen in approximately one third of all CMT patients (25,33), so RLS should not be considered as a separate entity. There are currently no reports addressing medical or surgical treatment of tremor associated with CMT.

III. MOTOR NEURON DISEASE

Involuntary movements may be seen in spinal muscular atrophy (SMA). Tremor-like movements have been described in patients with mild and moderate, but not severe, forms of SMA (34–36). These movements have been attributed to weakness (34) or fasciculations (35). In contrast, Spiro (36) called these movements "minipolymyoclonus." Minipolymyoclonus is a coarse, irregular tremor, seen predominantly in the hands. It is best demonstrated with the arms extended and fingers spread (37). Stress, fatigue, and anxiety affect the rate and amplitude of the movements (36). Minipolymyoclonus appears to be specific for SMA, assisting in distinguishing SMA from myopathies and other causes of hypotonic weakness in children. An interesting feature of these movements is that they usually produce coarse artifacts on electrocardiograms (ECG), especially from the limb leads (38,39). Finding such spikes on a routine ECG can be a clue in diagnosis.

Tremor is a characteristic manifestation of X-linked bulbospinal neuropathy, also known as Kennedy disease (40). In one series, >80% of patients had postural tremor (41). Kennedy disease patients frequently have decreased lower extremity sensation and abnormal nerve conduction studies indicative of peripheral neuropathy. In contrast to CMT, Kennedy disease patients have proximal, not distal, weakness. Gynecomastia and facial/tongue fasciculations are helpful hints to the diagnosis, but are not present in all Kennedy disease patients.

IV. FOCAL PERIPHERAL NERVE LESIONS

Myokymia caused by peripheral nerve lesions can produce tremor-like movements. Streib (42) described involuntary movements of the 4th and 5th fingers produced in a patient with ulnar neuropathy at the wrist. These finger movements coincided with bursts of myokymia, detected on electromyography of the 3rd and 4th interosseous muscles.

REFERENCES

1. Thomas PK, Lascelles RG, Hallpike JF, Hewer RL. Recurrent and chronic relapsing Guillain-Barré polyneuritis. Brain 1969; 92:589–606.
2. Grand'Maison F, Feasby TE, Hahn AF, Koopman WJ. Recurrent Guillain-Barré syndrome. Clinical and laboratory features. Brain 1992; 115:1093–1106.
3. Dalakas MC, Teräväinen H, King Engel W. Tremor as a feature of chronic relapsing and dysgammaglobulinemic polyneuropathies. Arch Neurol 1984; 41:711–714.
4. Saperstein DS, Katz JS, Amato AA, Barohn RJ. Clinical spectrum of chronic acquired demyelinating polyneuropathies. Muscle Nerve 2001; 24:311–324.
5. Katz JS, Saperstein DS, Gronseth G, Amato AA, Barohn RJ. Distal acquired demyelinating symmetric neuropathy. Neurology 2000; 54:615–620.
6. Vrethem M, Larsson, von Schenck, Ernerudh J. Immunofixation superior to agarose elctropheresis in detecting small M-components in patients with polyneuropathy. J Neurol Sci 1993; 120:93–98.
7. Nobile-Orazio E, Latov N, Hays AP, Takatsu M, Abrams GM, Sherman WH, Miller JR, Messito MJ, Saito T, Tahmoush A. Neuropathy and anti-MAG antibodies without detectable serum M-protein. Neurology 1984; 34:218–221.
8. Smith IS, Kahn SN, Lacey BW, King RH, Eames RA, Whybrew DJ, Thomas PK. Chronic demyelinating neuropathy associated with benign IgM paraproteinaemia. Brain 1983; 106:169–195.
9. Mendell JR, Sahenk Z, Whitaker JN, Trapp BD, Yates AJ, Griggs RC, Quarles RH. Polyneuropathy and IgM monoclonal gammopathy: studies on the pathogenetic role of anti-myelin-associated glycoprotein antibody. Ann Neurol 1985; 17:243–254.
10. Nobile-Orazio E, Marmiroli P, Baldini L, Spagnol G, Barbieri S, Moggio M, Polli N, Polli E, Scarlato G. Peripheral neuropathy in macroglobulinemia: incidence and antigen-specificity of M proteins. Neurology 1987; 37:1506–1514.
11. Yeung KB, Thomas PK, King RH, Waddy H, Will RG, Hughes RA, Gregson NA, Leibowitz S. The clinical spectrum of peripheral neuropathies associated with benign monoclonal IgM, IgG and IgA paraproteinaemia. Comparative clinical, immunological and nerve biopsy findings. J Neurol 1991; 238:383–391.
12. Leger JM, Younes-Chennoufi AB, Zuber M, Bouche P, Jauberteau MO, Dormont D, Danon F, Baumann N, Brunet P. Frequency of central lesions in polyneuropathy associated with IgM monoclonal gammopathy: an MRI, neurophysiological and immunochemical study. J Neurol Neurosurg Psychiatry 1992; 55:112–115.

13. Smith IS. The natural history of chronic demyelinating neuropathy associated with benign IgM paraproteinaemia. A clinical and neurophysiological study. Brain 1994; 117:949–957.

14. Bain PG, Britton TC, Jenkins IH, Thompson PD, Rothwell JC, Thomas PK, Brooks DJ, Marsden CD. Tremor associated with benign IgM paraproteinaemic neuropathy. Brain 1996; 119:789–799.

15. Barbieri S, Nobile-Orazio E, Baldini L, Fayoumi Z, Manfredini E, Scarlato G. Visual evoked potentials in patients with neuropathy and macroglobulinemia. Ann Neurol 1987; 22:663–666.

16. Hawke SH, Hallinan JM, McLeod JG. Cranial magnetic resonance imaging in chronic demyelinating polyneuropathy. J Neurol Neurosurg Psychiatry 1990; 53:794–796.

17. Brooks DJ, Jenkins IH, Bain P, Colebatch JG, Thompson PD, Findley LJ, Marsden CD. A comparison of the abnormal patterns of cerebellar activation associated with neuropathic and essential tremor. Neurology 1992; 42(suppl 3):423.

18. Jenkins IH, Bain PG, Colebatch JG, Thompson PD, Findley LJ, Frackowiak RS, Marsden CD, Brooks DJ. A positron emission tomography study of essential tremor: evidence for overactivity of cerebellar connections. Ann Neurol 1993; 34:82–90.

19. Colebatch JG, Findley LJ, Frackowiak RS, Marsden CD, Brooks DJ. Preliminary report: activation of the cerebellum in essential tremor. Lancet 1990; 336:1028–1030.

20. Weide R, Heymanns J, Koppler H. The polyneuropathy associated with Waldenstrom's macroglobulinaemia can be treated effectively with chemotherapy and the anti-CD20 monoclonal antibody rituximab. Br J Haematol 2000; 109:838–841.

21. Pestronk A, Florence J, Miller T, Choksi R, Al-Lozi MT, Levine TD. Treatment of IgM antibody associated polyneuropathies using rituximab. J Neurol Neurosurg Psychiatry 2003; 74:485–489.

22. Renaud S, Gregor M, Fuhr P, Lorenz D, Deuschl G, Gratwohl A, Steck AJ. Rituximab in the treatment of polyneuropathy associated with anti-MAG antibodies. Muscle Nerve 2003; 27:611–615.

23. Ruzicka E, Jech R, Zarubova K, Roth J, Urgosik D. VIM thalamic stimulation for tremor in a patient with IgM paraproteinaemic demyelinating neuropathy. Mov Disord 2003; 18:1192–1195.

24. Roussy G, Lévy G. Sept cas d'une maladie familiale particulière: troubles de la marche, pieds bots et aréflexie tendineuse généralisée, avec, accessoirement, légère maladresse des mains. Rev Neurol (Paris) 1926; 1:427–450.

25. Dyck PJ, Chance P, Lebo R, Carney JA. Hereditary motor and sensory neuropathy. In: Dyck PJ, Thomas PK, Griffin JW, Low PA, Poduslo JF, eds. Peripheral Neuropathy. Philadelphia: WB Saunders, 1993:1094–1136.

26. Lapresle J, Salisachs P. Onion bulbs in a nerve biopsy specimen from an original case of Roussy-Lévy disease. Arch Neurol 1973; 29:346–348.

27. Said G. Etude des fibres nerveuses isolées dans les névrites hypertrophiques primitives. Rev Neurol (Paris) 1976; 132:467–480.

28. Lapresle J. Postmortem study of case I of the original family of Roussy and Melle Levy. J Neurol Sci 1986; 74:223–230.

29. Thomas PK, Marques W Jr, Davis MB, Sweeney MG, King RH, Bradley JL, Muddle JR, Tyson J, Malcolm S, Harding AE. The phenotypic manifestations of chromosome 17p11.2 duplication. Brain 1997; 120:465–478.

30. Plante-Bordeneuve V, Guiochon-Mantel A, Lacroix C, Lapresle J, Said G. The Roussy-Lévy family: from the original description to the gene. Ann Neurol 1999; 46:770–773.

31. Senderek J, Hermanns B, Bergmann C, Boroojerdi B, Bajbouj M, Hungs M, Ramaekers VT, Quasthoff S, Karch D, Schroder JM. X-linked dominant Charcot-Marie-Tooth neuropathy: clinical, electrophysiological, and morphological phenotype in four families with different connexin32 mutations. J Neurol Sci 1999; 167:90–101.

32. Auer-Grumbach M, Strasser-Fuchs S, Wagner K, Korner E, Fazekas F. Roussy-Lévy syndrome is a phenotypic variant of Charcot-Marie-Tooth syndrome IA associated with a duplication on chromosome 17p11.2. J Neurol Sci 1998; 154:72–75.

33. Cardoso FE, Jankovic J. Hereditary motor-sensory neuropathy and movement disorders. Muscle Nerve 1993; 16:904–910.

34. Byers RK, Banker BQ. Infantile muscular atrophy. Arch Neurol 1961; 5:140–164.

35. Dubowitz V. Nonprogressive neurogenic muscular atrophy with "voluntary fasciculation." Proc Roy Soc Med 1964; 57:117.

36. Spiro AJ. Minipolymyoclonus. A neglected sign in childhood spinal muscular atrophy. Neurology 1970; 20:1124–1126.

37. Moosa A, Dubowitz V. Spinal muscular atrophy in childhood. Two clues to clinical diagnosis. Arch Dis Child 1973; 48:386–388.

38. Russman BS, Fredericks EJ. Use of the ECG in the diagnosis of childhood spinal muscular atrophy. Arch Neurol 1979; 36:317–318.

39. Dawood AA, Moosa A. Hand and ECG tremor in spinal muscular atrophy. Arch Dis Child 1983; 58:376–378.

40. Kennedy WR, Alter M, Sung JH. Progressive proximal spinal and bulbar muscular atrophy of late onset. A sex-linked recessive trait. Neurology 1968; 18:671–680.

41. Sperfeld AD, Karitzky J, Brummer D, Schreiber H, Haussler J, Ludolph AC, Hanemann CO. X-linked bulbospinal neuronopathy: Kennedy disease. Arch Neurol 2002; 59:1921–1926.

42. Streib EW. Distal ulnar neuropathy as a cause of finger tremor: a case report. Neurology 1990; 40:153–154.

20

Posttraumatic Tremor

Jennifer S. Hui and Mark F. Lew

University of Southern California, Los Angeles, California, USA

I. INTRODUCTION

While tremor following traumatic injury to the central nervous system (CNS) is a well-accepted phenomenon (1–3), peripheral injuries have received increasing consideration as a cause of posttraumatic tremor (4,5). The pathophysiological mechanisms underlying tremor following trauma are not yet clearly defined, even in cases where a specific lesion can be identified. This chapter will focus on tremor arising from both central and peripheral injuries, with an emphasis on clinical features, pathophysiology, and management.

II. CENTRAL INJURY

A. Epidemiology

There have been few epidemiologic studies examining the frequency of posttraumatic tremor, despite numerous case reports and series (6–13). Retrospective surveys have suggested that tremor, followed by dystonia, is the most common movement disorder following closed head injury (14,15). Although most often seen after severe head trauma, tremor has been reported in cases of mild head injury without loss of consciousness (7,9,14).

In a series of 158 patients with mild to moderate head trauma defined as a Glasgow Coma Score (GCS) of ≥9, sixteen (10.1%) were determined to have a movement disorder, the majority (15/16) reporting tremor. The tremor was transient in all but two patients, resolving in weeks or months following the injury. The two remaining patients reported persistent, nondisabling symptoms four to six years after their head injury (14). Despite the paucity of epidemiologic data, tremor following mild head injury is most likely a rare occurrence, with recall bias tending to overestimate the prevalence detected in retrospective studies.

Most often, posttraumatic tremor is the delayed sequelae of severe head trauma, typically a deceleration injury from an automobile accident (1,6). Most patients are comatose for days to weeks with significant brainstem injury, and continue to have multiple cognitive and motor deficits on recovery. The frequency of tremor following severe head injury has been reported as high as 45% in a retrospective survey of children with severe head injury; however, the presence of tremor in this study was not confirmed by interview or examination (16). In a separate study of adults with head trauma resulting in a GCS score of ≤8, posttraumatic tremor was found in 42/221 (19%) patients (15). Persistent tremor was reported in 9%. Compared with those without movement disorders, patients with kinetic tremor or dystonia had a significantly lower initial GCS score, and were more likely to have generalized brain edema and focal cerebral lesions on initial head computed tomography (CT). The location of these focal lesions was not reported.

B. Clinical Features

Several types of tremor have been reported following head injury, implying damage to a variety of motor circuits. In cases of minor head trauma, posttraumatic tremors are generally transient and non-disabling, characterized as similar to enhanced physiologic or essential tremor (14). Biary et al. (9) reported seven cases of tremor following mild head injury without prolonged loss of consciousness and with normal brain imaging. Tremor began several weeks after the injury, and was described as postural and kinetic, with occasional myoclonic jerks involving the limbs and occasionally the head (9).

Conversely, tremor following severe head injury can cause significant functional disability, and is often associated with other neurologic deficits and coexistent movement disorders. In a series of 35 patients with tremor as a result of severe head trauma, psychological/cognitive alterations were seen in 91%, dysarthria in 86%, oculomotor nerve deficits in 69%, and truncal ataxia in 91% (17). For reasons that are poorly understood, tremor is often delayed weeks to months after the accident, with one report of tremor onset 23 years after brainstem trauma (6,10,18,19). In a series of eight patients in a coma up to three weeks following their injury, tremor was delayed one to 18 months from the time of their accident (20).

The most commonly described tremor after severe head injury is a combination of kinetic and rest tremor, likely a result of lesions in the cerebellar outflow and striatonigral pathways. Although the terms "midbrain tremor" and "rubral tremor" have been used to describe this type of tremor, its nomenclature remains controversial, as lesions elsewhere have resulted in similar movements (21–23). The Movement Disorder Society has recently adopted the term "Holmes tremor" after its first descriptor, with the proposed criteria including: 1) the presence of rest, intention, and often a postural tremor, 2) low frequency, usually <4.5 Hz and rarely >5.5 Hz, and 3) a variable delay (usually 4 weeks to 2 years) between lesion onset and tremor (24). The tremor has a proximal distribution, with the less predominant rest component resembling a parkinsonian tremor, and the kinetic component worsening with goal-directed movement (1). This is generally considered a symptomatic tremor that can reach amplitudes of >10 cm. It is often interrupted with myoclonic-like jerks, which may in fact represent exaggerations of the underlying tremor rhythm (11).

Reports of tremor following isolated trauma to the brainstem are rare, but offer a unique opportunity to observe the sequelae of well-circumscribed lesions (Fig. 20.1). Kremer et al. (25) were one of the first to describe a coarse tremor following presumed midbrain injury, in which dysarthria, limb ataxia, and ophthalmoparesis were prominent features. Samie et al. (6) reported three cases of localized trauma to the midbrain, after which course flapping tremors developed an average of 10.6 months postinjury. The tremor in all three cases diminished after weeks to months. Singular cases of coexistent rest tremor and dystonia have been described after direct penetrating injury to the cerebral peduncle, subthalamic area, and thalamus (26,27). A delayed-onset cerebellar syndrome with ataxia and intention tremor has been reported after unilateral thalamic and midbrain lesions from trauma or stroke (18).

C. Pathophysiology

The pathophysiology of posttraumatic tremor is not well understood, with multiple etiologies and localizations likely playing a role. Several types of tremor

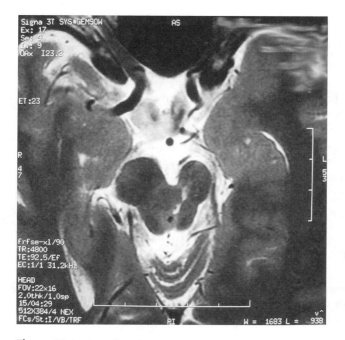

Figure 20.1 Localized brainstem injury in a patient with right-sided hemi-parkinsonism, rest and intention tremor following a motor vehicle accident.

may be seen in the same patient along with evidence of diffuse brain injury, making tremor analysis imprecise. Deuschl et al. (28) identified four fundamental tremor mechanisms: 1) expression of intrinsic mechanical properties of the limb, 2) reflex-activated tremor, 3) oscillation from a central pattern generator, and 4) malfunction of feed-forward loops in the cerebellum. The latter two mechanisms appear to be involved in cases of centrally-induced posttraumatic tremors, which fall clinically into the categories of Holmes tremor, cerebellar tremor, or dystonic tremor (24).

Holmes tremor can result from varying lesions in the brainstem, cerebellum, or thalamus. In all cases, however, there is evidence of dual interruption of both the cerebellothalamic and dopaminergic nigrostriatal systems, raising the possibility that Holmes tremor is actually a combination of two different tremors. This concept is clinically consistent with the presence of both rest and intention components, with some hypothesizing an interaction between the cerebellar and basal ganglia circuits in producing a tremor that is distinct from "pure" lesions of either system (28).

Several neuroimaging studies support this localization. Krauss et al. (29) demonstrated lesions of the dentatothalamic pathways in 22 of 25 instances of posttraumatic tremor using magnetic resonance imaging (MRI). In two of three patients with a resting parkinsonian tremor, lesions extending to the substantia nigra were found (29). In a separate positron emission tomography (PET) study of six patients with midbrain injury and tremor, Remy et al. (8) found markedly decreased [^{18}F]-fluorodopa uptake in the striatum without significant changes in D2-specific binding. This decrease was greater than that seen in idiopathic Parkinson's disease, suggesting presynaptic dopaminergic denervation as a result of trauma (8).

Midbrain lesions are an identified hallmark of diffuse axonal injury (DAI), a frequent finding in rapid deceleration trauma (30–32). The radiological presentation of DAI is that of generalized brain edema, with subsequent development of corpus callosal atrophy and ventricular enlargement (15,29). The development of kinetic tremors was significantly correlated to the presence of generalized brain edema on initial CT, perhaps serving as a marker for underlying midbrain injury as a cause of Holmes tremor (15).

Since lesions of the cerebellar cortex do not result in tremor, posttraumatic cerebellar tremor likely arises from damage to the deep cerebellar nuclei (dentate or globose-emboliform) or their efferents (33). The etiology of cerebellar outflow tremor involves the interruption of the superior cerebellar peduncle and dentato-rubral fibers, causing a disruption in the timing of agonist/antagonist muscle activation normally controlled by feed-forward loops (12,28,34). The mechanism of dystonic tremor remains unclear, but along with dystonia itself, it is thought to be localized to the basal ganglia (28).

The variable delay between head injury and symptom onset has been observed in other movement disorders (35), and may conceivably represent the slow resolution of inflammatory or oxidative damage, remyelination, or other mechanisms of neuronal reorganization (2). It has been hypothesized that there is a delayed development of a "second lesion" of the striatonigral system superimposed on an existing static cerebellar lesion, causing a Holmes type tremor (10,28). Newmark and Richards (19) invoked a trans-synaptic mechanism in which altered cortical input from a parietal lobe injury resulted in persistent basal ganglia hypometabolism over 13 years.

D. Posttraumatic Parkinsonism

Although there has not been substantial evidence to support trauma as a cause of idiopathic Parkinson's disease (36,37), severe or repeated head trauma can give rise to symptoms of parkinsonism. Reports of parkinsonism after a single head injury are rare, usually occurring in the context of direct damage to the midbrain and substantia nigra as a result of penetrating trauma or hemorrhage (26,27,38). In cases of unilateral brainstem injury, patients can present with contralateral hemiparkinsonism (Fig. 20.1). Tremor in these instances is usually not prominent. In contrast, tremor is the most common feature of parkinsonism from repeated head trauma, termed pugilistic encephalopathy, or the "punch drunk" syndrome of boxers (39). This well-defined progressive syndrome of ataxia, dementia, and parkinsonism is often accompanied by symptoms of dysarthria, seizures, or behavioral changes (39,40). Both a parkinsonian resting tremor and cerebellar intention tremor may be present. An estimated 17–20% of boxers develop symptoms of posttraumatic encephalopathy, with risk factors including length of career, number of bouts, and professional vs. amateur boxing (39,41).

The etiology of posttraumatic parkinsonism stems from presumed midbrain injury as a result of shearing forces produced by repeated rotational impacts to the head (42). Pathologically, there is depigmentation of the substantia nigra, although cortical neurofibrillary tangles provide evidence of more diffuse involvement. Furthermore, possession of the APOEε4 allele may promote amyloid deposition in the face of chronic head trauma (43). Levodopa responsiveness in posttraumatic parkinsonism is less predictable than in idiopathic Parkinson's disease (2,3). Thalamotomy has been used in selected cases (2,44).

E. Treatment

There have been no controlled trials of treatment for posttraumatic tremor. Importantly, spontaneous remission is possible, and was reported in over half of tremor cases after a mean follow up of 3.9 years following severe head injury (15). One reasonable approach has been to treat resting tremor with dopaminergic therapy, assuming midbrain damage to the striatonigral system. However, response to levodopa has been disappointing. Other conventional tremor medications have been used with varying success, with some disabling cases necessitating surgical intervention. Our review of 21 cases from the English literature reveals the most effective pharmacologic treatments in those tremors which responded to medical management (Table 20.1).

All classes of medication have been used, ranging from anti-cholinergics and anti-epileptics to beta-blockers, benzodiazepines, and dopaminergic compounds. Remy et al. (8) described six cases of "rubral" tremor which responded to levodopa therapy. Although tremor improved in all cases, results were variable and delayed up to several weeks, with two patients experiencing complete resolution of tremor, two patients with good response, and two patients with partial response (reduction in intensity of tremor, alleviation of rest component only). Mechanical damping using computer-generated viscous loads was shown in one case to reduce large amplitude kinetic tremor. While cumbersome, the authors suggest that this method may be more effective than simple inertial loading (weighting down the extremities) (45). Botulinum toxin injections may offer temporary relief (46).

Ventrolateral (VL) thalamotomy may be required for improvement of posttraumatic tremor, but at the risk of significant side effects. Long-term follow-up (mean 10.5 years) in one series of 35 patients yielded persistent improvement of tremor in 88%, with marked improvement in 65% (17). However, side effects such as increased dysarthria, truncal ataxia, and hemiballismus were seen in 38% on follow-up, and may be a relative contraindication to surgery if present preoperatively (20). A delay to surgery of one year has been proposed, given

Table 20.1 Individual Case Reports of Pharmacologic Treatments for Centrally-Induced Posttraumatic Tremor

Case	Source	Location of injury[a]	Tremor type	Effective treatment	Ineffective treatment
1	Aisen (64)	Not reported	Rest, kinetic	Glutethimide 1250 mg/d	Not reported
2	Biary (9)	None detected	Postural, kinetic, jerking	Clonazepam 2 mg/d	Propranolol
3	Biary	None detected	Postural, kinetic, jerking	Clonazepam 1.5 mg/d	Propranolol, primidone
4	Biary	None detected	Postural, kinetic	Propranolol 400 mg/d	Not reported
5	Biary	None detected	Postural, kinetic	Clonazepam 2 mg/d	Propranolol, primidone
6	Ellison (65)	Not reported	Postural, kinetic	Propranolol 60 mg/d	Not reported
7	Fernandez (66)	R midbrain, cerebral peduncle, substantia nigra, red nucleus, SCP	Rest, kinetic, postural	Benztropine 3 mg/d	Amantadine, valproic acid, L-dopa, pimozide, perphenazine, mexiletine, carbamazepine, baclofen, phenobarbital, clozapine
8	Harmon (67)	R red nucleus	Rest, kinetic	L-dopa 1500 mg/d, carbemazepinc 600 mg/d	Primidone, amantadine, propranolol
9	Krack (10)	R SCP, dorsal midbrain, substanitia nigra	Rest, intention, postural	Trihexyphenidyl 6 mg/d	Clonazepam
10	Newmark (19)	L parietal cortex, L basal ganglia	Rest, kinetic	Trihexyphenidyl 6 mg/d	L-dopa, baclofen, primidone
11	Obeso (11)	Not reported	Kinetic, postural, myoclonic jerking	Valproic acid 800 mg/d, propranolol 80 mg/d	Not reported

(continued)

Table 20.1 Continued

Case	Source	Location of injury[a]	Tremor type	Effective treatment	Ineffective treatment
12	Remy (8)	R substantia nigra, red nucleus, thalamus	Rest, intention, postural	L-dopa 600 mg, benserazide 150 mg	Not reported
13	Remy	Upper cerebral peduncle	Rest, intention, postural	L-dopa 300 mg, benserazide 75 mg, piribedil 120 mg	Not reported
14	Remy	L substantia nigra, red nucleus	Rest, postural	L-dopa 600 mg, benserazide 150 mg, bromocriptine 7.5 mg	Not reported
15	Remy	R substantia nigra, red nucleus, thalamus	Rest	L-dopa 500 mg, benserazide 125 mg, piribedil 300 mg	Not reported
16	Remy	R upper cerebral peduncle, thalamus	Rest, intention, postural	L-dopa 500 mg, benserazide 125 mg	Not reported
17	Remy	L substantia nigra, red nucleus, subthalamic region	Rest, intention, postural	L-dopa 600 mg, benserazide 150 mg	Not reported
18	Rondot (27)	L cerebral peduncle	Rest, intention, postural	L-dopa 300 mg/d, benserazide 75 mg/d, piribedil 120 mg/d	L-dopa, benserazide
19	Sandyk (68)	Not reported	Intention	Nadolol 80 mg/d	Not reported

[a]As demonstrated on MRI or CT.

Note: R = right, L = left, SCP = superior cerebellar peduncle, L-dopa = levodopa.

the possibility for spontaneous remission (20). Recently, high frequency thalamic stimulation has been introduced as an equally satisfactory treatment modality, with the added benefit of fewer and reversible side effects (47). Notably, the VL thalamus is an effective target not only for treatment of posttraumatic tremor, but also for tremor of various etiologies, raising the possibility of this site as the "final common pathway" for tremor.

III. PERIPHERAL INJURY

The existence of tremor and other movement disorders following peripheral trauma continues to be a topic of debate (48,49). Arguments against such a phenomenon include a lack of understanding of a suitable mechanism to explain the movement, difficulty in proving causality, and the scarcity of reports given the great number of peripheral injuries which occur, what some have termed the "denominator" problem (49). Nevertheless, there has been growing interest and scientific evidence supporting peripheral injury as a cause of movement disorders, particularly dystonia. The evidence for tremor follows in a similar vein.

A. Epidemiology and Clinical Features

The incidence of tremor following peripheral injuries has not been systematically studied, but Jankovic et al. (48) proposed a set of criteria for more accurate diagnosis of peripherally-induced movement disorders: 1) The trauma is severe enough to cause local symptoms for at least two weeks or requiring medical attention within two weeks of injury, 2) the initial manifestation of the movement disorder is anatomically related to the site of injury, and 3) the onset of the movement disorder is within days to months (up to 1 year) after the injury (48). Jankovic and Van Der Linden (5) used these criteria to select 23 subjects with suspected movement disorders induced by peripheral trauma from a database of 3500 patients (5). The latency between injury and movement onset ranged from one day to one year. Eighteen patients had focal dystonia, and five patients had tremor. Fifteen of the 23 patients (2/5 patients with tremor) had "predisposing factors" for the development of a movement disorder, including the use of neuroleptics, premature birth, family or personal history of essential tremor, or acquired immunodeficiency syndrome (AIDS) related complex. The authors suggested a central susceptibility to altered afferent input as a possible explanation.

In a separate study of 28 patients with peripherally-induced parkinsonism and tremor using the same inclusion criteria, a majority (21/28) developed symptoms within two months of peripheral injury (4). Seventeen had tremor without parkinsonism, most commonly postural tremor, although rest tremor was also present. The remainder developed resting tremor with unilateral rigidity and bradykinesia, which spread bilaterally to include postural instability, and in one case, the development of levodopa-induced motor fluctuations. In fact, all patients with parkinsonism and 9/17 (53%) patients with tremor alone experienced worsening or anatomic spread in their symptoms, suggesting a progression of the underlying insult, or continuing remodeling of central pathways. Predisposing factors were also present in 48% of this series, with nine patients having a family history of essential tremor.

Whiplash injury has been implicated as a cause of tremor and neck dystonia. Ellis (50) reported six cases of kinetic arm tremor, often associated with pain, following minor whiplash injury. A coarse postural tremor was described by Hashimoto et al. (51) after a four meters fall onto the ground, hitting the head and neck. Tremor following prolonged hand or wrist immobilization has also been reported, although in both cases, a low amplitude tremor was present before the cast or splint-requiring injury (52,53).

B.   Tremor and Complex Regional Pain Syndrome

The association of tremor with pain after peripheral injury has led to the question of whether movement disorders are a manifestation of complex regional pain syndrome (CRPS), previously referred to as reflex sympathetic dystrophy (RSD) or causalgia (54–56). The controversial nature of this association is raised by Verdugo and Ochoa (57) in a series of 58 patients referred for management of CRPS with abnormal movements. Tremor was present in 15%, and muscle spasms and dystonia in 60%. All patients exhibited at least one pseudo-neurologic sign, such as give-way weakness, disappearance with distraction, normalization with psychotherapy, and video surveillance documentation of malingering, leading the authors to conclude that the movements were psychogenic.

Schott (54), on the other hand, drew parallels between the pain and abnormal movements of causalgia, noting the shared features of delayed onset and anatomic spread beyond the site of initial injury, suggesting a common etiology for both. A specific analysis of tremor in 21 patients with RSD demonstrated a similar appearance to enhanced physiologic tremor, supported by a predictable response to weight loading (55). Tremor was alleviated with successful sympathetic blockade and upon recovery from RSD, indicating a possible relation between sympathetic activity and tremor. A similar phenomenon was seen in a selected population of 43 patients with RSD and abnormal movements, in which the tremor of 31 patients was relieved by sympathetic blockade (56).

C.   Pathophysiology

The pathophysiologic mechanisms of tremor following peripheral injury remain speculative; however, existing hypotheses invoke both central and peripheral mechanisms. Jankovic et al. (2,48) has postulated a central nervous system predisposition to the development of abnormal movements, perhaps through certain susceptibility genes such as the family of heat-shock proteins. A compelling observation for an underlying susceptibility is the high prevalence of "predisposing factors" exhibited among populations with peripherally-induced movement disorders, albeit in uncontrolled series (4,5). Neuroplasticity also plays an important role in mediating central nervous system adaptation to altered peripheral sensory input. These mechanisms are responsible for changes in cortical somatosensory maps in response to amputation and correction of syndactyly in both animals and humans (58–61). The same factors affecting change in cortical structures may apply to reorganization in the basal ganglia, giving rise to movement disorders indistinguishable from those of central origin. These precise mechanisms, however, have yet to be fully elucidated.

Peripherally, tremor analysis with electromyography (EMG) and weight loading has supported a reflex-activated mechanism underlying the tremor (51,55). The sympathetic nervous system has additionally been implicated as a trigger for tremor due to its potential role in CRPS. Deuschl et al. (55) proposed that the enhanced physiologic tremor of CRPS arises from the sympathetic sensitization of muscle spindles, causing an enhanced gain of reflexes. This enhanced excitability may be mediated by release of substance P from nociceptive fibers. Schwartzman and Kerrigan (56) also suggested that substance P, which has been shown to cause prolonged depolarization of motor neurons in the spinal cord, may interact with the sympathetic nervous system to cause the dystonia seen in CRPS (62,63).

Treatment for tremor induced by peripheral trauma has not been standardized, and response to conventional drugs for spasticity and tremor has been inconsistent. Case reports have utilized benzodiazepines, anti-convulsants, lioresal, and even levodopa. Sympathetic blockade has also been shown to alleviate tremor associated with CRPS.

IV. CONCLUSION

Posttraumatic tremor continues to be a challenging diagnosis with still undefined treatments. Although the concept of tremor following central injury is generally accepted, peripherally-induced tremor remains a controversial issue. Nevertheless, major advances in our understanding of the etiology of posttraumatic tremor have been made in the last decade, expanding our opportunities for developing targeted therapies for this disabling symptom.

REFERENCES

1. Krauss JK, Jankovic J. Head injury and posttraumatic movement disorders. Neurosurgery 2002; 50(5):927–940.
2. Jankovic J. Post-traumatic movement disorders: central and peripheral mechanisms. Neurology 1994; 44:2006–2014.
3. Koller WC, Wong GF, Lang A. Posttraumatic movement disorders: a review. Mov Disord 1989; 4(1):20–36.

4. Cardoso F, Jankovic J. Peripherally induced tremor and parkinsonism. Arch Neurol 1995; 52:263–270.
5. Jankovic J, Van Der Linden C. Dystonia and tremor induced by peripheral trauma: predisposing factors. J Neurol Neurosurg Psychiatry 1988; 51:1512–1519.
6. Samie MR, Selhorst JB, Koller WC. Post-traumatic midbrain tremors. Neurology 1990; 40:62–66.
7. Vanhatalo S, Paetau R. Posttraumatic tremor and arnold chiari malformation: no sign of compression, but cure after surgical decompression. Mov Disord 2000; 15(3):581–583.
8. Remy P, de Recondo A, Defer G, Loc'h C, Amarenco P, Plante-Bordeneuve V, Dao-Castellana M-H, Bendriem B, Crouzel C, Clanet M, Rondot P, Samson Y. Peduncular 'rubral' tremor and dopaminergic denervation: a PET study. Neurology 1995; 45:472–477.
9. Biary N, Cleeves L, Findley L, Koller WC. Post-traumatic tremor. Neurology 1989; 39:103–106.
10. Krack P, Deuschl G, Kaps M, Warnke P, Schneider S, Traupe H. Delayed onset of 'rubral tremor' 23 years after brainstem trauma. Mov Disord 1994; 9(2):240–241.
11. Obeso JA, Narbona J. Post-traumatic tremor and myoclonic jerking. J Neurol Neurosurg Psychiatry 1983; 46(8):488.
12. Haggard P, Miall RC, Wade D, Fowler S, Richardson A, Anslow P et al. Damage to cerebellocortical pathways after closed head injury: a behavioural and magnetic resonance imaging study. J Neurol Neurosurg Psychiatry 1995; 58:433–438.
13. Zijlmans J, Booij J, Valk J, Lees A, Horstink M. Posttraumatic tremor without parkinsonism in a patient with complete contralateral loss of the nigrostriatal pathway. Mov Disord 2002; 17(5):1086–1088.
14. Krauss JK, Trankle R, Kopp K-H. Posttraumatic movement disorders after moderate or mild head injury. Mov Disord 1997; 12(3):428–431.
15. Krauss JK, Trankle R, Kopp K-H. Post-traumatic movement disorders in survivors of severe head injury. Neurology 1996; 47:1488–1492.
16. Johnson SLJ, Hall DMB. Post-traumatic tremor in head injured children. Arch Dis Child 1992; 67:227–228.
17. Krauss JK, Mohadjer M, Nobbe F, Mundinger F. The treatment of posttraumatic tremor by stereotactic surgery. J Neurosurg 1994; 80:810–819.
18. Louis ED, Lynch T, Ford B, Paul G, Bressman SB, Fahn S. Delayed-onset cerebellar syndrome. Arch Neurol 1996; 53:450–454.
19. Newmark J, Richards TL. Delayed unilateral post-traumatic tremor: localization studies using single-proton computed tomographic and magnetic resonance spectroscopy techniques. Mil Med 1999; 164(1):59–64.
20. Andrew J, Fowler CJ, Harrison MJG. Tremor after head injury and its treatment by stereotaxtic surgery. J Neurol Neurosurg Psychiatry 1982; 45:815–819.
21. Qureshi F, Morales A, Elble RJ. Tremor due to infarction in the ventrolateral thalamus. Mov Disord 1996; 11(4):440–459.
22. Lee MS, Marsden CD. Movement disorders following lesions of the thalamus or subthalamic region. Mov Disord 1994; 9(5):493–507.
23. Miwa H, Hatori K, Kondo T, Imai H, Mizuno Y. Thalamic tremor: case reports and implications of the tremor-generating mechanism. Neurology 1996; 46:75–79.
24. Deuschl G, Bain P, Brin M, Committee AHS. Consensus statement of the Movement Disorder Society on tremor. Mov Disord 1998; 13(suppl 3):2–23.

25. Kremer M, Russell WR, Smyth GE. A mid-brain syndrome following head injury. J Neurol Neurosurg Psychiatry 1947; 10:49–60.
26. Krauss JK, Trankle R, Raabe A. Tremor and dystonia after penetrating diencephalic-mesencephalic trauma. Park Rel Disord 1997; 3(2):117–119.
27. Rondot P, Bathien N, de Recondo J, Gueguen B, Fredy D, de Recondo A et al. Dystonia-parkinsonism syndrome resulting from a bullet injury in the midbrain. J Neurol Neurosurg Psychiatry 1994; 57:658.
28. Deuschl G, Raethjen J, Lindemann M, Krack P. The pathophysiology of tremor. Muscle Nerve 2001; 24:716–735.
29. Krauss JK, Wakhloo AK, Nobbe F, Trankle R, Mundinger F, Seeger W. Lesions of dentatothalamic pathways in severe post-traumatic tremor. Neurol Res 1995; 17:409–416.
30. Adams JH, Doyle D, Ford I, Gennarelli TA, Graham DI, Mclellan DR. Diffuse axonal injury in head injury: definition, diagnosis, and grading. Histopathology 1989; 15:49–59.
31. Adams JH, Graham DI, Gennarelli TA, Maxwell WL. Diffuse axonal injury in non-missile head injury. J Neurol Neurosurg Psychiatry 1991; 54:481–483.
32. Rosenblum WI, Greenberg RP, Seelig JM, Becker DP. Midbrain lesions: frequent and significant prognostic feature in closed head injury. Neurosurgery 1981; 9:613–620.
33. Cole JD. Hemispheric lesions and tremor. In: Findley LJ, Koller WC, eds. Handbook of Tremor Disorders. New York: Marcel Dekker, 1995:429–441.
34. Vidailhet M, Jedynak C-P, Pollak P, Agid Y. Pathology of symptomatic tremors. Mov Disord 1998; 13(suppl 3):49–54.
35. Scott BL, Jankovic J. Delayed-onset progressive movement disorders after static brain lesions. Neurology 1996; 46:68–74.
36. Factor SA, Sanchez-Ramos J, Weiner WJ. Trauma as an etiology of parkinsonism: a historical review of the concept. Mov Disord 1988; 3:30–36.
37. Williams DB, Annegers JF, Kokmen E, O'Brien PC, Kurland LT. Brain injury and neurologic sequelae. Neurology 1991; 41:1554–1557.
38. Bhatt M, Desai J, Mankodi A, Elias M, Wadia N. Posttraumatic akinetic-rigid syndrome resembling Parkinson's disease: a report on three patients. Mov Disord 2000; 15(2):313–317.
39. Factor SA. Posttraumatic parkinsonism. In: Stern MB, Koller WC, eds. Parkinsonian Syndromes. New York: Marcel Dekker Inc., 1993:95–110.
40. Jordan BD. Neurologic aspects of boxing. Arch Neurol 1987; 44:453–459.
41. Jordan BD. Chronic traumatic brain injury associated with boxing. Semin Neurol 2000; 20(2):179–185.
42. Lampert PW, Hardman JM. Morphological changes in brains of boxers. JAMA 1984; 251(20):2676–2679.
43. Jordan BD, Relkin NR, Ravdin LD, Jacobs AR, Bennett A, Gandy S. Apolipoprotein E ε 4 associated with chronic traumatic brain injury in boxing. JAMA 1997; 278(2):136–140.
44. Niizuma H, Kwak R, Ohyama H, Ikeda S, Ohtsuki T, Saso S. Stereotactic thalamotomy for postapoplectic and posttraumatic involuntary movements. Appl Neurophysiol 1982; 45:295–298.
45. Aisen ML, Arnold A, Baiges I, Maxwell S, Rosen M. The effect of mechanical damping loads on disabling action tremor. Neurology 1993; 43:1346–1350.
46. Jankovic J, Schwartz K. Botulinum toxin treatment of tremors. Neurology 1991; 41:1185–1188.

47. Broggi G, Brock S, Franzini A, Geminiani G. A case of posttraumatic tremor treated by chronic stimulation of the thalamus. Mov Disord 1993; 8(2):206–208.
48. Jankovic J. Can peripheral trauma induce dystonia and other movement disorders? Yes! Mov Disord 2001; 16(1):7–12.
49. Weiner WJ. Can peripheral trauma induce dystonia? No! Mov Disord 2001; 16(1):13–22.
50. Ellis SJ. Tremor and other movement disorders after whiplash type injuries. J Neurol Neurosurg Psychiatry 1997; 63:110–112.
51. Hashimoto T, Sato H, Shindo M, Hayashi R, Ikeda S. Peripheral mechanisms in tremor after traumatic neck injury. J Neurol Neurosurg Psychiatry 2002; 73:585–587.
52. Herbaut AG, Soeur M. Two other cases of unilateral essential tremor, induced by peripheral trauma. J Neurol Neurosurg Psychiatry 1989; 52(10):1213.
53. Cole JD, Illis LS, Sedgwick EM. Unilateral essential tremor after wrist immobilization: a case report. J Neurol Neurosurg Psychiatry 1989; 52:286–290.
54. Schott GD. Induction of involuntary movements by peripheral trauma: an analogy with causalgia. Lancet 1986; 2(8509):712–716.
55. Deuschl G, Blumberg H, Lucking CH. Tremor in reflex sympathetic dystrophy. Arch Neurol 1991; 48:1247–1252.
56. Schwartzman RJ, Kerrigan J. The movement disorder of reflex xympathetic dystrophy. Neurology 1990; 40:57–61.
57. Verdugo RJ, Ochoa JL. Abnormal movements in complex regional pain syndrome: assessment of their nature. Muscle Nerve 2000; 23:198–205.
58. Clark SA, Allard T, Jenkins WM, Merzenck MM. Receptive fields in the body surface map in adult cortex defined by temporally correlated inputs. Nature 1988; 332:444–445.
59. Ramachandran VS. Behavioral and magnetoencephalographic correlates of plasticity in the adult human brain. Proc Natl Acad Sci 1993; 90:10413–10420.
60. Roricht S, Meyer B-U, Niehous L, Brandt SA. Long-term reorganization of motor complex outputs after arm amputation. Neurology 1999; 53:106–111.
61. Cohen LG, Bandinelli S, Findley TW, Hallet M. Motor reorganization after an upper limb amputation in man. Brain 1991; 114:615–627.
62. Koniski S, Otsuka M. The effects of substance P and other peptides on spinal neurons of the frog. Brain Res 1974; 65:397–410.
63. Henry JL. Effects of substance P on functionally identified units in cat spinal cord. Brain Res 1976; 114:439–451.
64. Aisen ML, Holzer M, Rosen M, Dietz M, McDowell F. Glutethimide treatment of disabling action tremor in patients with multiple scelrosis and traumatic brain injury. Arch Neurol 1991; 48:513–515.
65. Ellison PH. Propranolol for severe post-head injury action tremor. Neurology 1978; 28:197–199.
66. Fernandez HH, Freidman JH, Centofanti JV. Benedikt's syndrome with delayed-onset rubral tremor and hemidystonia: a complication of tic douloureux surgery. Mov Disord 1999; 14(4):695–697.
67. Harmon RL, Long DF, Shrtz J. Treatment of post-traumatic midbrain tresting-kinetic tremor with combined levodopa/carbidopa and carbamazepine. Brain Inj 1991; 5(2):213–218.
68. Sandyk R. Nadolol in posttraumatic intention tremor. J Neurosurg 1986; 64(1):162.

21

Infectious Tremor

Dee E. Silver

Scripps Memorial Hospital and Coastal Neurological Medical Group, Inc., La Jolla, California, USA

Infectious diseases or syndromes can be the primary etiology of tremor of any type and can be a confounding factor for an established tremor. Infectious diseases can also enhance or lower the threshold for physiological tremor and pathological tremor (1).

Determination of tremor type and phenomenology allows for understanding, classification, and possibly treatment. In tremor related to infection the treatment of the primary infection is crucial for the treatment management. As in most neurological diseases an accurate history is paramount, especially in determining the existence of a prior chronic tremor or a chronic tremor now made worse by an infection. The physical exam and various techniques for documentation of the tremor are essential.

The history for an infectious entity is most important, especially as to prior exposure, procedures, symptoms, and possible immune deficiency states. Geographical issues, especially travel, may also be important. The tremor type of the infectious or postinfectious tremor is greatly varied but usually 4 to 11 Hz and is most commonly postural and sometimes kinetic. The commonly associated neuropathic postinfectious syndromes with tremor are associated with infectious diseases such as brucellosis, Lyme's disease, and rickettsial diseases (1).

Infectious diseases associated with tremor are probably many but the case studies, anecdotal reports, and series described are relatively few. The classification of these infectious diseases can be divided into bacterial, viral, prion, fungal, parasitic, rickettsial, mycoplasma, and parainfectious. Also, infectious diseases as an etiology of tremor can be considered as to the location of the infection in the brain. These can be considered as a structural lesion or an inflammatory lesion or direct infectious localized process.

Often in infectious syndromes monitoring laboratory data such as a comprehensive metabolic panel, complete blood count (CBC), sed rate, C-reactive protein, liver function tests, and creatine phosphokinase (CPKs) tests will be of benefit to help determine if an infectious syndrome is present or to monitor its onset or progression.

Inflammatory infectious syndromes with diffuse and/or localized involvement of the central nervous system may be related to tremors of various types. Meningitis of any type; tuberculous, bacterial or viral, may be associated with a tremor. This may be related to an inflammatory infectious process that involves the cerebellar-brainstem-thalamic pathways. Tremors also may be related to some localized toxin that is associated with the infection and is directed at certain neurons or groups of neurons. Abscess, localized inflammation, or encephalitis, which is associated with actual pathogenic cell involvement, can be a cause of tremor. In viral syndromes cells or groups of cells can be made dysfunctional by direct invasion of the cells. Encephalitis, especially the viral and postviral syndromes, can be diffused or localized, and involve cells or groups of cells that may be related to tremor etiology.

Animal models for the study of infectious syndromes and tremor are limited. There is no known knockout mouse for the study of postural or kinetic tremor even though there are now genetic studies that show essential tremor in some cases genetically can be located on 3q13 and 2p24 (1). Studies with viruses in mice, rats, and pigs have given some insight as to genetic and infectious factors for tremor. In many studies there appears to be a "double hit," that is, a host gene or genes control susceptibility of the animal model to having induced tremor by a virus or some other agent. Porcine circovirus (PVC), especially PVC441 in mice, showed a dose and age dependence for tremor induction (2). Certain genetic mice were resistant to PVC441-induced tremor, and this supports a genetic control over which mice develop tremor induced by PVC441 virus. Pigs develop congenital tremors (CP type A2) associated with the PVC virus and abnormal myelin and occur in regional farm outbreaks (3). Pigs with tremor had more widely distributed viral infection in the brain and spinal cord, especially in large neurons. Even though some pigs had no tremor they were infected to a lesser extent. Polymerase chain reaction (PCR) analysis demonstrated only PCR type II and not PCR type I in all pigs infected. PCRV has been associated with a post-weaning multisystemic wasting syndrome in pigs. It seems to be related to the congenital tremor in pigs type A2, and is classified as PCV I and PCV II. In Spain, pigs with CP did not show evidence of PCV I or PCV II (4). Recombinants of amphotropic murine leukemic virus are used in retroviral vector systems in many species including humans. They can induce a spongiform encephalomyelopathy in mice. This involves nerve and glial cells, has a microgliosis and an astrogliosis, and the mice have tremors, ataxia, spasticity, and later tetraparesis and death (5). Other viruses such as the bovine viral diarrhea (BVD) virus have been associated with tremors in cattle. Rickettsia-like organisms have been associated with large outbreaks of death of ocean crabs, and prior to their death they develop a robust tremor (6). Enterovirus71(EV71) and other strains of enterovirus like the polio virus are major neurotrophic viruses and cause serious neurological consequences. EV71 isolated from human fatal encephalitis, meningitis, and hand-foot-and-mouth disease, were injected into Cynomolgus monkeys intraspinally, and the monkeys developed severe neurological manifestations (7). The clinical picture included flaccid paralysis, tremor, and ataxia and the virus was in the spinal cord, brainstem, cerebellar cortex, and cerebrum.

There is some evidence that neurotoxins associated with infection may cause neurological disorders. These neurotoxins may be localized to involve certain areas of the brain which are associated with tremor abnormalities. The Gordon phenomenon (tremor, ataxia, paralysis), with loss of Purkinje cells in the cerebellum, has been duplicated by the injection of human eosinophil extracts in guinea pigs (8). The eosinophil neurotoxin and not the Angiostrongylus cantonensis (a parasite) was responsible for the clinical picture and the development of the tremor, ataxia, and paralysis in the guinea pigs.

Bacterial infection presents neurologically as meningitis, encephalitis, encephalomyelitis, localized infection, or an abscess. Parameningeal infection can also evolve into any of the above diseases. Parameningeal infections are infections of the epidural area, sinuses, or other infections located in or around the meninges. The tremors are usually postural or kinetic but also infrequently resting. Meningitis involves many parts of the brain with both diffuse infection and inflammation but also resultant toxins which can be diffuse or localized, as can also be seen with bacterial encephalitis and encephalomyelitis. Any of the bacterial agents causing meningitis may have associated tremor but the less fulminating clinical course will allow the development of and observation of more subtle signs such as tremor. *Streptococcus, Escherichia coli, listeria,* and *staphylococcus* are the usual bacteria that occur in neonates. *Neisseria, streptococcus,* and *staphylococcus* occur later in childhood and adulthood. Lyme's disease, brucellosis, leptospirosis, and *Listeria* all may be present with any of the above syndromes and tremor. Tuberculosis as a meningitis not uncommonly has an associated tremor. If a granuloma is in the midbrain, a clinical presentation such as Holmes tremor may occur.

Reports of the *Helicobacter pylori* infection inducing tremor, aphasia, and stuttering are documented (9). *E. coli* O157:H7 infection associated with hemorrhagic colitis has a documented heterogeneous neurological syndrome including an action tremor (10). The neurological symptoms were thought to be induced by the verotoxin elaborated by the *E. coli.*

Syphilis, in the secondary and tertiary forms, is the great masquerader not unlike Lyme's disease and brucellosis. Syphilis can present with many varied neurological signs and symptoms. Tremor of various types, but especially postural tremor, are associated with syphilis. Recently labial, lingual, and orthostatic tremors have been documented in tertiary syphilis (11). The spirochete *Borrelia* has been associated with an encephalomyelitis and resultant tremor.

Postinfectious bacterial syndromes, most notably post-streptococcal movement disorders, have been widely described and recognized as a heterogeneous spectrum involving dyskinetic movements but also emotional disorders in at least 50% of cases. The dyskinetic movement disorders were reported in 40 patients with chorea ($n = 20$), motor tics ($n = 16$), dystonia ($n = 5$), tremor ($n = 3$), stereotypies ($n = 2$), opsoclonus ($n = 2$), and myoclonus ($n = 1$) (12). Typhoid fever and typhus can be associated with tremor and this has been well documented. Cat scratch fever and Whipple's disease can present with neurological manifestations that are very heterogeneous and involve tremor. In addition, many tropical diseases can result in tremor (13).

Viral syndromes, primarily meningitis, and encephalitis are associated with parkinsonism and movement disorders including tremor (14). Von Economo's encephalitis of the 1914–1921 period is a well-known viral syndrome that was associated with acute extrapyramidal signs and symptoms (14).

The encephalitic forms are more likely to have tremor since the parenchymal areas or cell groups, probably in the basal ganglia, brainstem, and cerebellum, are involved by inflammatory changes, direct viral cellular involvement, or possibly by toxins. Focal or diffuse signs with altered mental status and seizures help differentiate encephalitis from meningitis. Knowing the likely viral group involved may help with diagnosis of the neurological signs and symptoms. It is also important for the consideration of possible treatment. There are some important historical aspects for helping clinically to determine the virus or the group of viruses. Community outbreaks, exposure to animals, birds, or insects (mosquitoes/ticks), season of the year, travels, and prior infections over the last several weeks may help with the identification of a viral group. Since Herpes and human immunodeficiency virus (HIV) syndromes are more commonly related to tremors, the sexual and/or drug history is important. Also, postinfectious acute disseminated encephalomyelitis (ADEM) may be associated with tremor and is diagnosed by the latency time from the acute illness, the clinical picture, and the neurological syndrome. In ADEM there may be a variety of movement disorders and tremors. Polio and nonpolio enteroviruses such as ECHO virus and coxsackie virus presenting as meningitis and/or encephalitis may have associated tremor. Tremor in patients with arbovirus syndromes may also be observed. Herpes simplex virus (HSV), most noticeably HSV-1, HSV-2, cytomegalo virus (CMV), Epstein-Barr virus (EBV), Human herpes virus-6 (HHV-6), and Herpes B have been associated with tremor. A careful history and physical along with a cerebral spinal fluid (CSF) analysis with PCR is very helpful in making an accurate viral diagnosis and possible treatment plan.

Polio is not seen often clinically in the developed countries because of the vaccination programs but a case with tremor and paralysis was reported in a child with agammaglobulinemia (15).

Children with congenital, or more likely acquired, CMV, rubella, and HSV develop infantile spasms (convulsions) and longstanding tremors and a poor outcome neurologically (16). Encephalitic and meningitic involvement with clinical hepatitis usually precedes the clinical onset of the hepatitis and tremor often follows the onset of a viral hepatitis. The peripheral nerve disorders, neuro-psychological dysfunction, and Guillain-Barré syndromes associated with hepatitis may occur at any stage of the viral hepatitis in both B and non-B infections (17). The neurological clinical features are a result of either or both the direct viral invasion of the neural cells or an immune complex-mediated cell damage (17). HHV-6 is seen as a viral meningoencephalitis in humans but is now recognized as an important pathogen in immunocompromised hosts and is associated with tremor in these patients (18). EBV has been reported as an etiology of an acute cerebellitis associated with nausea and vomiting, ataxia, myoclonus, and tremor of the head and all or some of the four extremities (19). ECHO 5 virus with encephalitis has been associated with resting tremor (20).

HIV and neurological syndromes associated with HIV are on the rise in the developed countries, but especially in the third world countries, most noticeably Africa. In a review from 1986 to 1999, 2460 HIV-positive inpatients were seen in Rio de Janeiro. Forty three percent of the cases had neurological abnormalities (21). Of these 14 had secondary parkinsonism. The parkinsonism was thought to be related to encephalitic HIV itself (12), toxoplasmosis of the midbrain (1), and metoclopramide (1). Six had hemichorea/hemiballismus mostly due to toxoplasmosis of the basal ganglia. Four had myoclonus related to toxoplasmosis and HIV encephalopathy. Two had painful legs and moving toes related to axonal neuropathy oftentimes associated with HIV. One had hemidystonia related to toxoplasmosis of the basal ganglia. One had Holmes' tremor related to toxoplasmosis and tuberculosis of the midbrain and cerebellum. HIV can be associated with any movement disorder, and a treatable opportunistic infection such as toxoplasmosis must be ruled out, as must a mass lesion. Confounding medications such as dopamine antagonists must also be considered. Cardoso, in a Brazilian movement disorder center, noted that 58% of patients with autoimmune deficiency syndrome (AIDS) developed tremor, parkinsonism, or other extrapyramidal features (22). Hyperkinesis such as hemiballismus-hemichorea and tremor were the most common, but dystonia, chorea, myoclonus, tics, paroxysmal dyskinesias, and parkinsonism were also seen. Most hyperkinesias were associated with lesions by infections such as toxoplasmosis, which were usually located in the basal ganglia region. There was a consideration that HIV infection itself with direct cellular involvement and cell dysfunction could lead to dopaminergic dysfunction and parkinsonism. Infections, like toxoplasmosis, have to be aggressively treated with sulfadiazine and pyrimethamine, and the HIV treated with highly active antiretroviral therapy (HAART). Various therapies can be tried for the AIDS-related movement disorders but these are generally disappointing and ineffective. Aggressive early HAART may prevent the development of neurological dysfunction and movement disorders and also may benefit the symptomatic control of the movement disorders. A study in Tanzania noted that in 135 AIDS patients with clinical neurological symptoms, 19% of the patients had incoordination and tremor, 54% had dementia, 21% had areflexia, and 19% had pyramidal tract signs (23). Several studies have documented, in children and adults with HIV, slowed motor activity and reduced alternating movement testing. But it was noted that there were normal tremor peak frequencies as compared to controls in these studies. It seems to be the case that these abnormalities appear before abnormal structural changes (MRIs are normal); hence, cell changes in the basal ganglia occur before any clinical findings (24). Also, abnormal motor function tests may indicate early basal ganglia involvement even with normal MRIs. In patients with HIV dementia the MRI may show basal ganglia lesions despite tremor-peak-frequencies being normal in reference to controls (25).

The AIDS dementia complex is often anticipated clinically by motor and behavioral dysfunction. Motor abnormalities are often tremor, weakness, ataxia, and loss of fine motor coordination. HIV neuropathy, as occurs in many neuropathies, may be associated with postural tremor. Case reports of isolated postural tremor revealing HIV infection have been published (26).

Human T-cell lymphotropic virus type I (HTLV-I) has often been associated with clinical neuropathy, primarily sensory, and is often associated with an action tremor, atrophy, weakness, and spastic or non-spastic paraparesis or quadriparesis (myelopathy) (14).

ECHO 5 virus encephalitis has been associated with a transient Parkinson-like tremor with myoclonus and complete recovery in six years. The pathological changes are cellular (cytopathic) with loss of organelles and viral particles in astrocytes without inflammatory changes (27).

Inkoo and Tahyna viruses present with fever and neurological infection in which the latter has a septic meningitis and encephalitis. Encephalitis usually occurred in reported cases in three to seven days of the illness and had a heterogeneous clinical picture but often involved a generalized tremor (28). Lassa fever with acute encephalopathy in nine cases had confusion followed by tremor in seven cases with associated seizures and coma (29).

Any virus that presents with meningitis and/or encephalitis can have a postural tremor. Eastern and western equine, St. Louis and Japanese B encephalitis can each have associated parkinsonism and postural tremor. Some may even have a resting tremor (14). West Nile certainly has multiple neurological abnormalities by history and exam predominantly from the diffuse picture that can occur pathologically and also from the loss of anterior horn cells which may bring about tremor and other related symptoms. Tremor occured in 94%, myoclonus in 31% and Parkinson's disease in 69% of West Nile virus-seropositive patients. Movement disorders persisted for at least eight months in one third of the patients (30).

Fungal infections, probably because of a meningeal and inflammatory pathology, can be associated with tremor. *Cryptococcus* and *Coccidioides* are often likely to be associated with a mass or multiple masses resulting in tremor.

If the mass is located in the basal ganglia it may result in a postural tremor. Case reports of midbrain masses secondary to a fungus such as neuroparacoccidio-idomycosis have resulted in Holmes' tremor (31). Parasitic diseases such as toxoplasmosis as described above are seen in immune compromised patients and in HIV-positive patients. They are also seen in nonimmune compromised patients. The clinical picture is parkinsonism and postural tremor or Holmes' tremor, related to a lesion in the basal ganglia or midbrain. Diffuse toxoplasmosis has also been associated with tremor. Other parasitic infections such cysticercosis or equina coccus can act as a mass lesion also and depending on the site of the lesion may give some form of tremor. Rickettsial diseases such as Rocky Mountain spotted fever clinically have been associated with tremors, as has Q fever (14).

Generalized microsporidiosis presents as an encephalopathy often with fever, seizures, quadriparesis, and tremor. Recovery can be dramatic after treating with albendazol (32).

Malaria has an acute clinical picture which appears as an infectious syndrome and may have neurological symptoms early and later. A discreet "transient neurological syndrome" that occurs after recovery from the severe infection is called post-malarial neurological syndrome (PMNS). Nineteen of 124 treated had PMNS mainly associated clinically with confusion, seizures, and psychosis with one reporting tremor (33).

A typhoid epidemic in New Guinea from 1984 to 1990 in hospitalized patients showed a mortality rate of 10–15%, and cerebellar tremor and hearing loss were frequent neurological findings (34).

Chediak-Higashi syndrome is of uncertain etiology but can present as a tremor, gait disturbance, and later with parkinsonism and mental impairment (14). Creutzfeldt-Jakob disease (CJD), a prion disease that has three forms—sporadic, familial—and infectious (mad cow disease), is associated with myoclonus, dyskinesias, and in some cases also tremor (35). However, the predominant clinical features of CJD disease are usually behavior changes and dementia, but tremor may be seen early.

Episodic disseminated inflammation of the CNS has an unknown etiology and is difficult to differentiate from acute disseminated encephalomyelitis (ADE) and sometimes from multiple sclerosis (MS). The clinical picture is heterogeneous but tremor, ataxia, and dysmetria are seen along with paresis and mental changes (36). The diagnosis is helped by MRIs and treatment is steroids.

In summary, infections can be the primary etiology of tremor or they can exacerbate a pre-existing tremor. The history is important especially to the prior existence of a tremor and the existence of an infection or symptoms of an infection. Classifying the type of tremor and ruling out comorbidity or drugs that lower the threshold for tremor is important. The treatment is usually primarily based upon treatment and management of the infectious syndrome but later, if there is a residual tremor, standard pharmacological therapeutics for tremor such as propranolol, primidone, topiramate, or benzodiazepines may be used.

REFERENCES

1. Mark M. Tremor disorders. Continuum 2004; 10(3):113–127.
2. Kai K, Mitsuno K et al. Factors affecting indication of neurological disorders in mice by PVC viruses and the sequence of env-LTR region of PVC441. Leukemia 1997; 11(suppl 3):236–238.
3. Stevenson GW, Kuipel M et al. Tissue distribution and genetic typing of porcine circoviruses in pigs with naturally occurring congenital tremors. J Vet Diagn Invest 2001; 13(1):57–62.
4. Kennedy S, Segales J. Absence of evidence of porcine circovirus infection in piglets with congenital tremors. J Vet Diagn Invest 2003; 15(2):51–56.
5. Munk C, Lohler J et al. Amphotropic murine leukemia viruses induce spongiform encephalomyelopathy. Proc Natl Acad Sci USA 1997; 94(1):5837–5842.
6. Wang W, Gu Z. Rickettsial-like organisms associated with tremor disease and mortality of the chinese mitten crab eriocheir sinensis. Dis Aquat Organ 2002; 48(2):149–153.
7. Nagoti N, Shimizic H et al. Pyramidal and extrapyramidal involvement in experimental infections of cynomolgus monkeys with enterovirus 71. J Med Virol 2002; 67(2):207–216.
8. Perez O, Capron M et al. Angiostrongylus cantonensis: role of eosinophils in the neurotoxic syndrome (Gordon-like Phenomenon). Exp Parasitol 1989; 68(4):403–413.
9. Tsao JW, Shad JA et al. Tremor, aphasia, and stuttering associated with helicobacter pylori infection. Am J Med 2004; 116(3):211–212.
10. Hamano S, Nakaniski Y et al. Neurological manifestations of hemorrhagic colitis in the outbreak of escherichia coli O157:H7 infection in Japan. Asta Paediatr 1993; 82(5):454–458.
11. Brotman DJ, Foluhi M. Syphilis and orthostatic tremor of the limbs. Lancet 2000; 356(9243):1734.
12. Dale RC, Heyman I, Surtus RA et al. Dyskinesias and associated psychiatric disorders following streptococcal infection. Arch Dis Child 2004; 89(7):604–610.
13. Kumar A. Movement disorders in the tropics. Parkinsonism Relat Disord 2002; 9(2):69–75.
14. Roos KL. Viral infections. In: Goetz CG (ed.) Textbook of Clinical Neurology, 2nd ed. Philadelphia, PA: Saunders. 2003:895–918.
15. Abo W, Chiba S et al. Paralytic poliomyelitis in a child with agammaglobulinemia. Eur J Pediatr 1979; 132(1):11–16.
16. Riikonen R. Infantile spasms: infectious disorders. Neuropediatrics 1993; 24(5):274–280.
17. Apstein MD, Koff E et al. Neuropsychological dysfunction in acute viral hepatitis. Digestion 1979; 19(6):349–358.
18. Woshida H, Matsunaga K et al. HHV-6 Meningoencephalitis successfully treated with gansiclovir in a patient who underwent allogenic bone marrow transplantation from an HLA-identical sibling. Int J Hematol 2002; 75(4):421–425.
19. Teive HA, Zavala JA et al. Acute cerebellitis caused by Epstein-Barr virus: case report. Arq Neuropsiquiatr 2001; 59(3-A):616–618.
20. Foncin JF, Maurin J et al. Curable ECHO 5 viral encephalitis. clinical, electroencephalographic, virologic, and ultrastructural study. Ann Med Interne (Paris) 1977; 128(4):335–343.

21. Mallos JP, Rosso AA et al. Movement disorders in 28 HIV-infected patients. Arq Neuropsiquiatr 2002; 60(3-A):525–530.
22. Cardoso F. HIV-related Movement disorders: epidemiology, pathogenesis, and management. CMS Drugs 2002; 16(10):663–668.
23. DeCork KM. Neurological disorders in AIDS and HIV diseases in the northern zone of Tanzania. WHO AIDS Tech Bull 1989; 2:157–158.
24. Arendt G, Hefter H et al. Motor dysfunction in HIV-infected patients without clinically detectable central nervous deficit. J Neurol 1990; 237(6):362–368.
25. Arendt G, Hefter H et al. New Electrophysiological findings on the incidence of brain involvement in clinically and neurologically asymptomatic HIV infections. Eeg Emgz 1989; 20(4):280–287.
26. Petiot T, Vighetto A et al. Isolated postural tremor revealing HIV-1 infection. J Neurol 1993; 240(8):507–508.
27. Foncin JF, Maurin J et al. Curable ECHO 5 virus encephalitis. clinical, electroencephalographic, virological, and ultrastructural study. Ann Med Interni (Paris) 1977; 128(4):335–343.
28. Demikhov VG, Chaitsev VG. Neurological characteristics of diseases caused by inkoo and tahyna viruses. Vopr Virusol 1995; 40(1):21–25.
29. Cummins D, Bennett D et al. Lassa fever encephalopathy: clinical and laboratory findings. J Trop Med Hyg 1992; 95(3):1997–2001.
30. Sejvar JJ, Haddab MB, Tierney BC et al. Neurological manifestations and outcome of West Nile virus infection. JAMA 2003; 290(4):511–515.
31. Teive HA, Zanatta A et al. Holmes' tremor and neuro paracoccidioidomycosis: a case report. Mov Disord 2002; 17(6):1392–1394.
32. Vasquez TO, Rodriquez H et al. Generalized microsporidiosis caused by encephalitozoon Sp in pediatric patients with burton's disease. Bol Chil Parasitol 2001; 56(1–2):16–21.
33. Nguyen TH, Day NP et al. Postmalarial neurological syndrome. Lancet 1996; 348(9032):917–921.
34. Richens J. Typhoid in the Highlands of Papua New Guinea 1984–1990: a hospital-based perspective. PNG Med J 1995; 38(4):305–314.
35. Cardoso F. Infectious and transmissible movement disorders. In: Jankovic J, Tolosa E (eds.) Parkinson's Disease and Movement Disorders, 4th ed. Philadelphia, PA: Lippincott, Williams & Wilkins. 2002:584–595.
36. Lopez-Pison J, Garcia-Bodega O et al. Episodic disseminated inflammation of the CNS. Case makes review over a 13-year period. Rev Neural 2004; 38(5):405–410.

22

Intracranial Lesions and Tremor

Hubert H. Fernandez and Michael S. Okun

University of Florida, Gainesville, Florida, USA

I. INTRODUCTION

A tremendous number of reports of brain lesions resulting in tremor have been described in the literature (1–52). Advances in imaging and other diagnostic techniques have improved the recognition and reporting of lesions that result in tremor. As a result of this improved technology, a myriad of diseases and pathologies from many intracranial regions have been reported to result in almost every type of tremor. Although most intracranial lesions still follow the "general rules" regarding localization, pathophysiology, and corresponding tremor phenomenology such as basal ganglia lesions resulting in a contralateral resting 4–7 Hz tremor, cerebellar lesions resulting in a slow ipsilateral intention tremor, and midbrain lesions resulting in a contralateral resting, postural, and intention tremor, there have been occasional exceptions to the established notion of tremor pathophysiology. This should, however, be cautiously interpreted. Localization by imaging may be only as good as the technological modality used. An ipsilateral tremor from a large basal ganglia lesion does not definitively exclude a small contralateral lesion missed by a computed tomography (CT) scan. Magnetic resonance imaging (MRI) may better expose a lesion's anatomical devastation. Functional (or "pressure") effects of the lesions on contiguous or contralateral areas that more intuitively explain a patient's tremor phenomenology may not be fully appreciated. Only recent case reports have considered the "vascular effects" of intracranial lesions on distant brain regions through magnetic resonance angiography (MRA). With regard to intracranial infectious and neoplastic lesions, tremor resulting from slow infiltration, co-infection, edema, distant metastasis, and antibody/paraneoplastic phenomena, may be missed or misinterpreted despite contrast enhancement.

A variety of treatments have been utilized to control tremors resulting from cerebral lesions. All of these treatments have had variable success (2,51,53–62). However, descriptions of tremor treatment, success, and failure largely depend on the prognosis and treatment of the primary etiology and the degree of functional disability from the tremor. In some cases, tremor is only an incidental finding in a malignant encephalopathic syndrome, while in others it may be the presenting or most disabling feature of the disease or syndrome. Thus, in some reports the tremor type and its treatment is described in detail, while in others it is vaguely mentioned.

This chapter is divided into the broad etiologic categories of intracranial lesions: neoplastic, infectious, vascular, demyelinating, and miscellaneous causes. Each of these categories is discussed based on the phenomenology or clinical presentation of the tremor (i.e., resting/parkinsonian, postural, intentional), the identified anatomical localization, the postulated mechanistic hypothesis, and the response to treatment.

II. NEOPLASTIC LESIONS

A. Resting and/or Parkinsonian Tremor

Most resting tremors, with or without the associated features of parkinsonism, usually resulted from lesions affecting the contralateral basal ganglia (63–66). An example was a 66-year-old woman who presented with a three year history of progressive, pure right-sided hemiparkinsonism manifested by a right-hand resting tremor and right-sided bradykinesia (64). MRI revealed a non-enhancing polycystic mass in the left midbrain. Positron emission tomography (PET) revealed striatal hypometabolism that was restricted to the left side. The tumor was an astrocytoma. Her symptoms markedly improved with levodopa. Similarly, Singer et al. (65) reported a levodopa-responsive 66-year old woman who presented with blepharospasm, left-sided tremor and bradykinesia from a right mesencephalic arachnoid cyst. Bilaterally decreased striatal fluorodopa uptake was present on PET scan.

Not all tumor-induced resting tremors were reported to primarily involve the midbrain or basal ganglia (67–69). Moreover, they were not all located contralateral to the symptomatic side (70). A 14-year-old boy with an immature teratoma of the pineal gland was described to have parkinsonism. Diagnostic evaluation, however, revealed hydrocephalus, with the teratoma lesion extending to the thalamus. He was treated with levodopa and amantadine but marked improvement was only observed with shunt placement (67). A 44-year-old woman with a right frontal meningioma presented with resting tremor, rigidity, and bradykinesia of the left arm and leg. A CT scan showed a high-density mass of the right frontal lobe, but with marked surrounding edema probably causing compression of the basal ganglia. Prior to surgery, treatment with bromocriptine and levodopa was effective but the symptoms ultimately resolved with surgical resection of the tumor (68). Finally, Krauss et al. (70) reported a 47-year-old woman with a low-grade astrocytoma located in the right basal ganglia extending into the subthalamic area. Although she presented with left hemiparesis, she developed right-sided (ipsilateral) resting tremor and also right hemichorea. The authors postulated that the hemiparesis contralateral to the basal ganglia lesion might have had a "conditioning effect" on the appearance of her ipsilateral movement disorders.

Similarly, not all tremor-inducing tumors with a basal ganglia or thalamic location uniformly presented with resting or parkinsonian tremors. In a series of 225 patients with astrocytomas of the basal ganglia and thalamus, 20 had movement disorders. Of these 20, tremor was observed in 12 patients (71,72). Only five patients had parkinsonism with resting tremor, though tremor was also noted in these reports to be present with action. Ten patients had unilateral tremor, which in two was only present with action. Two other patients in this series had action and postural tremor, and six had a combined resting-postural-intention tremor. In nine of these patients, the tumor involved the thalamus. In the tenth, the tumor was predominantly located in the pallidum and putamen, sparing the thalamus, but exerting considerable compression on it. In one patient the tumor was located mainly in the red nucleus and in another the astrocytoma extended from the thalamus to the quadrigeminal plate. Tremor disappeared in three patients, improved to some degree in five, fluctuated in one, and did not change in two.

B. Intention and Cerebellar Tremor

Most tumors that cause tremor with intention, especially if accompanied by cerebellar features, were situated in the cerebellum, its peduncles, or at the level of the fourth ventricle (73–75). Additionally, intention tremors have also been described with bilateral thalamic tumors, and in particular childhood astrocytomas (76,77). Most of these cases were associated with ventricular dilatation/hydrocephalus and cerebellar features including progressive ataxia, slurred speech and nystamus. Attempts at treatment were most often disappointing.

Interestingly, a single case report was described in a 49-year-old man with a large epidermoid cyst in the left frontal lobe who presented with both parkinsonian and cerebellar tremors (78). Histological examination at necropsy revealed widespread granulomatous meningitis and ependymitis, cerebellar degeneration with marked loss of Purkinje cells, resulting from what the authors believe was dissemination throughout the subarachnoid space of the degredative products of the epidermoid cyst.

Treatment of these cases was variable including different pharmacologic and surgical approaches. One interesting treatment involved a single case report of improvement in action tremor from an acoustic neuroma with concomitant improvement of severe facial pain when treated with chronic cortical stimulation (75). The electrode was placed over the inferior part of the precentral region to stimulate at the level of the cortical representation of the face. Differential effects on pain and tremor were observed when parameters of stimulation were varied, suggesting different mechanisms for the relief of pain and tremor. The authors postulated that the positive observation could be the result of inhibition of subcortical structures which were involved in tremor.

C. Holmes Tremor

Most of the reported tumor-induced Holmes-type tremors were situated in the midbrain (56,79). However, a "tremor at rest in the left arm aggravated by intentional movement" was described in a boy with bilateral thalamic astrocytoma (77) and a "combined resting-postural-intention tremor" was described in six patients also with astrocytomas predominantly affecting the thalamus (71).

Pharmacotherapy has not been effective for these tremors. Thalamotomy (56) and thalamic stimulation (59) of the nucleus ventrointermedius (VIM) were reported to provide significant improvement in tumor-induced tremors especially in the midbrain.

D. Other Tremor Types

Non-specific unilateral tremors have been described, with gliomatosis cerebri which diffusely involved the cerebral hemispheres (80), an ependymal cyst in the paraventricular area (81), a meningioma of the anterior part of the falciform process (82), and in Hodgkin's disease involving the temporal region (83).

Cortical tremor, a rare movement disorder with the electrophysiological characteristics of cortical reflex myoclonus, has been described in a 76-year-old man with a meningioma over the right frontal cortex (84).

"Exertional tremor" was described in an 18-year old woman resulting from a posterior fossa arachnoid cyst. Leg tremor developed only during vigorous exercise, after 3–4 minutes of playing basketball, and gradually was relieved with rest. The exertional tremor resolved after decompression of the posterior fossa arachnoid cyst (85).

III. INFECTIOUS INTRACRANIAL LESIONS

Infections, whether intracranial or systemic, may present with tremors as part of their clinical spectrum, with or without an identified intracranial lesion. Tremors induced by infections with diffuse brain pathology or those without an identified intracranial lesion will be described briefly. Of these, the most reported are those associated with human immunodeficiency virus (HIV). Patients with HIV type 1 infection may develop hyperkinetic or hypokinetic movement disorders such as hemichorea-ballismus, myoclonus, dystonia, tremor, and parkinsonism. Tremor may be the presenting manifestation of the HIV infection (86), part of the clinical spectrum of advanced "HIV-dementia" (87), or result from an opportunistic process in the brain affecting the thalamus or basal ganglia (88,89). Parkinsonism and tremor can result from dopaminergic dysfunction resulting from HIV, or the use of anti-dopaminergic drugs (86,90). Rarely, trimethropim/sulfamethoxazole, an antibiotic often used in HIV, has been reported to cause tremor (91–93). The management involves recognition and treatment of opportunistic infections, symptomatic treatment of the movement disorder, and the use of highly active antiretroviral therapy (HAART). Cerebral toxoplasmosis in patients with HIV infection is often treated with the combination of sulfadiazine and pyrimethamine. Symptomatic treatment of the movement disorder, especially tremor and parkinsonism, is often disappointing. Preliminary data suggest that HAART may be helpful in the control and prevention of movement disorders in HIV patients (90).

Cerebral toxoplasmosis can also occur in patients with other immunodeficient states. Non-specific tremor was reported as part of a meningoencephalitis syndrome in a patient following stem cell transplantation for chronic myelogenous leukemia (94).

Among the viruses, tremor has been reported as part of brainstem encephalitis in enetrovirus 71 infections in children (95), meningo-encephalitis in West Nile virus infections (96), Inkoo and Tahyna viruses (97), and Lassa fever encephalopathy (98). Cerebellar-type tremors in the setting of acute cerebellitis have been described in association with varicella-zoster virus, mumps, enterovirus, mycoplasma, and less commonly, Epstein-Barr virus (99). A similar cerebellar-type tremor has been reported in type 1 human T-cell lymphotropic virus (HTLV-1) (100,101), a retrovirus that more commonly gives rise to a broad spectrum of disorders such as T-cell leukemia/lymphoma, tropical spastic paraparesis, uveitis, arthritis, polymyositis, and peripheral neuropathy. An extrapyramidal tremor with cerebellar ataxia has been described in tick-borne encephalitis (102).

Among the treponemas, "tremor of the tongue and hands" (103) and "orthostatic limb shaking," presumably representing recurrent transient ischemic attacks from an aortic aneurysm (104), were reported in syphilitic infections.

Cerebellar ataxia and tremor have been described in central nervous system tuberculosis (105). Neuroimaging revealed meningeal enhancement in 53%, tuberculoma in 50%, and occasionally hydrocephalus, infarction, or bleeding.

A postural and/or intention tremor may be part of the clinical picture of post-malaria neurological syndrome (PMNS), usually associated with encephalopathy, aphasia, myoclonus, convulsions, or ataxia, or as patients recover from an acute falciparum malaria infection (106,107).

Among infections with an identified specific intracranial lesion or pathology, resting tremors, associated with ataxia, sleepiness, hyperesthesia, and slurred speech had been described with bilateral edema of the basal ganglia and cerebellar peduncles in an echovirus type 21 infection (108). After three months, MRI changes and clinical symptoms resolved.

Holmes-type tremors from infectious etiologies have been reported in midbrain toxoplasma abcess (86,88,89), midbrain paracoccidioidomycosis (109), and cytomegalovirus infection involving the thalamus, basal ganglia, and external capsule following liver transplantation (110). Levodopa, clonazepam, and trihexyphenidyl were all tried without significant benefit.

Finally, tremors were reported to occur as part of an acute encephalopathy associated with bilateral striatal necrosis from a herpes simplex type 1 infection (111) or bilateral thalamic necrosis from a mycoplasma pneumoniae infection (112). In both cases, tremor improved with corticosteroid therapy.

IV. VASCULAR LESIONS

The majority of vascular lesions resulting in tremor are the result of stroke or intracranial hemorrhage (1–52). The clinical manifestation is ultimately the result of the pathophysiological influence of these lesions on the basal ganglia and on other intracranial structures. In some cases, that is, vascular parkinsonism (113–115), it may be hypothesized that the tremor is the result of the lesion's effect upon the direct and indirect basal ganglia pathways. However in the majority of cases of lesion-induced tremor, the pathophysiology remains unclear.

There have been many reports of tremors resulting from stroke and intracranial hemorrhage. A literature search of "stroke" and "tremor" yielded 118 well described cases published between 1982 and 2003, however, there were only seven cases of tremor related to cavernous angioma and arterio-venous malformations (AVM). A detailed review of these cases yields some useful information regarding the presentation of these tremors (see Tables 22.1 and 22.2). The vast majority of cases present with postural-action tremors. Occasionally, vascular parkinsonism may present with a resting tremor. Most patients with vascular parkinsonism present with lower body parkinsonism, rigidity, bradykinesia, and a gait disorder (113–115). Although there have been reported cases of

Table 22.1 Strokes and Intracerebral Hemorrhages Reported Between 1982 and 2003 to be Associated with Tremor ($n = 118$ Cases)

Author	Year	N	Rest	Postural/intention	Location	Etiology	Associated features	Treatment
Negata (1)	1982	1	(−)	(−)	Midbrain	Stroke	Head tremor	
Berkovic (2)	1984	3	(+)	(+)	Midbrain	Stroke	Dystonia, Holmes tremor	Levodopa
Bogousslavsky (4)	1986	1	(−)	(+)	Anterior choroidal artery	Stroke	Hemiataxia, sensory loss	
Schlitt (5)	1986	1	(−)	(+)	Thalamus	ICH	Appendicular tremor, weakness	Thalamotomy
Nagaratnam (6)	1988	1	(−)	(+)	Multiple lacunes	Stroke		
Arunabh (7)	1992	1	(−)	(+)	Caudate nucleus	Stroke	Blepharospasm, hemifacial spasm	
Kim (8)	1992	3	(+)	(−)	Caudate nucleus, Thalamus	Stroke		
Ferbert (9)	1993	4	(−)	(+)	Thalamus ($n = 2$), others unknown ($n = 2$)	Stroke	Dystonia	Some spontaneous resolution
Lee (10)	1993	1	(+)	(−)	Thalamus, internal capsule	Stroke		
Mano (11)	1993	2	(−)	(+)	Thalamus	ICH		Cerulitide
Milandre (12)	1993	1	(−)	(+)	Thalamus	Stroke		
Mossuto-Agatiello (13)	1993	1	(+)	(+)	Thalamus	Stroke	Holmes tremor	Incidental stroke
Okuda (14)	1993	1	(−)	(+)	Midbrain	Stroke	Intranuclear ophthalmoplegia, Ataxia	
Defer (15)	1994	1	(+)	(+)	Midbrain	Stroke		Levodopa

(continued)

Table 22.1 *Continued*

Author	Year	N	Rest	Postural/ intention	Location	Etiology	Associated features	Treatment
Dove (16)	1994	1	(−)	(+)	Parietal/occipital	ICH		Metoprolol
Ghika (17)	1994	3	(−)	(+)	Posterior choroidal (thalamic)	Stroke	Ataxia, tremor, dystonia, myoclonus and chorea	
Kim (18)	1994	1	(−)	(+)	Left frontal	Stroke	Primary writing tremor	
Moroo (19)	1994	5	(−)	(+)	Thalamus, pulvinar in one patient	Stroke	Chorea, Holmes tremor	
Otto (20)	1995	1	(−)	(−)	Bilateral thalamic, midbrain	Stroke	Head tremor	
Finsterer (21)	1996	1	(−)	(−)	Bilateral cerebellar	Stroke	Head tremor	
Louis (22)	1996	5	(−)	(+)	Cerebellar, brainstem	Stroke/ Trauma	Delayed cerebellar syndrome	
Miwa (23)	1996	2	(+)	(+)	Thalamus	Stroke		
Qureshi (24)	1996	1	(−)	(+)	Thalamus	Stroke		
Ghika-Schmid (25)	1997	3	(−)	(+)	Middle and posterior cerebral artery	Stroke		
Imai (26)	1997	1	(−)	(+)	Midbrain	Stroke		
Moroo (27)	1997	1	(−)	(+)	Parietal	Stroke		
Ghika (28)	1998	5	(−)	(+)	Parietal	Stroke	Parietal motor syndrome	
Schulze-Bonhage (29)	1998	1	(−)	(+)	Parietal	Stroke	Focal motor seizures	

Author (Ref)	Year	N			Location	Etiology	Description	Treatment
van Zagten (30)	1998	4	(+)	(−)	White matter lacunes	Stroke	Post-Stroke Parkinsonism	
Brannan (31)	1999	1	(−)	(−)	Striatum	Stroke		
Endo (32)	1999	2	(+)	(−)	Cerebellar	ICH, Stroke		
Fernandez (33)	1999	1	(+)	(+)	Midbrain	Stroke	Holmes tremor, dystonia, Benedikts syndrome	
Kalita (34)	1999	1	(+)	(−)	Midbrain	Stroke	Head tremor, cryptococcal meningitis	Antifungals
Kao (35)	1999	1	(+)	(−)	Thalamus, subthalamus	Stroke	Myoclonus	Resolved
Soler (36)	1999	1	(+)	(−)	Thalamus	Stroke		
Yanagisawa (37)	1999	1	(+)	(−)	Brainstem, superior peduncle, dentate	Stroke	Palatal tremor	
Benamer (38)	2000	1	(+)	(−)	Putamen	Stroke		Ondansetron
Cho (39)	2000	1	(+)	(+)	Anterior thalamus	Stroke	Dystonic tremor	
Frates (40)	2001	1	(+)	(+)	Superior cerebellar, thalamus, basal ganglia	Stroke		Levodopa
Kim (41)	2001	35	(+)	(−)	Thalamus	ICH, Stroke	Dystonia, athetosis, chorea	
Kim (42)	2001	6	(−)	(+)	Anterior cerebral artery, SMA	Stroke	Parkinsonian syndrome	
Lehericy (43)	2001	6	(+)	(−)	Thalamus	Stroke		
Tan (44)	2001	1	(+)	(−)	Bilateral paramedian and cerebellar infarcts	Stroke	Complex movement disorder	
Tan (45)	2001	2	(+)	(+)	Bilateral thamalus	Stroke	Holmes tremor	

Note: ICH, intracerebral hemorrhage; SMA, supplementary motor area.

Table 22.2 Cavernous Malformations, AVM's and Intracerebral Hemorrhages Reported Between 1982 and 2003 to be Associated with Tremor (*n* = 7 Cases)

Author	Year	N	Rest	Postural/ intention	Location	Etiology	Associated features	Treatment
Krings (50)	2003	1	(−)	(+)	Pontine	Cavernous	Palatal tremor	
Samadani (51)	2003	1	(+)	(+)	Midbrain	Cavernous	Chorea	Thalamic stimulation
Ohara (49)	2002	1	(−)	(+)	Cerebellum	Cavernous	Cerebellar signs	
Weng (48)	2000	1	(+)	(+)	Midbrain	Cavernous	Holmes tremor	
Leung (47)	1999	1	(−)	(+)	Midbrain	Cavernous	Holmes tremor	
Krauss (46)	1999	1	(−)	(+)	Frontal lobe	AVM	Cortical tremor	Thalamotomy
Koshimura (52)	1996	1	(−)	(−)	Basal ganglia/ posterior fossa	AVM	Head tremor	

Note: AVM, arteriovenous malformation.

resting tremors after stroke (8,10,30) this is a rare occurrence unless the resting tremor is part of a Holmes-type tremor (2). These tremors may also be associated with dystonia and other movement disorders (2,13,33,45). Additionally, they may be associated with a head tremor as are other vascular lesions particularly when involving the cerebellum, brainstem, or thalamus (1,21,34,44). Virtually all of the different movement disorder phenomenologies (e.g., dystonia, ataxia, chorea, myoclonus, etc.) may present with tremor as an accompanying feature.

The neuroanatomical location of vascular lesions resulting in tremor is as variable as the phenomenology. Lesions of the frontal, parietal, occipital, brainstem, cerebellum, and all subcortical structures have been reported to result in tremor (1–45,116,117). Although most of the lesions are associated with large or small vessel disease in the middle cerebral artery territories, other vascular territories have also been reported, including the anterior (42) and posterior cerebral arteries (25), the basilar and penetrating arteries (19,20,33,34), and the anterior (4) and posterior choroidal artery (28) distributions.

The neuroanatomical location of a lesion may occasionally be helpful in clarifying phenomenology. Examples of this include the Holmes tremors often seen with brainstem pathology, head tremor seen with brainstem and cerebellar pathology, chorea and other movement disorders seen with thalamic pathology, and parkinsonism (often without tremor) seen with multiple lacunar states (see Table 22.1). However, as discussed previously, in tremors which result from lesions, phenomenology does not always predict location or pathology.

Treatment for tremors resulting from vascular lesions has been in general inconsistent and disappointing. There are few reports of success, including carbidopa/levodopa, beta blockers, anticholinergics, benzodiazepines, anticonvulsants, ondansetron, and other oral agents (2,11,16,40,53–56,59,61). These may prove to be useful in dampening and in rare cases eliminating tremor. Additionally, there have been reports of tremor with acute stroke that has resolved on follow-up without treatment. For post-stroke Holmes tremors, one medication that has been consistently used, and perhaps should be tried in all patients, is high dose (i.e., >1 g/day) carbidopa/levodopa.

Patients with severe tremors which are refractory to medications may consider surgical therapies. There are no prospective randomized trials of surgical therapies for post-stroke tremor, however, there are individual case reports of thalamotomy and thalamic deep brain stimulation being useful in this setting (51,55–58,60,62,118–123). Because of the variability of lesion size and location in post-stroke and post-hemorrhage tremor, the optimal site and procedure for surgical interventions may be different in individual patients.

V. DEMYELINATING LESIONS

There are several causes of demyelinating disease resulting in tremor including acute disseminated encephalomyelitis (124,125), neuropathies [such as IGM paraproteinemia (126–130), chronic inflammatory demyelinating neuropathy

(131,132), acute inflammatory demyelinating neuropathy (133)], and multiple sclerosis (MS). The most commonly encountered cause of tremor from cerebral demyelination is MS (134). Estimated in some series as occurring in as high as 75% of cases, MS tremor can be both disabling and difficult to treat (135).

Phenomenologically these patients usually present with postural or postural-action tremors. The tremor can involve the head, trunk, limbs or a combination of multiple body parts (134,136–141). Some authors have referred to the large amplitude postural tremor seen in MS as a classic "wing beating" tremor (139–141). MS does not usually present with a true Holmes tremor or with an isolated resting tremor (134,136), although patient positioning may contribute to the visual image of a resting tremor. It is important to separate tremor from cerebellar dysfunction, but this is often not a straightforward task.

Since lesions may have a relapsing-remitting course, the exact neuroanatomical region responsible for MS-induced tremor can be challenging to pinpoint. Autopsy studies have implicated multiple regions (134,136), and likely the genesis of this tremor is a disruption of the neurophysiology of one or more basal ganglia pathways. Cerebellar lesions are thought to be involved in postural-intention tremors in MS.

Many treatments have been directed at MS tremor, with little or no effect (136,137,139–144). Although the course of a patient's disease may fluctuate, the majority of MS patients do not experience waning of their tremor while in remission. It is unclear whether interferon or other immunomodulation therapies have any effect on tremor. Several therapies have been directed at MS tremor with mixed and often unsatisfactory results, including isoniazid, glutethimide, clonazepam, carbamazepine, dilantin, primidone, hyoscine, tetra-hydrocannibol, ondansetron, propranolol, alcohol, weights for the wrists, and physical therapy (136,137,139–144). Occasionally, surgical therapies such as thalamic deep brain stimulation or thalamotomy have resulted in improvement in MS tremor (145–149).

VI. IATROGENIC ETIOLOGIES

Rarely, tremor has been reported in patients after radiation of intracranial lesions. A single case report described a 20-year-old woman with a vascular hamartoma in the pineal region who underwent radiotherapy, whereupon a unilateral low-frequency resting and intention tremor later developed. Following resection of the lesion, the tremor resolved. The authors hypothesized that the tremor was secondary to radiation-induced tumor shrinkage and distortion of the mesencephalon (150). Similarly, six autopsy-proven cases of post-radiation pathology characterized by swelling and loss of the myelin sheath in the white matter, with resulting brain atrophy, were reported to clinically present with subacute, progressive mental status change, akinesia, and "tremor-like involuntary movement" several months after radiation therapy for residual or recurrent brain tumors (151).

Finally, movement disorders, including tremor, have been described following craniocerebral surgery (152,153). In one series of 14 patients who suffered from movement disorders after craniocerebral or spinal surgery, in all but two patients, the movement disorder became manifest only after a delay. Dystonic movements developed in eight patients, unilateral tremors in three patients, unilateral facial myokymia in one patient, and hemichorea in two patients. The mean delay of onset of tremor was five weeks. Lesions of the dentatothalamic outlflow were identified in the patients with tremor. Medical treatment rendered only limited benefit and occasionally, these post-operative tremors were transient. A single case report of a 59-year-old woman who developed an isolated transient pill-rolling resting tremor one month post-operatively after a frontal meningioma resection was described (153). The tremor spontaneously disappeared after eight weeks. The authors postulated that perioperative factors such as local ischemia, disturbed venous drainage, or diffuse hypoxia related to events associated with general anesthesia may have caused impaired nigrostriatal transmission bilaterally leading to the transient rest and postural tremor in the patient.

REFERENCES

1. Nagata H, Kamo H, Kato T, Kameyama M, Toyoshima M. Tremor-like involuntary movements in head due to midbrain infarction. Rinsho Shinkeigaku 1982; 22(6):521–525.
2. Berkovic SF, Bladin PF. Rubral tremor: clinical features and treatment of three cases. Clin Exp Neurol 1984; 20:119–128.
3. Tashiro K, Sawamura Y, Matsumoto A, Hamada T, Moriwaka F, Shima K. Clinical studies on multiple lacunar state. No To Shinkei 1984; 36(5):475–480.
4. Bogousslavsky J, Regli F, Delaloye B, Delaloye-Bischoff A, Uske A, Despland PA. Hemiataxia and ipsilateral sensory deficit. Infarct in the area of the anterior choroidal artery. Crossed cerebellar diaschisis. Rev Neurol (Paris) 1986; 142(8–9):671–676.
5. Schlitt M, Brown JW, Zeiger HE, Galbraith JG. Appendicular tremor as a late complication of intracerebral hemorrhage. Surg Neurol 1986; 25(2):181–184.
6. Nagaratnam N, Ghougassian DF, Lewis-Jones M. The shaking limb—a lacunar syndrome. Postgrad Med J 1988; 64(750):311–312.
7. Arunabh, Jain S, Maheshwari MC. Blepharospasm hemifacial spasm and tremors possibly due to isolated caudate nucleus lesions. J Assoc Physicians India 1992; 40(10):687–689.
8. Kim JS. Delayed onset hand tremor caused by cerebral infarction. Stroke 1992; 23(2):292–294.
9. Ferbert A, Gerwig M. Tremor due to stroke. Mov Disord 1993; 8(2):179–182.
10. Lee MS, Lee SA, Heo JH, Choi IS. A patient with a resting tremor and a lacunar infarction at the border between the thalamus and the internal capsule. Mov Disord 1993; 8(2):244–246.
11. Mano Y, Nakamuro T, Takayanagi T, Mayer RF. Ceruletide therapy in action tremor following thalamic hemorrhage. J Neurol 1993; 240(3):144–148.

12. Milandre L, Brosset C, Gabriel B, Khalil R. Transient involuntary movement disorders and thalamic infarction. Rev Neurol (Paris) 1993; 149(6–7):402–406.
13. Mossuto-Agatiello L, Puccetti G, Castellano AE. "Rubral" tremor after thalamic haemorrhage. J Neurol 1993; 241(1):27–30.
14. Okuda B, Tachibana H, Sugita M, Maeda Y. Bilateral internuclear ophthalmoplegia, ataxia, and tremor from a midbrain infarction. Stroke 1993; 24(3):481–482.
15. Defer GL, Remy P, Malapert D, Ricolfi F, Samson Y, Degos JD. Rest tremor and extrapyramidal symptoms after midbrain haemorrhage: clinical and ^{18}F-dopa PET evaluation. J Neurol Neurosurg Psychiatry 1994; 57(8):987–989.
16. Dove CA, Vezzetti D, Escobar N. Metoprolol for action tremor following intracerebral hemorrhage. Arch Phys Med Rehabil 1994; 75(9):1011–1014.
17. Ghika J, Bogousslavsky J, Henderson J, Maeder P, Regli F. The "jerky dystonic unsteady hand": a delayed motor syndrome in posterior thalamic infarctions. J Neurol 1994; 241(9):537–542.
18. Kim JS, Lee MC. Writing tremor after discrete cortical infarction. Stroke 1994; 25(11):2280–2282.
19. Moroo I, Hirayama K, Kojima S. Involuntary movements caused by thalamic lesion. Rinsho Shinkeigaku 1994; 34(8):805–811.
20. Otto S, Buttner T, Schols L, Windmeier DT, Przuntek H. Head tremor due to bilateral thalamic and midbrain infarction. J Neurol 1995; 242(9):608–610.
21. Finsterer J, Muellbacher W, Mamoli B. Yes/yes head tremor without appendicular tremor after bilateral cerebellar infarction. J Neurol Sci 1996; 139(2):242–245.
22. Louis ED, Lynch T, Ford B, Greene P, Bressman SB, Fahn S. Delayed-onset cerebellar syndrome. Arch Neurol 1996; 53(5):450–454.
23. Miwa H, Hatori K, Kondo T, Imai H, Mizuno Y. Thalamic tremor: case reports and implications of the tremor-generating mechanism. Neurology 1996; 46(1):75–79.
24. Qureshi F, Morales A, Elble RJ. Tremor due to infarction in the ventrolateral thalamus. Mov Disord 1996; 11(4):440–444.
25. Ghika-Schmid F, Ghika J, Regli F, Bogousslavsky J. Hyperkinetic movement disorders during and after acute stroke: the Lausanne Stroke Registry. J Neurol Sci 1997; 146(2):109–116.
26. Imai N, Hara A, Miyata K, Terayama Y, Ishihara N. A case of midbrain infarction with ipsilateral hand tremor. No To Shinkei 1997; 49(11):1033.
27. Moroo I, Hirayama K, Nakajima M. Delayed onset postural tremor caused by parietal lesion. Mov Disord 1997; 12(6):1098–1100.
28. Ghika J, Ghika-Schmid F, Bogousslavky J. Parietal motor syndrome: a clinical description in 32 patients in the acute phase of pure parietal strokes studied prospectively. Clin Neurol Neurosurg 1998; 100(4):271–282.
29. Schulze-Bonhage A, Ferbert A. Cortical action tremor and focal motor seizures after parietal infarction. Mov Disord 1998; 13(2):356–358.
30. van Zagten M, Lodder J, Kessels F. Gait disorder and parkinsonian signs in patients with stroke related to small deep infarcts and white matter lesions. Mov Disord 1998; 13(1):89–95.
31. Brannan T, Yahr MD. Focal tremor following striatal infarct—a case report. Mov Disord 1999; 14(2):368–370.
32. Endo K, Mito T, Kano T et al. Contralateral cerebellar infarction after aneurysmal clipping with pterional craniotomy: report of two cases. No Shinkei Geka 1999; 27(7):659–665.

33. Fernandez HH, Friedman JH, Centofanti JV. Benedikt's syndrome with delayed-onset rubral tremor and hemidystonia: a complication of tic douloureux surgery. Mov Disord 1999; 14(4):695–697.

34. Kalita J, Bansal R, Ayagiri A, Misra UK. Midbrain infarction: a rare presentation of cryptococcal meningitis. Clin Neurol Neurosurg 1999; 101(1):23–25.

35. Kao YF, Shih PY, Chen WH. An unusual concomitant tremor and myoclonus after a contralateral infarct at thalamus and subthalamic nucleus. Kaohsiung J Med Sci 1999; 15(9):562–566.

36. Soler R, Vivancos F, Munoz-Torrero JJ, Arpa J, Barreiro P. Postural tremor after thalamic infarction. Eur Neurol 1999; 42(3):180–181.

37. Yanagisawa T, Sugihara H, Shibahara K, Kamo T, Fujisawa K, Murayama M. Natural course of combined limb and palatal tremor caused by cerebellar-brain stem infarction. Mov Disord 1999; 14(5):851–854.

38. Benamer HT, Russell AJ, Hadley DM, Grosset DG. Unilateral arm tremor as the sole feature of ischemic stroke: a 5-year follow up. Mov Disord 2000; 15(2):346–347.

39. Cho C, Samkoff LM. A lesion of the anterior thalamus producing dystonic tremor of the hand. Arch Neurol 2000; 57(9):1353–1355.

40. Frates EP, Burke DT, Chae H, Ahangar B. Post-stroke violent adventitial movement responsive to levo-dopa/carbi-dopa therapy. Brain Inj 2001; 15(10): 911–916.

41. Kim JS. Delayed onset mixed involuntary movements after thalamic stroke: clinical, radiological and pathophysiological findings. Brain 2001; 124(Pt 2):299–309.

42. Kim JS. Involuntary movements after anterior cerebral artery territory infarction. Stroke 2001; 32(1):258–261.

43. Lehericy S, Grand S, Pollak P et al. Clinical characteristics and topography of lesions in movement disorders due to thalamic lesions. Neurology 2001; 57(6):1055–1066.

44. Tan EK, Chan LL, Auchus AP. Complex movement disorders following bilateral paramedian thalamic and bilateral cerebellar infarcts. Mov Disord 2001; 16(5):968–970.

45. Tan H, Turanli G, Ay H, Saatci I. Rubral tremor after thalamic infarction in childhood. Pediatr Neurol 2001; 25(5):409–412.

46. Krauss JK, Kiriyanthan GD, Borremans JJ. Cerebral arteriovenous malformations and movement disorders. Clin Neurol Neurosurg 1999; 101(2):92–99.

47. Leung GK, Fan YW, Ho SL. Rubral tremor associated with cavernous angioma of the midbrain. Mov Disord 1999; 14(1):191–193.

48. Weng YH, Kao PF, Tsai CH, Yen TC, Lu CS. Dopamine deficiency in rubral tremor caused by midbrain hemangioma: case report. Changgeng Yi Xue Za Zhi 2000; 23(8):485–491.

49. Ohara K, Shinjo T, Nishii R, Takeda K, Kokai M, Morita Y. A case of intra-axial multiple cavernous angiomas, presented with dementia and cerebellar signs. Seishin Shinkeigaku Zasshi 2002; 104(7):585–594.

50. Krings T, Foltys H, Meister IG, Reul J. Hypertrophic olivary degeneration following pontine haemorrhage: hypertensive crisis or cavernous haemangioma bleeding? J Neurol Neurosurg Psychiatry 2003; 74(6):797–799.

51. Samadani U, Umemura A, Jaggi JL, Colcher A, Zager EL, Baltuch GH. Thalamic deep brain stimulation for disabling tremor after excision of a midbrain cavernous angioma. Case report. J Neurosurg 2003; 98(4):888–890.

52. Koshimura I, Takeda N, Ohtomo T et al. A 32-year-old man who developed a posterior fossa mass 12 years after the radiation therapy for cerebellar arteriovenous malformation. No To Shinkei 1996; 48(1):81–89.

53. Chen JJ, Swope DM. Essential tremor: diagnosis and treatment. Pharmacotherapy 2003; 23(9):1105–1122.

54. Deuschl G, Wilms H, Krack P, Wurker M, Heiss WD. Function of the cerebellum in Parkinsonian rest tremor and Holmes' tremor. Ann Neurol 1999; 46(1):126–128.

55. Deuschl G, Bain P. Deep brain stimulation for tremor [correction of trauma]: patient selection and evaluation. Mov Disord 2002; 17(suppl 3):S102–S111.

56. Kim MC, Son BC, Miyagi Y, Kang JK. Vim thalamotomy for Holmes' tremor secondary to midbrain tumour. J Neurol Neurosurg Psychiatry 2002; 73(4):453–455.

57. Li JY, Chen G, Zhuang P, Li YJ. Neuroelectrophysiological basis and surgical treatment of essential tremor. Zhongguo Yi Xue Ke Xue Yuan Xue Bao 2003; 25(2):207–209.

58. Miyagi Y, Shima F, Ishido K, Moriguchi M, Kamikaseda K. Posteroventral pallidotomy for midbrain tremor after a pontine hemorrhage. Case report. J Neurosurg 1999; 91(5):885–888.

59. Pahwa R, Lyons KE. Essential tremor: differential diagnosis and current therapy. Am J Med 2003; 115(2):134–142.

60. Romanelli P, Bronte-Stewart H, Courtney T, Heit G. Possible necessity for deep brain stimulation of both the ventralis intermedius and subthalamic nuclei to resolve Holmes tremor. Case report. J Neurosurg 2003; 99(3):566–571.

61. Serrano-Duenas M. Use of primidone in low doses (250 mg/day) versus high doses (750 mg/day) in the management of essential tremor. Double-blind comparative study with one-year follow-up. Parkinsonism Relat Disord 2003; 10(1):29–33.

62. Zervas NT, Horner FA, Pickren KS. The treatment of dyskinesia by stereotxic dentatectomy. Confin Neurol 1967; 29(2):93–100.

63. Rousseaux M, Parent M, Lesoin F et al. Rhythmical myoclonus and tremor at rest disclosing mesencephalic metastasis. Rev Neurol (Paris) 1990; 146(4):283–287.

64. Yoshimura M, Yamamoto T, Iso-o N et al. Hemiparkinsonism associated with a mesencephalic tumor. J Neurol Sci 2002; 197(1–2):89–92.

65. Singer C, Schatz NJ, Bowen B et al. Asymmetric predominantly ipsilateral blepharospasm and contralateral parkinsonism in an elderly patient with a right mesencephalic cyst. Mov Disord 1998; 13(1):135–139.

66. Bosch J, Vilalta J, Tintore M, Ortega A, Montalban X, Codina A. Parkinsonian hemi-syndrome as the initial manifestation of supratentorial cystic hemangioblastoma in a patient with Von Hippel-Lindau disease. Rev Neurol 1998; 26(150):221–223.

67. Dolendo MCLT, Tat OH, Chong QT, Timothy LK. Parkinsonism as an unusual presenting symptom of pineal gland teratoma. Pediatr Neurol 2003; 28(4):310–312.

68. Lu CS, Chang CN. Hemiparkinsonism in a patient with frontal meningioma. J Formos Med Assoc 1992; 91(12):1216–1218.

69. Husag L, Wieser HG, Probst C. Extrapyramidal symptoms in meningiomas. Schweiz Arch Neurol Neurochir Psychiatr 1975; 116(2):257–279.

70. Krauss JK, Pohle T, Borremans JJ. Hemichorea and hemiballism associated with contralateral hemiparesis and ipsilateral basal ganglia lesions. Mov Disord 1999; 14(3):497–501.

71. Krauss JK, Nobbe F, Wakhloo AK, Mohadjer M, Vach W, Mundinger F. Movement disorders in astrocytomas of the basal ganglia and the thalamus. J Neurol Neurosurg Psychiatry 1992; 55(12):1162–1167.

72. Krauss JK, Braus DF, Mohadjer M, Nobbe F, Mundinger F. Evaluation of the effect of treatment on movement disorders in astrocytomas of the basal ganglia and the thalamus. J Neurol Neurosurg Psychiatry 1993; 56(10):1113–1138.

73. Fiume D, Gazzeri G, Spallone A, Santucci N. Epidermoid cysts of the fourth ventricle. Surg Neurol 1988; 29(3):178–182.

74. Ibayashi N, Ueda S, Uchibori M, Hirakawa K. A case of cerebellar neuroblastoma. No Shinkei Geka 1987; 15(4):459–463.

75. Nguyen JP, Pollin B, Feve A, Geny C, Cesaro P. Improvement of action tremor by chronic cortical stimulation. Mov Disord 1998; 13(1):84–88.

76. Gudowius S, Engelbrecht V, Messing-Junger M, Reifenberger G, Gartner J. Diagnostic difficulties in childhood bilateral thalamic astrocytomas. Neuropediatrics 2002; 33(6):331–335.

77. Di Rocco C, Iannelli A. Bilateral thalamic tumors in children. Childs Nerv Syst 2002; 18(8):440–444.

78. Tomlinson BE, Walton JN. Granulomatous meningitis and diffuse parenchymatous degeneration of the nervous system due to an intracranial epidermoid cyst. J Neurol Neurosurg Psychiatry 1967; 30(4):341–348.

79. Pahwa R, Lyons KE, Kempf L, Wilkinson SB, Koller WC. Thalamic stimulation for midbrain tremor after partial hemangioma resection. Mov Disord 2002; 17(2):404–407.

80. Jayawant S, Neale J, Stoodley N, Wallace S. Gliomatosis cerebri in a 10-year-old girl masquerading as diffuse encephalomyelitis and spinal cord tumour. Dev Med Child Neurol 2001; 43(2):124–126.

81. Bejar JM, Kepes J, Koller WC. Hemiballism and tremor due to ependymal cyst. Mov Disord 1992; 7(4):370–372.

82. El'ner AM, Gabibov GA, Lobkova EF. Unusual tremor in a patient with a local lesion of the brain. Zh Nevropatol Psikhiatr Im S S Korsakova 1984; 84(4):530–533.

83. Ogata H, Karikomi M, Araki T, Uchiyama G. A case of intracranial involvement of Hodgkin's disease. Radiat Med 1993; 11(5):210–213.

84. Wang HC, Hsu WC, Brown P. Cortical tremor secondary to a frontal cortical lesion. Mov Disord 1999; 14(2):370–374.

85. Heller AC, Kellogg J, Delashaw J, Camicioli R. Posterior fossa arachnoid cyst associated with an exertional tremor. Mov Disord 2000; 15(4):746–749.

86. De Mattos JP, Rosso AL, Correa RB, Novis S. Involuntary movements and AIDS: report of seven cases and review of the literature. Arq Neuropsiquiatr 1993; 51(4):491–497.

87. Gray F. Dementia and human inmmunodeficiency virus infection. Rev Neurol (Paris) 1998; 154(suppl 2):S91–S98.

88. Pezzini A, Zavarise P, Palvarini L, Viale P, Oladeji O, Padovani A. Holmes' tremor following midbrain Toxoplasma abscess: clinical features and treatment of a case. Parkinsonism Relat Disord 2002; 8(3):177–180.

89. Daras M, Koppel BS, Samkoff L, Marc J. Brainstem toxoplasmosis in patients with acquired immunodeficiency syndrome. J Neuroimaging 1994; 4(2):85–90.

90. Cardoso F. HIV-related movement disorders: epidemiology, pathogenesis and management. CNS Drugs 2002; 16(10):663–668.

91. Slavik RS, Rybak MJ, Lerner SA. Trimethoprim/sulfamethoxazole-induced tremor in a patient with AIDS. Ann Pharmacother 1998; 32(2):189–192.
92. Van Gerpen JA. Tremor caused by trimethoprim-sulfamethoxazole in a patient with AIDS. Neurology 1997; 48(2):537–538.
93. Aboulafia DM. Tremors associated with trimethoprim-sulfamethoxazole therapy in a patient with AIDS: case report and review. Clin Infect Dis 1996; 22(3):598–600.
94. Gonzalez MI, Caballero D, Lopez C et al. Cerebral toxoplasmosis and Guillain-Barre syndrome after allogeneic peripheral stem cell transplantation. Transpl Infect Dis 2000; 2(3):145–149.
95. Huang CC, Liu CC, Chang YC, Chen CY, Wang ST, Yeh TF. Neurologic complications in children with enterovirus 71 infection. N Engl J Med 1999; 341(13):936–942.
96. Sejvar JJ, Haddad MB, Tierney BC et al. Neurologic manifestations and outcome of West Nile virus infection. Jama 2003; 290(4):511–515.
97. Demikhov VG, Chaitsev VG. Neurologic characteristics of diseases caused by Inkoo and Tahyna viruses. Vopr Virusol 1995; 40(1):21–25.
98. Cummins D, Bennett D, Fisher-Hoch SP, Farrar B, Machin SJ, McCormick JB. Lassa fever encephalopathy: clinical and laboratory findings. J Trop Med Hyg 1992; 95(3):197–201.
99. Teive HA, Zavala JA, Iwamoto FM, Bertucci-Filho D, Werneck LC. Acute cerebellitis caused by Epstein-Barr virus: case report. Arq Neuropsiquiatr 2001; 59(3-A):616–618.
100. Carod-Artal FJ, del Negro MC, Vargas AP, Rizzo I. Cerebellar syndrome and peripheral neuropathy as manifestations of infection by HTLV-1 human T-cell lymphotropic virus. Rev Neurol 1999; 29(10):932–935.
101. Castillo LC, Gracia F, Roman GC, Levine P, Reeves WC, Kaplan J. Spinocerebellar syndrome in patients infected with human T-lymphotropic virus types I and II (HTLV-I/HTLV-II): report of 3 cases from Panama. Acta Neurol Scand 2000; 101(6):405–412.
102. Duniewicz M. Clinical picture of Central European tick-borne encephalitis (author's transl). MMW Munch Med Wochenschr 1976; 118(49):1609–1612.
103. Pavlovic DM, Milovic AM. Clinical characteristics and therapy of neurosyphilis in patients who are negative for human immunodeficiency virus. Srp Arh Celok Lek 1999; 127(7–8):236–240.
104. Brotman DJ, Fotuhi M. Syphilis and orthostatic shaking limbs. Lancet 2000; 356(9243):1734.
105. Kurisaki H. Central nervous system tuberculosis with and without HIV infection—clinical, neuroimaging, and neuropathological study. Rinsho Shinkeigaku 2000; 40(3):209–217.
106. Nguyen TH, Day NP, Ly VC et al. Post-malaria neurological syndrome. Lancet 1996; 348(9032):917–921.
107. Schnorf H, Diserens K, Schnyder H et al. Corticosteroid-responsive postmalaria encephalopathy characterized by motor aphasia, myoclonus, and postural tremor. Arch Neurol 1998; 55(3):417–420.
108. Freund A, Zass R, Kurlemann G, Schuierer G, Ullrich K. Bilateral oedema of the basal ganglia in an echovirus type 21 infection: complete clinical and radiological normalization. Dev Med Child Neurol 1998; 40(6):421–424.

109. Teive HA, Zanatta A, Germiniani FM, Almeida SM, Werneck LC. Holmes' tremor and neuroparacoccidioidomycosis: a case report. Mov Disord 2002; 17(6):1392–1394.
110. Coelho JC, Wiederkehr JC, Cat R et al. Extrapyramidal disorder secondary to cytomegalovirus infection and toxoplasmosis after liver transplantation. Eur J Pediatr Surg 1996; 6(2):110–111.
111. Yamamoto K, Chiba HO, Ishitobi M, Nakagawa H, Ogawa T, Ishii K. Acute encephalopathy with bilateral striatal necrosis: favourable response to corticosteroid therapy. Eur J Paediatr Neurol 1997; 1(1):41–45.
112. Ashtekar CS, Jaspan T, Thomas D, Weston V, Gayatri NA, Whitehouse WP. Acute bilateral thalamic necrosis in a child with Mycoplasma pneumoniae. Dev Med Child Neurol 2003; 45(9):634–637.
113. Winikates J, Jankovic J. Clinical correlates of vascular parkinsonism. Arch Neurol 1999; 56(1):98–102.
114. Jankovic J. Lower body (vascular) parkinsonism. Arch Neurol 1990; 47(7):728.
115. FitzGerald PM, Jankovic J. Lower body parkinsonism: evidence for vascular etiology. Mov Disord 1989; 4(3):249–260.
116. Alexander GE, DeLong MR, Strick PL. Parallel organization of functionally segregated circuits linking basal ganglia and cortex. Annu Rev Neurosci 1986; 9:357–381.
117. Alexander GE, Crutcher MD, DeLong MR. Basal ganglia-thalamocortical circuits: parallel substrates for motor, oculomotor, "prefrontal" and "limbic" functions. Prog Brain Res 1990; 85:119–146.
118. Goto S, Kunitoku N, Hamasaki T, Nishikawa S, Ushio Y. Abolition of postapoplectic hemichorea by Vo-complex thalamotomy: long-term follow-up study. Mov Disord 2001; 16(4):771–774.
119. Goldman MS, Kelly PJ. Symptomatic and functional outcome of stereotactic ventralis lateralis thalamotomy for intention tremor. J Neurosurg 1992; 77(2):223–229.
120. Andrew J, Fowler CJ, Harrison MJ, Kendall BE. Post-traumatic tremor due to vascular injury and its treatment by stereotactic thalamotomy. J Neurol Neurosurg Psychiatry 1982; 45(6):560–562.
121. Tronnier VM, Fogel W, Krause M et al. High frequency stimulation of the basal ganglia for the treatment of movement disorders: current status and clinical results. Minim Invasive Neurosurg 2002; 45(2):91–96.
122. Lozano AM. Vim thalamic stimulation for tremor. Arch Med Res 2000; 31(3):266–269.
123. Hubble JP, Busenbark KL, Wilkinson S et al. Effects of thalamic deep brain stimulation based on tremor type and diagnosis. Mov Disord 1997; 12(3):337–341.
124. Nishikawa M, Ichiyama T, Hayashi T, Ouchi K, Furukawa S. Intravenous immunoglobulin therapy in acute disseminated encephalomyelitis. Pediatr Neurol 1999; 21(2):583–586.
125. Nishimura A, Fuchigami T, Izumi H, Okubo O, Takahashi S, Harada K. A case of early-onset acute disseminated encephalomyelitis. No To Hattatsu 1997; 29(5):396–400.
126. Ruzicka E, Jech R, Zarubova K, Roth J, Urgosik D. VIM thalamic stimulation for tremor in a patient with IgM paraproteinaemic demyelinating neuropathy. Mov Disord 2003; 18(10):1192–1195.
127. Saverino A, Solaro C, Capello E, Trompetto C, Abbruzzese G, Schenone A. Tremor associated with benign IgM paraproteinaemic neuropathy successfully treated with gabapentin. Mov Disord 2001; 16(5):967–968.

128. Cai Z, Cash K, Swift J et al. Focal myelin swellings and tomacula in anti-MAG IgM paraproteinaemic neuropathy: novel teased nerve fiber studies. J Peripher Nerv Syst 2001; 6(2):95–101.

129. Nobile-Orazio E, Meucci N, Baldini L, Di Troia A, Scarlato G. Long-term prognosis of neuropathy associated with anti-MAG IgM M-proteins and its relationship to immune therapies. Brain 2000; 123(Pt 4):710–717.

130. Bain PG, Britton TC, Jenkins IH et al. Tremor associated with benign IgM paraproteinaemic neuropathy. Brain 1996; 119(Pt 3):789–799.

131. Busby M, Donaghy M. Chronic dysimmune neuropathy. A subclassification based upon the clinical features of 102 patients. J Neurol 2003; 250(6):714–724.

132. Matsuda M, Ikeda S, Sakurai S, Nezu A, Yanagisawa N, Inuzuka T. Hypertrophic neuritis due to chronic inflammatory demyelinating polyradiculoneuropathy (CIDP): a postmortem pathological study. Muscle Nerve 1996; 19(2):163–169.

133. Grand'Maison F, Feasby TE, Hahn AF, Koopman WJ. Recurrent Guillain-Barre syndrome. Clinical and laboratory features. Brain 1992; 115(Pt 4):1093–1106.

134. Alusi SH, Glickman S, Aziz TZ, Bain PG. Tremor in multiple sclerosis. J Neurol Neurosurg Psychiatry 1999; 66(2):131–134.

135. Deuschl G, Bain P, Brin M. Consensus Statement of the Movement Disorder Society on Tremor. Ad Hoc Scientific Committee. Mov Disord 1998; 13(suppl 3):2–23.

136. Alusi SH, Worthington J, Glickman S, Bain PG. A study of tremor in multiple sclerosis. Brain 2001; 124(Pt 4):720–730.

137. Mao CC, Gancher ST, Herndon RM. Movement disorders in multiple sclerosis. Mov Disord 1988; 3(2):109–116.

138. Minagar A, Sheremata WA, Weiner WJ. Transient movement disorders and multiple sclerosis. Parkinsonism Relat Disord 2002; 9(2):111–113.

139. Hallett M, Lindsey JW, Adelstein BD, Riley PO. Controlled trial of isoniazid therapy for severe postural cerebellar tremor in multiple sclerosis. Neurology 1985; 35(9):1374–1377.

140. Hallett M. Isoniazid and action tremor in multiple sclerosis. J Neurol Neurosurg Psychiatry 1985; 48(9):957.

141. Sabra AF, Hallett M, Sudarsky L, Mullally W. Treatment of action tremor in multiple sclerosis with isoniazid. Neurology 1982; 32(8):912–913.

142. Albrecht H, Schwecht M, Pollmann W, Parag D, Erasmus LP, Konig N. Local ice application in therapy of kinetic limb ataxia. Clinical assessment of positive treatment effects in patients with multiple sclerosis. Nervenarzt 1998; 69(12):1066–1073.

143. Feys P, Romberg A, Ruutiainen J et al. Assistive technology to improve PC interaction for people with intention tremor. J Rehabil Res Dev 2001; 38(2):235–243.

144. Gbadamosi J, Buhmann C, Moench A, Heesen C. Failure of ondansetron in treating cerebellar tremor in MS patients—an open-label pilot study. Acta Neurol Scand 2001; 104(5):308–311.

145. Critchley GR, Richardson PL. Vim thalamotomy for the relief of the intention tremor of multiple sclerosis. Br J Neurosurg 1998; 12(6):559–562.

146. Hooper J, Taylor R, Pentland B, Whittle IR. A prospective study of thalamic deep brain stimulation for the treatment of movement disorders in multiple sclerosis. Br J Neurosurg 2002; 16(2):102–109.

147. Matsumoto J, Morrow D, Kaufman K et al. Surgical therapy for tremor in multiple sclerosis: an evaluation of outcome measures. Neurology 2001; 57(10):1876–1882.

148. Montgomery EB Jr, Baker KB, Kinkel RP, Barnett G. Chronic thalamic stimulation for the tremor of multiple sclerosis. Neurology 1999; 53(3):625–628.
149. Wishart HA, Roberts DW, Roth RM et al. Chronic deep brain stimulation for the treatment of tremor in multiple sclerosis: review and case reports. J Neurol Neurosurg Psychiatry 2003; 74(10):1392–1397.
150. Pomeranz S, Shalit M, Sherman Y. "Rubral" tremor following radiation of a pineal region vascular hamartoma. Acta Neurochir (Wien) 1990; 103(1–2):79–81.
151. Asai A, Matsutani M, Kohno T et al. Subacute brain atrophy after radiation therapy for malignant brain tumor. Cancer 1989; 63(10):1962–1974.
152. Krauss JK, Borremans JJ, Pohle T, Godoy N. Movement disorders following nonfunctional neurosurgery. J Neurosurg 1999; 90(5):883–890.
153. Wenning GK, Luginger E, Sailer U, Poewe W, Donnemiller E, Riccabona G. Postoperative parkinsonian tremor in a patient with a frontal meningioma. Mov Disord 1999; 14(2):366–368.

23

Drug- and Toxin-Induced Tremor

John C. Morgan and Kapil D. Sethi

Medical College of Georgia and Department of Veterans Affairs Medical Center, Augusta, Georgia, USA

Tremor is a common adverse effect of prescribed drugs. It also occurs following exposure to various environmental or occupational toxins and poisons. Given that tremor is a prevalent condition that may exist in patients not on medications, it is often difficult to determine if a drug is responsible for a patient's tremor. Occasionally, neurological examination is performed prior to and after starting a drug making assumptions about causality more tenable. In addition, some patients are on multiple drugs that can cause or exacerbate tremor and identifying a single drug as the culprit is often difficult. In this chapter we will attempt to identify the drugs and toxins most commonly associated with inducing or exacerbating tremors.

The major classes of drugs associated with tremor are listed in Table 23.1. The most common form of drug-induced tremor is enhanced physiological tremor due to various drugs including sympathomimetics or antidepressants. Different drugs can cause different types of tremors varying from resting (neuroleptics) to postural (numerous) to intention (alcohol and lithium). Typically, drug-induced tremors are rapid in onset and dramatically improve or resolve with discontinuing the offending drug, unlike organic forms of tremor.

I. ANTIARRHYTHMICS

Amiodarone is a class III antiarrhythmic and is the most common drug in this class that induces tremor. Reports of amiodarone-induced tremors first appeared

Table 23.1 Major Classes of Drugs Which Induce or Exacerbate Tremors

Drug class	Major drugs associated with tremor
Antiarrhythmics	Amiodarone
Antibiotics/antivirals	Trimethoprim/sulfa, vidarabine
Antidepressants/mood stabilizers	Amitriptyline, SSRIs, lithium
Antiepileptics	Valproate, tiagabine
Bronchodilators	Albuterol, salmeterol
Chemotherapeutics	Tamoxifen, α-interferon
Drugs of abuse	Alcohol, cocaine, nicotine, amphetamine, MDMA
Gastrointestinal drugs	Metoclopramide, cimetidine
Hormones	Thyroxine, epinephrine
Immunosuppressants	Tacrolimus, cyclosporine
Methylxanthines	Theophylline, caffeine
Neuroleptics	Haloperidol, cinnarizine
Poisons/toxins	Organochlorine pesticides, lead, mercury, dioxin, Cnidirian venom, scorpion venom, tremorogenic mycotoxins

Note: SSRIs, selective serotonin reuptake inhibitors; MDMA, 3,4-methylenedioxy-methamphetamine (ecstasy).

in the French literature (1) followed by a report in the English language literature in 1974 (2). Since these initial reports, amiodarone has been associated with tremors in numerous reports. In one large series up to 36% of patients suffered neurological problems, predominantly tremor and ataxia (3). Other studies have found that <10% of patients treated with amiodarone complained of tremor (4). Two other studies demonstrated that 39% and 30% of patients complained of tremor (5,6).

Amiodarone-induced tremor is frequently postural and intentional and resembles essential tremor, usually presenting in the 6–10 Hz range (5). The tremor can emerge at any time in therapy and typically improves within two weeks with dose reduction or after stopping the drug (5). Keeping the dose of the drug lower (200 mg/day) appears to provide good arrhythmia control while minimizing side effects (7). In one study propranolol provided some tremor reduction in two patients that remained on chronic amiodarone therapy (5).

Amiodarone can cause both hypothyroidism and hyperthyroidism. Given that hyperthyroidism can cause tremor, this should be eliminated as a secondary cause of tremor in amiodarone-treated patients. The mechanism of amiodarone-induced tremor is unknown; however the drug is known to have a toxic effect on mitochondrial function, including inhibiting β-oxidation of fatty acids at lower concentrations (100 μM) and inhibiting the electron transport chain at higher concentrations (200 μM) (8).

Other antiarrhythmics may also cause tremor. Procainamide, a Class IA antiarrhythmic, was reported to cause severe postural and intention tremor in the arms as well as the head in an 82-year-old man being treated for ventricular premature complexes (9). This tremor emerged within hours of initial treatment, resolved on discontinuation, and recurred with re-challenge in a dose-dependent fashion (9). Mexiletine, a Class IB antiarrhythmic, is also associated with neurological side effects including tremor, dizziness and memory loss in up to 10% of patients (10). Tremor was associated with increasing plasma levels of mexiletine in two other studies (11,12). The mechanism of tremor induction by antiarrhythmics is unknown.

II. ANTIBIOTICS/ANTIVIRALS/ANTIFUNGALS

Antibiotics, antivirals, and antifungals are widely prescribed. There are few reports of tremor secondary to these drugs. Trimethoprim-sulfamethoxazole (TMP-SMX) is reported to cause significant tremor in patients with acquired immunodeficiency syndrome (AIDS) (13–15). Interestingly, tremors typically have occurred in patients undergoing treatment of *Pneumocystis carinii* pneumonia (13–15). It appears to cause both resting and postural tremor, with resolution typically occurring within several days after discontinuing the drug (13,14). There is also one report of action and postural tremor interfering with writing in an immunocompetent man undergoing treatment with TMP-SMX (16). The mechanism of TMP-SMX-induced tremor is unknown, however,

Van Gerpen (14) proposed that this drug may indirectly reduce catecholamine and indolamine synthesis through inhibition of dihydrofolate reductase, leading to tremors.

Vidarabine (Ara-A) was frequently used for treatment of various viral infections in the past. Vidarabine was associated with development of intention tremors followed by gross tremors in two patients treated for herpes zoster, complicating therapy for solid malignant tumors (17). One patient eventually died and the other patient developed a chronic pain syndrome. Other authors have also reported a propensity for this drug to cause tremor (18). The tremor was dramatic in one patient undergoing treatment for herpes simplex encephalitis and resolved after discontinuing the drug (19). Tremor and other side effects were greatest when patients were treated with 20 mg/kg per day relative to lower doses and typically emerged 5–7 days after initiating therapy with the drug (20).

Acyclovir, an antiviral drug, was associated with tremor in five of six patients undergoing bone marrow transplantation within a median of eight days after beginning therapy and resolving within a median of 13 days after therapy (21). In another study of 35 patients with neuropsychiatric symptoms during acyclovir therapy, 11 patients had associated tremors (22). Tremor and other neuropsychiatric manifestations appear more commonly in the elderly and in patients with renal dysfunction (22). Tremor is typically dose-related and usually resolves in several days after discontinuing acyclovir therapy (22).

Amphotericin B is an antifungal drug that was associated with a parkinsonian syndrome (including rest tremor) in three children undergoing treatment for aspergillosis without central nervous system (CNS) involvement (23). Amphotericin B was also associated with tremors and leukoencephalopathy in patients undergoing treatment for focal, disseminated, and nervous system mycotic infections (24). Ketoconazole also induced tremor in an elderly man taking an oral 200 mg dose (25). The tremor was associated with a complex clinical picture of dysarthria and weakness of the extremities starting within one hour after ingesting the drug and resolving within 24 hours. This recurred on rechallenge with the same dose and resolved within hours (25). Tremor was also reported in one patient in a series of 31 bone marrow transplant patients taking fluconazole for candida prophylaxis/treatment and quickly resolved after discontinuing the drug (26).

III. ANTIDEPRESSANTS/MOOD STABILIZERS

Tricyclic antidepressants (TCAs) have been in use for many decades and remain viable agents for numerous conditions including depression, headaches, pain syndromes, and multiple other ailments. Amitriptyline can cause a disabling postural tremor of the hands (27). Recent research has demonstrated that amitriptyline enhances the central component of physiological tremor (28). Of 15 patients treated with amitriptyline, five had an increase in postural tremor (28). While clinically-rated postural tremor was increased in only five of 15 patients, accelerometry demonstrated an increase in tremor amplitude in all 15 patients who were treated with amitriptyline (28). While postural tremor can be a reason for discontinuing amitriptyline therapy (29,30), clinically significant tremor occurs in a minority of patients and this can improve during continued therapy (28,31). Tremor as a side effect is not limited to amitriptyline and can be caused by other TCAs (32,33). There is evidence in one report that imipramine-induced tremor responds to a beta-adrenergic blocking agent (33).

Selective serotonin reuptake inhibitors (SSRIs) are widely used to treat depression, anxiety and multiple other conditions. They have largely replaced TCAs in the treatment of depression due to various reasons including safety profile in the setting of overdose. SSRI-induced tremor is probably the most common movement disorder induced by these drugs (34,35). It is estimated that new-onset tremor occurs in 20% of patients (36,37).

One report describes 21 patients who developed fluoxetine-induced tremors at a mean dose of 26 mg/day (38). The tremors emerged at a mean latency of 54 days following introduction of the drug and the frequency was typically 6–12 Hz (38). The tremors were typically postural in nature, however, resting and action tremor did occur. In half of these patients the tremor remitted within one month after discontinuing fluoxetine, while in the remaining patients, the tremor persisted for at least 15 months (38). Another report demonstrated similar findings in a 40-year-old woman who was prescribed fluoxetine for depression (39). She developed coarse tremors in both hands/arms, interfering with activities of daily living one month after starting fluoxetine therapy. This resolved within one week of discontinuing the drug and recurred on rechallenge (39).

SSRI withdrawal syndrome is characterized by tremulousness, irritability, anxiety, paresthesias, and a multitude of other symptoms. This syndrome can occur in withdrawal states with any SSRI, but is probably more common with SSRIs with shorter half-lives such as fluvoxamine or paroxetine (40).

Tremor is the most common movement disorder due to lithium, and lithium-induced tremor is one of the most commonly seen drug-induced tremors (41). While the true prevalence of lithium-induced tremor is unknown, one review of the literature estimated from an analysis of 1000 patients in several studies that 27% of lithium-treated patients develop tremors, with studies showing wide variability from 4% to 65% (42). The exact number of patients discontinuing treatment due to lithium-induced tremor is unknown; however, one study found that 32% of patients felt that the tremor resulted in non-compliance and some disability (43). For the majority of patients, however, the tremor was mild and not disabling. One study demonstrated tremor was more common in men than women on chronic lithium therapy (44). In a study of 60 patients treated for bipolar disorder with lithium, men complained of tremor more frequently than women (54% vs. 26%, respectively) (45). Lithium-induced tremor may also occur more frequently in elderly patients (46,47).

The tremor induced by lithium is typically 8–12 Hz, falling into the category of enhanced physiological tremor and affecting mainly the hands (41). While tremor can occur in patients over a wide range of lithium levels (46), there may be a correlation of tremor with certain lithium levels in individual patients. Concomitant therapy with certain drugs such as antidepressants or valproate can potentiate the tremorogenic features of lithium (42). A quantitative study of tremor in lithium-maintained patients revealed significantly increased tremor in patients adding paroxetine or amitriptyline co-treatment, even after six weeks (48). Despite increased tremor in these patients, it did not appear to interfere with patient compliance (48,49). Tremor can also vary based upon the emotional state of the patient, with tremors becoming worse in patients with significant anxiety. Lithium-induced tremor can improve over time (47).

The mechanism of lithium-induced tremor is unknown. Given the tremor appears to be an enhancement of physiological tremor and given its response to beta-adrenergic blockade, multiple theories exist. The first step in treating someone with lithium-induced tremor is to try and reduce the dose or discontinue the drug. Valproate is another first line agent in the treatment of bipolar disorder, and this drug is also of significant tremorogenic potential.

While placebo-controlled trials have not been performed, it appears that the nonselective beta-adrenergic blocker propranolol is perhaps the most effective agent for lithium-induced tremor (50). Other beta-blockers may also be effective, but are less well studied. Primidone may also be an effective agent for lithium-induced tremor (50).

IV. ANTIEPILEPTICS

Valproic acid (VPA) is the most common antiepileptic (AED) associated with tremor. Given the wide use of VPA for epilepsy, migraine prophylaxis, and bipolar disorder, tremor due to this drug is one of the most common drug-induced tremors (51,52).

The clinical and electrophysiological features of VPA-induced tremor resemble essential tremor, and VPA may exacerbate underlying tremor conditions (53,54). While up to 25% of patients may complain of tremor due to VPA, up to 80% of patients may show evidence of tremor on accelerometry recordings (54). The tremor is typically action and postural, however rest tremor may occur along with head and truncal tremor (53,54). The tremor appears dose-related and dose reduction can improve VPA-induced tremor, usually within several weeks (53,54). If dose reduction is not possible, then propranolol (55), amantadine (55), or acetazolamide (56) appear to provide benefit for VPA-induced tremor.

There are few reports of tremor with other AEDs, however, tiagabine was associated with tremor as an adverse event in a dose-dependent manner. The incidence was highest in patients taking 56 mg of tiagabine per day compared with 32 mg or placebo (21%, 14%, 1%, respectively) (57). Gabapentin was associated with tremor in 6.8% of patients compared with 3.2% of patients on placebo as adjunctive therapy for epilepsy (58). Tremor was an adverse reaction in 4% of patients on monotherapy with oxcarbazapine compared with 0% on placebo in a controlled clinical trial (59). Tremor due to this drug caused 1.8% of patients to discontinue its use in clinical trials (59). Levetiracetam is not associated with an increased incidence of tremor in adjunctive epilepsy therapy trials (60). Lamotrigine was associated with tremor in 4% of patients (vs. 1% of patients on placebo) in adjunctive trials, however, there was not a significantly increased incidence of tremor in a placebo-controlled monotherapy trial (61). Lamotrigine was associated with a disabling tremor when added to VPA in one patient (62). Lamotrigine was also associated with inducing tremors, unsteadiness, and chorea in a child being treated for myoclonic jerks (63). Tremor is a frequent adverse event in patients taking zonisamide (1 in 100) as adjunctive therapy, however it was not more frequent than with placebo (64). Topiramate was associated with tremor in 9% of patients vs. 6% of patients on placebo in adjunctive therapy trials (65).

There is evidence that AEDs are useful in treating essential and other forms of tremor. Primidone is used extensively as a first line treatment of essential tremor (66). Carbamazepine was effective for cerebellar tremors in a small series (67). There are reports that gabapentin is effective in treating essential tremor (68–70) as well as orthostatic tremor (71,72). Topiramate, like primidone and gabapentin, is also used to treat essential tremor (73,74)

V. BRONCHODILATORS

Albuterol (salbutamol) is a β_2-adrenergic agonist widely prescribed for chronic obstructive pulmonary disease (COPD) and asthma and one of the most common drugs causing drug-induced tremor. Tremor is a common side effect with all β-adrenergic agonists. In large clinical trials 7–20% of patients complained of tremor due to inhaled albuterol with similar numbers of patients complaining of tremor due to inhaled isoproterenol (14%) (75,76). Tremor and other side effects appear dose related with β_2-adrenergic agonists (77).

Salmeterol, a newer β_2-adrenergic agonist with a significantly longer half-life, is associated with tremor in 1.7% of patients chronically treated with 50 μg twice daily (78). In single dose studies, however, 100 μg of salmeterol resulted in reports of tremor in 5.7% of patients (78). Tremor was reported in one of every 128 patients in a large United Kingdom cohort of 15,407 patients taking salmeterol (79). One in 256 patients discontinued salmeterol secondary to tremor (79). Fenoterol, another β_2-adrenergic agonist, is more likely to produce tremor than albuterol or terbutaline (80).

While the exact mechanism for tremor induction by β_2-adrenergic agonists is unknown, there is some evidence that β-agonists act through a peripheral mechanism at the level of the muscle. Supporting this hypothesis is an experiment by Foley et al. (81). When patients in this study were ischemically prevented from receiving an infusion of epinephrine in their arm, tremor did not occur in the ischemic arm (81). Adrenergic stimulation is thought to cause an imbalance between fast- and slow-twitch muscle groups in the extremities, leading to tremors. Tolerance develops with continued use of β-agonists.

VI. CHEMOTHERAPEUTICS

There are some reports of tremor associated with chemotherapy, however, no chemotherapeutic clearly stands out as a tremorogenic agent. Tamoxifen is an anti-estrogenic agent used in the treatment of breast cancer and in early studies the dose-limiting toxic effects of tamoxifen were neurological and consisted of tremor, hyperflexia, dysmetria, unsteady gait, and dizziness (82).

Thalidomide has emerged as a treatment for cutaneous lupus erythematosis and tremor was reported as an adverse event with this drug in one study (83). Thalidomide caused tremor in 36% (10/28) of patients with multiple myeloma when used alone and in 30% (12/40) of patients receiving combination therapy with dexamethasone (84). Other authors have reported thalidomide associated reversible dementia and rest tremor in an elderly man (85). Unlike thalidomide-associated neuropathy that is frequently irreversible, tremors associated with thalidomide therapy are mild and reversible (84,85).

Cytarabine (Ara-C) is common in many chemotherapy regimens for various cancers and is most commonly known to cause cerebellar toxicity manifested by nystagmus, dysarthria and ataxia (86). Intention tremor was noted in a four year old boy who inadvertently received Ara-C intrathecally for CNS relapse of acute lymphoblastic leukemia (87). As a clinical sign of Ara-C cerebellar toxicity, handwriting samples are followed during chemotherapy and fine motor skills and handwriting remain impaired following chemotherapy for acute lymphoblastic leukemia in children two years after treatment (88). Whether this represents cerebellar ataxia or tremor is not clear, however, intention tremor due to Ara-C appears underreported in the literature relative to other cerebellar findings. Ara-C appears to cause damage to cerebellar Purkinje cells in the lateral hemispheres in autopsied patients (89). The cerebellar toxicity can occur in 8–23% of patients depending on the dose, the age of the patient (older patients have greater risk of toxicity), and the presence of prior neurological dysfunction or hepatic abnormalities (86,90,91).

Ifosfamide was associated with transient neurotoxicity including tremor in one study using the drug for chemotherapy of malignant solid tumors in children (92). Vincristine is also associated with tremor in some patients, and caused a coarse tremor, nausea, emesis, nystagmus, and stupor in a 59-year-old woman inadvertently treated with vincristine in her Ommaya reservoir for acute lymphoblastic leukemia with meningeal involvement (93). Cisplatin was indirectly associated with mild tremor, muscle cramps, and twitching in some patients undergoing treatment for testicular cancer due to the drug causing hypomagnesemia (94).

VII. DRUGS OF ABUSE

While ethanol is helpful in the treatment of various movement disorders (myoclonus-dystonia and essential tremor), it is also associated with tremors of various types. Ethanol is reported to cause multiple forms of tremor: postural tremor as an acute/transient disorder, a "metabolic tremor" associated with alcoholic liver disease, a 3 Hz leg tremor and parkinsonian tremor associated with alcoholic cerebellar degeneration (95). Tremor secondary to portosystemic shunts can occur as well (95). Of 100 alcoholics who did not use ethanol for more than weeks, 47 had postural tremor while only 3% of 100 controls in the same study demonstrated postural tremor (96). Functional disability due to tremor occurred in only 17% of the alcoholic patients (96). Alcoholic tremor in these patients was at a slightly faster frequency relative to 50 patients with essential tremor (8.6 vs. 5.7 Hz), however propranolol improved alcoholic tremor more than essential tremor in this study (96).

Smoking has been associated with an increase in tremor amplitude by at least two-fold (97). Maternal smoking was also associated with tremor in a newborn infant (98). In another study of 33 patients from two age groups, cigarette smoking increased tremor significantly independent of age, sex, and anxiety levels (99). This effect was documented using electrophysiology and it appears that the effect is due to nicotine given that chewing gum containing 4 mg of nicotine increased tremor to the same degree as smoking two cigarettes (99,100). In contrast, nicotine or cigarette smoking appeared to improve tremor and other parkinsonian features in some small studies (101,102). In a randomized, double-blind, placebo-controlled clinical trial using transdermal nicotine in non-smokers with PD, there was no significant tremor benefit using either 17.5 mg or 35 mg patches over three weeks (103).

Ecstasy, 3,4-methylenedioxymethamphemtamine (MDMA), can cause a serotonin syndrome in some patients due to robust release of serotonin in the CNS after intoxication. One patient had sustained postural tremors of both upper extremities for at least 10 days after ingesting a single dose (104). Another chronic MDMA user developed parkinsonism associated with unilateral rest tremor as well as bilateral postural arm tremor (105). This patient's parkinsonism was levodopa-responsive and his parkinsonism responded to deep brain stimulation of the subthalamic nucleus (105). Cocaine can also cause chronic movement disorders including resting hand tremor and parkinsonism (106). In a study of cocaine-dependent patients, resting hand tremor did not remit even after three months of abstinence (107).

Amphetamine derivatives can cause tremors in humans, but perhaps this is better documented in animal models. Unanesthetized cats injected in the caudate nucleus with d-amphetamine developed significant tremors on repeated treatments (108). In a similar fashion, mice that were given a lethal dose of methamphetamine developed piloerection, agitation and tremors as a part of their symptomatology (109). Methylphenidate may also cause tremors and this drug in combination with desipramine appeared to cause tremor in twice as many children as either drug alone (110).

VIII. GASTROINTESTINAL DRUGS

Metoclopramide is a dopamine-receptor blocking agent that remains in relatively widespread use for gastroesophageal reflux disease and gastroparesis. Metoclopramide-induced tremor and parkinsonism are among the most common drug-induced movement disorders. This drug can induce a parkinsonian tremor (111) or an essential-like tremor that responds to ethanol (112). Metoclopramide-induced parkinsonism and tremor appears more common in patients with renal failure and the dose should be lowered in these patients (113).

Metoclopramide can also cause tardive tremors with predominantly postural and resting components (114,115). These tremors are typically larger in amplitude than parkinsonian tremor and interfere with activities of daily living. Tardive tremor typically responds to tetrabenazine or other neuroleptics, unlike parkinsonian tremor which is typically made worse by these agents (114). Metoclopramide may cause tremor by acting as a cholinomimetic tremorogen (116) or due to its dopamine-receptor blocking properties.

Cimetidine, a histamine H2 receptor antagonist, was shown to exacerbate tremors in three patients in one report (117). In the first patient, pre-existing action tremor was worsened and again worsened on rechallenge. In the second patient, action and postural tremors of 8–10 Hz were associated with concomitant use of metoclopramide and cimetidine. Seventy-two hours after discontinuing both drugs, treatment with 200 mg of intravenous cimetidine resulted in recurrence of the tremor. In the third patient, cimetidine worsened tremors in the setting of thyrotoxicosis. Propranolol treatment significantly improved tremor in all three patients (117). It was proposed that histaminergic pathways may normally be involved in suppression of physiological and essential tremors (117). Cimetidine was also shown to cause tremor in all rats injected with 200 μg of the drug into the lateral ventricles of the brain (118).

Cisapride is chemically related to metoclopramide, however, unlike metoclopramide, cisapride is largely devoid of central depressant or antidopaminergic effects (119). It stimulates release of acetylcholine from the myenteric plexus and may have 5HT-4 receptor agonist properties (119). Cisapride was frequently used in the United States for gastroesophageal reflux and gastroparesis until it was discovered that the drug could lead to life-threatening cardiac arrythmias in treated patients. This led to the FDA recall of this drug in July 2000. Cisapride aggravated parkinsonian tremor in two patients to the point of interfering with daily activities (120). This drug is known to cross the blood–brain barrier and was thought to possibly exacerbate tremors in these patients due to its influence on serotoninergic pathways (120). Misoprostol, a prostaglandin E1 analog used to treat gastric ulcers and other conditions, was associated with tremor and multiple other symptoms in the setting of acute toxicity (121). This occurred after an elderly woman accidentally ingested 3 mg of the drug (15× the maximum recommended dose) (121).

Bismuth salts were first reported to cause an encephalopathy with myoclonus and ataxia in 1974 (122,123). This condition was not uncommon in France and other European countries in the 1970s. While most features of bismuth encephalopathy are reversible, it was noted that tremor was both an acute and chronic problem associated with bismuth neurotoxicity in many patients (122). One report described a 54-year-old man who developed prolonged encephalopathy, myoclonus and coarse postural tremor due to bismuth subsalicylate toxicity (124).

While the mechanism of bismuth-induced encephalopathy and tremor is unknown, autopsy of three patients who died of this condition demonstrated higher levels of bismuth in grey matter relative to white matter (125). In another series of 12 autopsied patients dying of bismuth encephalopathy, perivenular lymphocytic infiltration and abundant intra-cytoplasmic lipofuscin was noted (126). In a mouse model of this condition, female mice injected intraperitoneally with bismuth subnitrate developed tremors, myoclonus, ataxia and convulsions and were found to have hydrocephalus and axonal swellings in the spinal cord at autopsy (127).

IX. HERBS/ALTERNATIVE MEDICINES/SPICES

Chinese star anise (*Illicium verum*) is a spice used in Caribbean and Hispanic cultures as a tea infusion for infant colic. There are numerous reports in the literature of star anise causing toxicity in treated infants manifested by tremors, jitteriness, myoclonus and seizures (128,129). These neurological symptoms appear to resolve within 24 hours (129). Some cases may represent contamination and poisoning with a more toxic form of star anise—Japanese star anise (*Illicium anisatum*) (128,129). Kava kava caused generalized tremors and rapidly progressive parkinsonism in a woman taking the herbal medicine for anxiety at a dose of 65 mg/day for 10 days (130). Blockade of dopamine receptors may be a mechanism by which this compound causes parkinsonism (130,131).

β-carbolines are found in nature in many plants and are used as an herbal medicine (132). Plants containing this compound are associated with numerous neurological side effects and are used as hallucinogens, abortifacients, and sexual stimulants (132). These compounds are also made in the body and are a normal part of proteinacious foods that have been heat-prepared (132). Higher blood and cerebrospinal fluid (CSF) levels of harman and norharman (both β-carbolines) are associated with Parkinson's disease (133,134) and elevated blood levels of harman were also present in essential tremor patients relative to a control group (135). Valerian root, which is used as an antianxiety and hypnotic drug, is known to cause numerous symptoms including tremor of the hands and feet in patients who were "toxic" (136). Yohimbine, an herb long-used for male erectile dysfunction was found to cause tremor in healthy subjects as a common side effect (137).

X. HORMONES

Of all hormones associated with tremor, excess thyroid hormone is perhaps the most well known, causing tremor in patients with hyperthyroidism and also causing tremor in patients ingesting excess levothyroxine. In one study of patients 75 or older with hyperthyroidism, 36% (9 out of 25) had tremor (138). The incidence of tremor in patients with thyrotoxic storm (severe, rapid decompensation associated with hyperthermia, tachycardia, and altered mental status) is perhaps universal; however, this feature is underreported (139). Thyroid storm can occur in patients following infection, radioactive iodine treatment, surgery, or administration of iodinated contrast media (139,140).

Tremor, myorhythmia, and myoclonus are characteristically associated with anti-thyroid antibodies and normal thyroid hormone levels in Hashimoto's encephalopathy (141,142). Tremor and myoclonus served as a harbinger of more significant CNS manifestations of stupor, coma and generalized tonic-clonic seizures in one patient (143).

Tremor is frequently noted in children or adults who overdose on levothyroxine (144,145). The dietary supplement tiratricol is frequently sold as a weight loss aid and resulted in symptomatic hyperthyroidism with tremor, nervousness and insomnia in one elderly patient (146). It appears that the peak tremor frequency in thyrotoxicosis is the same as that of physiological tremor in healthy subjects (147), however, the power of thyrotoxic tremor is increased (148). Thyrotoxic tremor responds to both β-adrenoreceptor blockade by nadolol as well as treatment of the thyrotoxicosis by carbimazole (148).

Tremor is commonly encountered in patients taking high-dose medroxyprogesterone acetate in advanced breast cancer (149). In a study of 3900 women using the injectable form of the drug for birth control, however, tremor is not listed as an adverse event in the package insert (150).

Epinephrine and norepinephrine are associated with tremor in patients with pheochromocytomas. Both epinephrine- and norepinephrine-secreting tumors were associated with tremors (151). Epinephrine and norepinephrine have been extensively studied and appear to act by enhancing physiological tremor at the level of the muscle (81,147). While the tremorogenic effects of epinephrine and norepinephrine have been known for decades, recently tremor was noted as a side effect in all children injected with the EpiPen® (epinephrine injectable for patients at risk for anaphylaxis) (152). Given these hormones act on β-adrenergic receptors at the level of the muscle, β-blockers help to reduce tremor.

Sodium calcitonin caused widespread tremor in one patient after injection (153). This occurred in a 35-year-old insulin dependent diabetic woman 90 minutes after her first subcutaneous injection of 100 IU of salmon calcitonin. The tremor was fine and affected the head, arms and legs and lasted for about one hour. This occurred with rechallenge and did not occur after injection of placebo (153). The tremor was not due to changes in calcium concentrations. The mechanism for tremor-induction by this drug is unknown.

XI. IMMUNOSUPPRESSANTS/IMMUNOMODULATORS

Calcineurin inhibitors such as cyclosporine and FK-506 (tacrolimus) are widely used in immunosuppressive transplant regimens to help prevent rejection of transplanted organs and as immunosuppressants in autoimmune disorders (cyclosporine–myasthenia gravis). These medications can have significant neurological side effects, including tremor. A review of cyclosporine neurotoxicity revealed that postural tremor is reported in up to 40% of patients with intention tremor being less frequent (154). The tremor typically begins after initiation of cyclosporine therapy and is frequently mild and generalized in nature (154). Higher blood levels of cyclosporine are correlated with tremor, however, some patients can experience tremor even with lower blood levels of the drug. Given metabolic disturbances due to hepatic or renal failure and treatment with other medications in most patients, tremor is frequently pre-existent (155). Cyclosporine tremor is typically mild to moderate and dose reduction is not always required (154).

FK-506 (tacrolimus) is also commonly used in immunosuppressive regimens and was associated with tremor in the first reports of neurological toxicity related to the drug following liver transplantation (156,157). Tremor was observed in 8 of 22 pediatric liver transplant patients on FK-506 (157) and occurred in 10 of 44 patients undergoing orthotopic liver transplantation in another study (156). The tremor associated with FK-506 therapy in the latter 10 patients was severe and affected the hands, interfering with handwriting and worsening with action (156). Decreasing the FK-506 dose resulted in tremor improvement, however several patients continued to have "fine, nonsignificant" tremors (156).

Tremor also occurs in non-transplant therapeutic settings with FK-506. Patients taking FK-506 at 3 mg/day for rheumatoid arthritis had tremor as a frequent side effect, occurring in 9% of 896 patients (158). Tremor also occurred as an adverse event in a randomized, placebo-controlled trial of FK-506 in the treatment of patients with fistulas related to Crohn's disease (159).

Tremor was the major neurological side effect in a trial of α-interferon for metastatic melanoma (160). Significantly increased action tremor occurred in 22% of patients in this trial (160). Myorhythmia manifesting as a slow facial tremor was associated with long-term α-2a-interferon use in a 49-year-old woman with chronic myelogenous leukemia (161). There is also a report of parkinsonism associated with α-interferon therapy for chronic myelogenous leukemia in a 79-year-old man (162). The tremorogenic action of this drug may be due to its inhibition of dopaminergic neural activity in mouse models (163).

XII. METHYLXANTHINES

Methylxanthines include theophylline, aminophylline, and caffeine. Theophylline and aminophylline are typically used in the treatment of COPD and asthma. Caffeine is widely consumed throughout the world. Aminophylline and theophylline lead to increased tremor. In 10 patients with essential tremor, intravenous aminophylline increased tremor on accelerometry (165).

In contrast to these reports, there is evidence that theophylline, an adenosine antagonist, may improve essential tremor (166). In one study, theophylline at 150 mg/day quantitatively reduced tremor to the same extent as 80 mg/day of propranolol (166). This effect was only evident after two weeks of therapy, while the reduction in tremor was evident within one week after initiating propranolol (166). Chronic administration of theophylline appeared to enhance GABA-induced NMDA receptor depolarization based upon experiments in mice and this was proposed as a possible mechanism of decreasing essential tremor (167).

Studies on caffeine and tremor have demonstrated that 2% of normal controls complained of tremor when drinking coffee (168). Essential tremor and Parkinson's disease patients complained that coffee worsened their tremors in 8% and 6% of patients, respectively (168). However, 325 mg of oral caffeine did not increase physiological, parkinsonian or essential tremor in formal clinical studies (168). Accelerometry studies have shown that 450 mg/day of caffeine appears to increase finger tremor in fasting patients but not in the same patients on their normal diet (169). In another accelerometry study, a dose of caffeine equal to two or three cups of coffee increased whole-arm tremor in normal subjects (170).

XIII. NEUROLEPTICS/DOPAMINE DEPLETING AGENTS

Neuroleptics (dopamine-receptor blocking agents) can cause resting and postural tremors. Tremor occurs most frequently as a part of drug-induced parkinsonism with these drugs, however, tardive tremor after prolonged neuroleptic therapy can occur as well (114). Tremor heralded onset of drug-induced parkinsonism with older neuroleptics in 35% of patients in a study of 3775 patients (171). Tremor typically began asymmetrically in one arm. In the same study, 60% of patients with drug-induced parkinsonism manifested tremor at some point during their illness (171). Fluphenazine and thioridazine were more likely than chlorpromazine to cause tremor in schizophrenics (172). Drug-induced parkinsonism has been discussed elsewhere by multiple authors (173–175).

Cinnarizine and flunarizine are vestibular sedatives not prescribed in the United States, however, they are frequently associated with drug-induced parkinsonism and postural/rest tremor (175). Up to 51% of patients with cinnarizine-induced parkinsonism may develop postural tremor with 37% having bilateral rest tremor (176). The tremorogenic action of these drugs is probably related to their ability to deplete dopamine presynaptically and block postsynaptic dopamine receptors (175).

Dopamine-depleting agents can cause tremor and parkinsonism as well. Tetrabenazine is not currently available in the United States but is used worldwide for hyperkinetic movement disorders and can cause tremors (177). Reserpine and methyldopa, like tetrabenazine, can cause parkinsonism and tremors in patients being treated for hypertension (178,179).

XIV. TOXINS

Multiple poisons, toxins, and venoms can cause tremors. Louis (180) identified numerous poisons/compounds that are known to cause tremor in animals and humans. Organochlorine pesticides are prevalent throughout the world and have been used in large amounts for the past 50 years. These compounds are tremorogenic in both animals and humans (181,182) and typically cause a tremor of 6–8 Hz (182,183). The tremor may occur immediately after a significant exposure or may appear several months later (182). Up to two-thirds of exposed chemical workers are affected with tremors in some studies (182–184). It is unknown how these compounds cause tremor, but they may act by interfering with GABA production (185), GABAergic neurotransmission (186), or cause neurodegeneration in the cerebellar cortex (187).

Mercury poisoning is characterized by the triad of tremor, behavioral changes, and gingivitis. Patients can be poisoned typically from inhaled mercury vapor (elemental or inorganic mercury) or by ingestion of contaminated foods (organic, methyl mercury compounds). Action tremors due to mercury exposure vary widely in frequency (4–16 Hz) (188–191). Patients can suffer with chronic action tremors in the setting of acute (189) or chronic low level exposures (192). Chronic exposure to inorganic mercury results in accumulation of mercury, with highest concentrations in the cerebellum and brainstem nuclei (193). This can lead to significant atrophy of the vermis and cerebellar hemispheres.

Lead, like mercury, is present in the environment in both organic and inorganic forms. Workers in printing, battery factories, gasoline manufacturing, and smelting are exposed to inorganic lead. Gasoline sniffers/huffers are also prone to develop side effects from lead exposure. Another very common cause of lead exposure and resultant encephalopathy in children is the presence of lead-based paints in many older homes. In acute organic lead intoxication, patients develop an encephalopathy with associated nausea and vomiting (194). In chronic exposure, lead can cause a chronic progressive disorder of which tremor is a significant feature (194). Lead appears to interfere with GABA uptake in the rat brain (195) and appears to cause degenerative changes in the cerebellum of rats and rabbits (196,197). Autopsy of patients with chronic exposure to organic lead revealed significant loss of Purkinje cells in the cerebellum (198).

Occupational exposure to manganese is linked with parkinsonism, tremor, postural instability, and incoordination in several settings (199,200). Manganese toxicity is perhaps most frequently seen in manganese miners, and neuropathology in this condition demonstrates cerebellar and basal ganglia damage (201). Manganese toxicity was reported to occur even in the setting of total parenteral nutrition in a 2-year-old girl (202). Characteristic magnetic resonance imaging (MRI) findings in patients with manganese toxicity include hyperintensity in the globus pallidus, striatum, and midbrain (202,203). Despite termination of exposure, extrapyramidal features may be irreversible and may even progress (203). The mechanism of manganese CNS toxicity is unclear, and positron emission tomography (PET) scans typically reveal normal presynaptic and post-synaptic nigrostriatal dopaminergic function (203).

Chronic exposure to organic solvents such as toluene, methanol, and carbon disulfide can also cause tremor. Chronic toluene (typically found in paint thinners) abuse causes tremor in many patients. The tremor is typically postural (5–6 Hz), worsens with action, and can be asymmetric and irreversible (204,205). T2-weighted MRI typically shows hypointensity in the basal ganglia and red nucleus (204). The mechanism of toluene-induced tremor is unknown; however, a VIM thalamotomy abolished tremor of the contralateral limb in one man (204).

Methanol intoxication can cause parkinsonism with mild tremor, hypo-phonia, rigidity, and bradykinesia (206). Other patients with chronic methanol poisoning can develop intention tremors, visual disturbances, and impaired coordination (207). Pathologically, patients can demonstrate cystic resorption of the putamen and the frontocentral subcortical white matter in addition to wide-spread neuronal damage in multiple other areas of the CNS (206).

Carbon disulfide is linked with tremor and parkinsonism in viscose rayon plant workers and grain industry workers exposed to fumigants containing this compound (208–210). Resting and action tremors can occur with carbon disul-fide exposure. An electrophysiological study of finger tremor in 19 chronically exposed grain workers demonstrated a tremor frequency typically in the 5–7 Hz range (209). MRI abnormalities in the subcortical white matter, basal ganglia, and brainstem as well as lack of levodopa response may help distinguish this entity from idiopathic Parkinson's disease (210). Single photon emission computed tomography (SPECT) scanning using the TRODAT-1 ligand [which binds to the dopamine transporter (DAT) in the striatum] may help differentiate between idiopathic Parkinson's disease (where DAT binding is reduced) and par-kinsonism due to carbon disulfide (where DAT binding may be normal) (210).

Cyanide intoxication can produce parkinsonism with resultant tremors (211,212). Acute cyanide poisoning causes CNS-mediated tremors in mice, and this may be due to modulation of intraneuronal calcium stores (211). There is also a report of rest tremor associated with exposure to monesin (an antiparasitic added to animal feed) (213). A farmer was exposed to large amounts of the compound through his skin one month prior to tremor onset. The tremor occurred both at rest and with action in the right hand and occasionally right leg, improving with trihexyphenidyl (213).

There is one report of dystonia and tremor associated with exposure to the polychlorinated phenol, 2,3,7,8-tetrachlorodibenzo-*p*-dioxin (214). In this report, 35 of 45 individuals exposed to this chemical as part of a railroad tank car clean-up six years earlier manifested postural and intention tremor on neurological examination (214). There was no family history of tremors in any of the patients, and each patient dated the onset of tremor to some time subsequent to the toxic exposure (214). The cause of dioxin-associated tremors in these patients is unknown.

MPTP, 1-methyl-4-phenyl-1,2,3,6-tetrahydropyridine is a toxin that is used extensively in laboratory models of Parkinson's disease. This toxin was identified as a contaminant in the attempted synthesis of a meperidine analog and caused parkinsonism and tremor following intravenous injection of the drug/toxin by abusers (215). A physiological study of MPTP-induced tremor revealed that MPTP-treated monkeys developed a postural and action tremor in the 10–16 Hz range as well as prolonged episodes of lower frequency (4–6 Hz) tremor (216).

Envenomation with cnidarian and scorpion venoms can produce tremors in patients, presumably due to catecholaminergic excess, and they frequently require treatment with antivenom and supportive therapies due to autonomic nervous system dysfunction (217–219). Latrodectism is the clinical syndrome patients experience following envenomation by widow family spiders (black widows, Australian redback spiders, others) (220). Patients experience significant localized pain, redness, and swelling with systemic effects of generalized limb pain, tremor, rigidity, sweating, paresthesias, and abdominal pain in some cases (220,221). In some studies tremor occurred in up to 29% of patients following widow spider bites (221). The toxic effects of these venoms are mediated largely by α-latrotoxin, a 120 kDa protein that induces neurotransmitter release by calcium-dependent and independent mechanisms leading to vesicle depletion (222).

Ingestion of mycotoxins is a well-recognized cause of tremor in dogs and other animals (223). This may occur in humans as well, as illustrated by the case of a young man who ingested moldy silage and subsequently developed mental status changes and tremor precipitated by movement, resolving in one week (224). Mycotoxins from *Penicillium cyclopium* were probably responsible for symptoms of food poisoning (gastralgia, diarrhea, dizziness, and malaise) secondary to contaminated dried persimmon in one report (225). When crude extracts of this fungus were injected into mice, diarrhea, tremor, and convulsions were observed before death (225).

XV. OTHER MISCELLANEOUS DRUGS

While most β-blockers typically improve various forms of tremor, pindolol is known to cause tremor in various settings. In one report, five patients ranging in age from 20 to 69 years received pindolol and developed fine tremor of the arms and hands (226). Another man initially developed "muscle twitches" of the legs at night followed by tremor of both hands while taking 30 mg of pindolol twice daily (227). Tremor onset was typically within hours or days and resolved completely within 24–72 hours after stopping the drug in most patients (226). Tremor appeared in patients taking as little as 2.5 mg daily or as high as 60 mg daily (226,227). The tremor appears mostly postural and action in nature and in one patient had a frequency of 6.7 Hz (227). A controlled trial of pindolol vs. propranolol in essential tremor patients demonstrated that pindolol actually increased tremor amplitude (228). One patient also developed chin tremor on reintroduction of pindolol in addition to postural and action tremors of the hands (227). The mechanism of pindolol-induced tremor is very likely to be its partial β-agonist activity, unlike other β-blockers (226,227).

Various reports have documented tremor in patients taking ephedrine, pseudoephedrine, and phenylpropanolamine (229–232). These drugs are/were typically found in over-the-counter cold and appetite suppressant preparations. They are known to have sympathomimetic activity and can cause tremor in various settings. Ephedrine (February 2004) and phenylpropanolamine (November 2000) were actually taken off the over-the-counter market in the United States due to serious risk of stroke, myocardial infarction, and death, with ephedrine and problems with phenylpropanolamine causing an increased risk of hemorrhagic stroke. Pseudoephedrine remains in use for colds and appetite suppression.

Tremor associated with exaltation and insomnia occurred in four patients taking a combination pill of ephedrine, caffeine, and other substances ("Elsinore pill") for weight loss (229). Tremor (frequently transient) occurred in 10 of 38 patients on the "Elsinore pill" compared to only two of 39 patients taking another appetite suppressant, diethylpropion, during the 12 week clinical trial (229). Acute amphetamine-like CNS effects were also noted in patients taking phenylpropanolamine, including tremor, agitation, restlessness, hallucinations (230). In another study of pseudoephedrine plus loratadine for allergic rhinitis, 39% of patients complained of tremor at some point during 14 days of therapy (231).

XVI. CONCLUSION

The list of drugs that induce or exacerbate tremors is growing larger each year. While the majority of drugs cause postural tremors, many drugs can also cause resting and intention tremors. Table 23.2 lists the major drugs associated with each tremor type. The data for this table are based on a compilation of the references above as well as the Consensus Statement on Tremor by the Movement Disorder Society (233).

Table 23.3 is a list of the most widely prescribed and used tremorogenic drugs in the United States today. While these drugs may cause tremors, it is

Table 23.2   Major Drugs Known to Cause Resting, Postural, and Action/Intention Tremors

Resting

Major category	*Typical examples*
Antibiotics/antivirals/antifungals	Trimethoprim/sulfa, amphotericin B
Antidepressants/mood stabilizers	SSRIs, lithium
Antiepileptics	Valproate
Chemotherapeutics	Thalidomide
Drugs of abuse	Cocaine, ethanol, MDMA
Gastrointestinal drugs	Metoclopramide
Hormones	Medroxyprogesterone
Neuroleptics/dopamine depleters	Haloperidol, thioridazine, cinnarizine, reserpine, tetrabenazine
Poisons/toxins	Manganese, lead, mercury, carbon disulfide

Postural

Major category	*Typical examples*
Antiarrhythmics	Amiodarone, mexiletine, procainamide
Antidepressants/mood stabilizers	Amitriptyline, lithium, SSRIs
Antiepileptics	Valproate
Bronchodilators	Albuterol, salmeterol
Chemotherapeutics	Tamoxifen, Ara-C, ifosfamide
Drugs of abuse	Cocaine, ethanol, MDMA, nicotine
Gastrointestinal drugs	Metoclopramide, cimetidine
Herbs	Kava-kava, star anise
Hormones	Thyroxine, calcitonin, medroxyprogesterone
Immunosuppressants	Tacrolimus, cyclosporine, α-interferon
Methylxanthines	Theophylline, caffeine
Neuroleptics/dopamine depleters	Haloperidol, thioridazine, cinnarizine, reserpine, tetrabenazine
Poisons/toxins	Manganese, lead, mercury, toluene, methanol, MPTP, cyanide, dioxin, various venoms, mycotoxins

Action/Intention

Major category	*Typical examples*
Antibiotics/antivirals/antifungals	Vidarabine
Antidepressants/mood stabilizers	Lithium
Bronchodilators	Albuterol, salmeterol
Chemotherapeutics	Ara-C, ifosfamide
Drugs of abuse	Ethanol
Hormones	Epinephrine
Immunosuppressants	Tacrolimus, cyclosporine
Poisons/toxins	Mercury, lead, manganese, methanol

Note: SSRIs, selective serotonin reuptake inhibitors; MDMA, 3,4-methylenedioxy-methamphetamine (ecstasy); MPTP, 1-methyl-4-phenyl-1,2,3,6-tetrahydropyridine; Ara-C, cytosine arabinoside (cytarabine).

Table 23.3 Widely-Prescribed Tremorogenic Drugs

Drug	Treatment
Albuterol	Reduce frequency or discontinue use, longer-acting inhaled β-agonist may help
Amiodarone	Screen for hyperthyroidism, reduce dose to 200 mg/day if possible, β-blocker may help
Amitriptyline/ TCAs	Allow time to see if tremor will improve, discontinue use and switch to an SSRI, β-blocker may help
Caffeine	Reduce caffeine intake
Cyclosporine	Avoid toxic states and consider reducing dose, try another immunosuppressive agent
Ethanol	Abstinence, β-blockers, consider carbamazepine for intention tremors
Lithium	Check drug levels, reduce dose change medications (valproate, lamotrigine, etc.) β-blocker therapy (may worsen depression)
Metoclopramide	Discontinue use and observe consider using erythromycin for gastroparesis observe for signs of parkinsonism
Nicotine	Stop using all forms of tobacco or nicotine gum
SSRIs	Wait to see if tremor improves over time reduce dose if depression allows β-blockers (may worsen depression)
Tacrolimus (FK-506)	Reduce dose try another immunosuppressive agent
Valproate	Reduce dose change to another antiepileptic or mood stabilizer β-blockers

Note: TCAs, tricyclic antidepressants; SSRIs, selective serotonin reuptake inhibitors.

important to remember that many drugs exacerbate underlying tremors, and an underlying cause for tremor (essential tremor, Parkinson's disease, cerebellar dysfunction, psychogenic tremor) should be considered in each patient.

REFERENCES

1. Lhuillier M, Gouin B. [Amiodarone and trembling]. Nouv Presse Med 1972; 1:1844.
2. Lustman F, Monseu G. Letter: Amiodarone and neurological side-effects. Lancet 1974; 1(7857):568.
3. Morady F, Scheinman MM, Hess DS. Amiodarone in the management of patients with ventricular tachycardia and ventricular fibrillation. Pacing Clin Electrophysiol 1983; 6:609–615.

4. Coulter DM, Edwards IR, Savage RL. Survey of neurological problems with amiodarone in the New Zealand Intensive Medicines Monitoring Programme. N Z Med J 1990; 103:98–100.
5. Charness ME, Morady F, Scheinman MM. Frequent neurologic toxicity associated with amiodarone therapy. Neurology 1984; 34:669–671.
6. Harris L, McKenna WJ, Rowland E, Krikler DM. Side effects and possible contraindications of amiodarone use. Am Heart J 1983; 106:916–923.
7. Hilleman D, Miller MA, Parker R, Doering P, Pieper JA. Optimal management of amiodarone therapy: efficacy and side effects. Pharmacotherapy 1998; 18:138S–145S.
8. Fromerty B, Fisch C, Labbe G, Deggot C, Deschamps D, Berson A, Letteron P, Pessayre D. Amiodarone inhibits the mitochondrial β oxidation of fatty acids and produces microvesicular steatosis of the liver in mice. J Pharmacol Exp Ther 1990; 255:1371–1376.
9. Rubinstein A, Cabili S. Tremor induced by procainamide. Am J Cardiol 1986; 57:340–341.
10. Manolis AS, Deering TF, Cameron J, Estes NA 3rd. Mexiletine: pharmacology and therapeutic use. Clin Cardiol 1990; 13:349–359.
11. Peyrieux JC, Boissel JP, Leizorovicz A. Relationship between plasma mexiletine levels at steady-state. Presence of ventricular arrhythmias and side effects. Fundam Clin Pharmacol 1987; 1:45–57.
12. Ando K, Wallace MS, Braun J, Schulteis G. Effect of oral mexiletine on capsaicin-induced allodynia and hyperalgesia: a double-blind, placebo-controlled, crossover study. Reg Anesth Pain Med 2000; 25:468–474.
13. Borucki MJ, Matzke DS, Pollard RB. Tremor induced by trimethoprim-sulfamethoxazole in patients with acquired immunodeficiency syndrome (AIDS). Ann Intern Med 1988; 109:77–78.
14. Van Gerpen JA. Tremor caused by trimethoprim-sulfamethoxazole in a patient with AIDS. Neurology 1997; 48:537–538.
15. Floris-Moore MA, Amodio-Groton MI, Catalano MT. Adverse reactions to trimethoprim/sulfamethoxazole in AIDS. Ann Pharmacother 2003; 37:1810–1813.
16. Patterson RG, Couchenour RL. Trimethoprim-sulfamethoxazole-induced tremor in an immunocompetent patient. Pharmacotherapy 1999; 19:1456–1458.
17. Burdge DR, Chow AW, Sacks SL. Neurotoxic effects during vidarabine therapy for herpes zoster. Can Med Assoc J 1985; 132:392–395.
18. Cullis PA, Cushing R. Vidarabine encephalopathy. J Neurol Neurosurg Psychiatry 1984; 47:1351–1354.
19. Nadel AM. Vidarabine therapy for herpes simplex encephalitis. The development of an unusual tremor during treatment. Arch Neurol 1981; 38:384–385.
20. Ross AH, Julia A, Balakrishnan C. Toxicity of adenine arabinoside in humans. J Infect Dis 1976; 133(suppl):A192–A198.
21. Wade JC, Meyers JD. Neurologic symptoms associated with parenteral acyclovir treatment after marrow transplantation. Ann Intern Med 1983; 98:921–925.
22. Rashiq S, Briewa L, Mooney M, Giancarlo T, Khatib R, Wilson FM. Distinguishing acyclovir neurotoxicity from encephalomyelitis. J Intern Med. 1993; 234:507–511.
23. Mott SH, Packer RJ, Vezina LG, Kapur S, Dirndorf PA, Conry JA, Pranzatelli MR, Quinones RR. Encephalopathy with parkinsonian features in children following bone marrow transplantations and high-dose amphotericin B. Ann Neurol 1995; 37:810–814.

24. Ellis WG, Sobel RA, Nielsen SL. Leukoencephalopathy in patients treated with amphotericin B methyl ester. J Infect Dis 1982; 146:125–137.
25. Bulkowstein M, Mordish Y, Zimmerman DR, Sherman E, Berkovitch M. Ketoconazole-induced neurologic sequelae. Vet Hum Toxicol 2003; 45:239–240.
26. Quabeck K, Muller KD, Beelen DW, Dermoumi H, Kolbel M, Kraft J, Ansorg R, Schaefer UW. Prophylaxis and treatment of fungal infections with fluconazole in bone marrow transplant patients. Mycoses 1992; 35:221–224.
27. Watanabe S, Yokoyama S, Kubo S, Iwai H, Kuyama C. A double-blind controlled study of clinical efficacy of maprotiline and amitriptyline in depression. Folia Psychiatr Neurol Jpn 1978; 32:1–31.
28. Raethjen J, Lemke MR, Linderman M, Wenzelburger R, Krack P, Deuschl G. Amitriptyline enhances the central component of physiological tremor. J Neurol Neurosurg Psychiatry 2001; 70:78–82.
29. Smith WT, Glaudin V, Panagides J, Gilvary E. Mirtazapine vs. amitriptyline vs. placebo in the treatment of major depressive disorder. Psychopharmacol Bull 1990; 26:191–196.
30. Chouinard G. A double-blind controlled clinical trial of fluoxetine and amitriptyline in the treatment of outpatients with major depressive disorder. J Clin Psychiatry 1985; 46:32–37.
31. Fruensgaard K, Hansen CE, Korsgaard S, Nymgaard K, Vaag UH. Amoxapine vs. amitriptyline in endogenous depression. A double-blind study. Acta Psychiatr Scan 1979; 59:502–508.
32. Guelfi JD, Dreyfus JF, Pichot P. A double-blind controlled clinical trial comparing fluvoxamine with imipramine. Br J Clin Pharmacol 1981; 15(suppl 3):411S–417S.
33. Kronfol Z, Greden JF, Zis AP. Imipramine-induced tremor: effects of a beta-adrenergic blocking agent. J Clin Psychiatry 1983; 44:225–226.
34. Bharucha KJ, Sethi KD. Movement disorders induced by selective serotonin reuptake inhibitors and other antidepressants. In: Sethi KD, ed. Drug-Induced Movement Disorders. New York: Marcel Dekker, 2004:233–257.
35. Edwards JG, Anderson I. Systematic review and guide to selection of selective serotonin reuptake inhibitors. Drugs 1999; 57:507–533.
36. Wernicke JF. The side effect profile and safety of fluoxetine. J Clin Psychiatry 1985; 46:59–67.
37. Diaz-Martinez A, Benassinni O, Ontiveros A, Gonzalez S, Salin R, Basquedano G, Martinez RA. A randomized, open-label comparison of venlafaxine and fluoxetine in depressed outpatients. Clin Ther 1998; 20:467–476.
38. Serrano-Duenas M. Fluoxetine-induced tremor: clinical features in 21 patients. Parkinsonism Relat Disord 2002; 8:325–327.
39. Anand KS, Prasad A, Pradhan SC, Biswas A. Fluoxetine-induced tremors. J Assoc Physicians India 1999; 47:651–652.
40. Lejoyeux M, Ades J. Antidepressant discontinuation: a review of the literature. J Clin Psychiatry 1997; 58(suppl 7):11–15.
41. Factor SA. Lithium-induced movement disorders. In: Sethi KD, ed. Drug-Induced Movement Disorders. New York: Marcel Dekker, 2004:209–231.
42. Gelenberg AJ, Jefferson JW. Lithium tremor. J Clin Psychiatry 1995; 56:283–287.
43. Goodwin FK, Jamison KR. Medication compliance. In: Goodwin FK, Jamison KR, eds. Manic-Depressive Illness. New York: Oxford University Press, 1990:746–762.

44. Vestergaard P, Amidsen A, Shou M. Clinically significant side effects of lithium treatment. A survey of 237 patients in long-term treatment. Acta Psychiatr Scand 1980; 62:193–200.
45. Henry C. Lithium side-effects and predictors of hypothyroidism in patients with bipolar disorder: sex differences. J Psychiatry Neurosci 2002; 27:104–107.
46. Bech P, Thomsen J, Prytz S, Vendsborg PB, Zilstorff K, Rafaelsen OJ. The profile and severity of lithium-induced side effects in mentally healthy subjects. Neuropsychobiology 1979; 5:160–166.
47. Vestergaard P, Poulstrup I, Shou M. Prospective studies on a lithium cohort. 3. Tremor, weight gain, diarrhea, psychological complaints. Acta Psychiatr Scand 1988; 78:434–441.
48. Zaninelli R, Bauer M, Jobert M, Muller-Oerlinghausen B. Changes in quantitatively assessed tremor during treatment of major depression with lithium augmented by paroxetine and amitriptyline. J Clin Psychopharmacol 2001; 21:190–198.
49. Zubenko GS, Cohen BM, Lipinski JF. Comparison of metoprolol and propranolol in the treatment of lithium tremor. Psychiatry Res 1984; 11:163–164.
50. Goumentouk AD, Hurwitz TA, Zis AP. Primidone in drug-induced tremor. J Clin Psychopharmacol 1989; 9:451.
51. Morgan JC, Harrison MB. Antiepileptics. In: Factor SA, Weiner WJ, Lang AE, eds. Drug-Induced Movement Disorders, 2nd ed. New York: Blackwell (in press).
52. Kellett MW, Chadwick DW. Antiepileptic drug-induced movement disorders. In: Sethi KD, ed. Drug-Induced Movement Disorders. New York: Marcel Dekker, 2004:309–356.
53. Hyman NM, Dennis PD, Sinclair KG. Tremor due to sodium valproate. Neurology 1979; 29:1177–1180.
54. Karas BJ, Wilder BJ, Hammond EJ, Bauman AW. Valproate tremors. Neurology 1982; 32:428–432.
55. Karas BJ, Wilder BJ, Hammond EJ, Bauman AW. Treatment of valproate tremors. Neurology 1983; 33:1380–1382.
56. Lancman ME, Asconape JJ, Walker F. Acetazolamide appears effective in the management of valproate-induced tremor. Mov Disord 1994; 9:369.
57. Product Information, Gabatril®, Cephalon
58. Product Information, Neurontin®, Parke-Davis
59. Product Information, Trileptal®, Novartis
60. Product Information, Keppra®, UCB Pharma
61. Product Information, Lamictal®, GlaxoSmithKline
62. Reutens DC, Duncan JS, Patsalos PN. Disabling tremor after lamotrigine with sodium valproate. Lancet 1993; 342:185–186.
63. Das KB, Harris C, Smyth DP, Cross JH. Unusual side effects of lamotrigine therapy. J Child Neurol 2003; 18:479–480.
64. Product Information, Zonegran®, Elan
65. Product Information, Topamax®, Ortho-McNeil
66. Louis ED. Clinical practice. Essential tremor. N Engl J Med 2001; 345:887–891.
67. Sechi GP, Zuddas M, Piredda M et al. Treatment of cerebellar tremors with carbamazepine: a controlled trial with long-term follow-up. Neurology 1989; 39:1113–1115.
68. Merren MD. Gabapentin for treatment of pain and tremor: a large case series. South Med J 1998; 91:739–744.

69. Gironell A, Kulisevsky J, Barbanoj M et al. A randomized placebo-controlled comparative trial of gabapentin and propranolol in essential tremor. Arch Neurol 1999; 56:475–480.
70. Ondo W, Hunter C, Vuong KD et al. Gabapentin for essential tremor: a multiple-dose, double-blind, placebo-controlled trial. Mov Disord 2000; 15:678–682.
71. Onofrj M, Thomas A, Paci C et al. Gabapentin in orthostatic tremor: results of a double-blind crossover with placebo in four patients. Neurology 1998; 51:880–882.
72. Evidente VG, Adler CH, Caviness JN et al. Effective treatment of orthostatic tremor with gabapentin. Mov Disord 1998; 13:829–831.
73. Galvez-Jimenez N, Hargreave M. Topiramate and essential tremor. Ann Neurol 2000; 47:837–838.
74. Connor GS. A double-blind placebo-controlled trial of topiramate treatment for essential tremor. Neurology 2002; 59:132–134.
75. Product Information, Proventil®, Key Pharmaceuticals
76. Product Information, Albuterol sulfate, Astra USA
77. Rodrigo G, Rodrigo C. Metered dose inhaler salbutamol treatment of asthma in the ED: comparison of two doses with plasma levels. Am J Emerg Med 1996; 14:144–150.
78. Shrewsbury S, Hallett C. Salmeterol 100 microg: an analysis of its tolerability in single and chronic-dose studies. Ann Allergy Asthma Immunol 2001; 87:465–473.
79. Mann RD, Kubota K, Pearce G, Wilton L. Salmeterol: a study by prescription-event monitoring in a UK cohort of 15,407 patients. J Clin Epidemiol 1996; 49:247–250.
80. Wong CS, Pavord ID, Williams J, Britton JR, Tattersfield AE. Bronchodilator, cardiovascular, and hypokalemic effects of fenoterol, salbutamol, and terbutaline in asthma. Lancet 1990; 336(8728):1396–1399.
81. Foley TH, Marsden CD, Owen DA. Evidence for a direct peripheral effect of adrenaline on physiological tremor in man. J Physiol 1967; 189:65P–66P.
82. Trump DL, Smith DC, Ellis PG, Rogers MP, Schold SC, Winer EP, Panella TJ, Jordan VC, Fine RL. High-dose oral tamoxifen, a potential multidrug-resistance-reversal agent: phase I trial in combination with vinblastine. J Natl Cancer Inst 1992; 84:1811–1816.
83. Thomson KF, Goodfield MJ. Low-dose thalidomide is an effective second-line treatment in cutaneous lupus erythematosus. Dermatolog Treat 2001; 12:145–147.
84. Weber D, Rankin K, Gavino M, Delasalle K, Alexanian R. Thalidomide alone or with dexamethasone for previously untreated multiple myeloma. J Clin Oncol 2003; 21:16–19.
85. Morgan AE, Smith WK, Levenson JL. Reversible dementia due to thalidomide therapy for multiple myeloma. N Engl J Med. 2003; 348:1821–1822.
86. Baker WJ, Royer GL Jr, Weiss RB. Cytarabine and neurologic toxicity. J Clin Oncol 1991; 9:679–693.
87. Lafolie P, Lilliemark J, Bjork O, Aman J, Wranne L, Peterson C. Exchange of cerebrospinal fluid in accidental intrathecal overdose of cytarabine. Med Toxicol Adverse Drug Exp 1988; 3:248–252.
88. Reinders-Messelink HA, Schoemaker MM, Hofte M, Goeken LN, Kingma A, van den Briel MM, Kamps WA. Fine motor and handwriting problems after treatment for childhood acute lymphoblastic leukemia. Med Pediatr Oncol 1996; 27:551–555.
89. Dworkin LA, Goldman RD, Zivin LS, Fuchs PC. Cerebellar toxicity following high-dose cytosine arabinoside. J Clin Oncol 1985; 3:613–616.

90. Nand S, Messmore HL Jr, Patel R, Fisher SG, Fisher RI. Neurotoxicity associated with systemic high-dose cytosine arabinoside. J Clin Oncol 1986; 4:571–575.

91. Herzig RH, Hines JD, Herzig GP, Wolff SN, Cassileth PA, Lazarus HM, Adelstein DJ, Brown RA, Coccia PF, Strandjord S et al. Cerebellar toxicity with high-dose cytosine arabinoside. J Clin Oncol 1987; 5:927–932.

92. Pratt CB, Horowitz ME, Meyer WH, Etcubanas E, Thompson EI, Douglass EC, Wilimas JA, Hayes FA, Green AA. Phase II trial of ifosfamide in children with malignant solid tumors. Cancer Treat Rep 1987; 71:131–135.

93. Meggs WJ, Hoffman RS. Fatality resulting from intraventricular vincristine administration. J Toxicol Clin Toxicol 1998; 36:243–246.

94. Schilsky RL, Barlock A, Ozols RF. Persistent hypomagnesemia following cisplatin chemotherapy for testicular cancer. Cancer Treat Rep 1982; 66:1767–1769.

95. Neiman J, Lang AE, Fornazzari L, Carlen PL. Movement disorders in alcoholism: a review. Neurology 1990; 40:741–746.

96. Koller W, O'Hara R, Dorus W, Bauer J. Tremor in chronic alcoholism. Neurology 1985; 35:1660–1662.

97. Lippold OC, Williams EJ, Wilson CG. Finger tremor and cigarette smoking. Br J Clin Pharmacol 1980; 10:83–86.

98. Marthinsen L, Uges DR. Tremor in the newborn infant caused by maternal smoking. Ther Drug Monit 2002; 24:455.

99. Shiffman SM, Gritz ER, Maltese J, Lee MA, Schneider NG, Jarvik ME. Effects of cigarette smoking and oral nicotine on hand tremor. Clin Pharmacol Ther 1983; 33:800–805.

100. Zdonczyk D, Royse V, Koller WC. Nicotine and tremor. Clin Neuropharmacol 1988; 11:282–286.

101. Ishikawa A, Miyatake T. Effects of smoking in patients with early-onset Parkinson's disease. J Neurol Sci 1993; 117:28–32.

102. Fagerstrom KO, Pomerleau O, Giordani B, Stelson F. Nicotine may relieve symptoms of Parkinson's disease. Psychopharmacology (Berl) 1994; 116:117–119.

103. Vieregge A, Sieberer M, Jacobs H, Hagenah JM, Vieregge P. Transdermal nicotine in PD: a randomized, double-blind, placebo-controlled study. Neurology 2001; 57:1032–1035.

104. Demirkiran M, Jankovic J, Dean JM. Ecstasy intoxication: an overlap between serotonin syndrome and neuroleptic malignant syndrome. Clin Neuropharmacol 1996; 19:157–164.

105. O'Suilleabhain P, Giller C. Rapidly progressive parkinsonism in a self-reported user of ecstasy and other drugs. Mov Disord 2003; 18:1378–1403.

106. Daras M, Koppel BS, Atos-Radzion E. Cocaine-induced choreoathetoid movements ('crack dancing'). Neurology 1994; 44:751–752.

107. Bauer LO. Psychomotor and electroencephalographic sequelae of cocaine dependence. NIDA Res Monogr 1996; 163:66–93.

108. Baker WW, Zivanovic D, Malseed RT. Tremorogenic effects of intracaudate d-amphetamine and their suppression by dopamine. Arch Int Pharmacodyn Ther 1976; 223:271–281.

109. McKinney PE, Tomaszewski C, Phillips S, Brent J, Kulig K. Methamphetamine toxicity prevented by activated charcoal in a mouse model. Ann Emerg Med 1994; 24:220–223.

110. Pataki CS, Carlson GA, Kelly KL, Rapport MD, Biancaniello TM. Side effects of methylphenidate and desipramine alone and in combination in children. J Am Acad Child Adolesc Psychiatry 1993; 32:1065–1072.

111. Kataria M, Traub M, Marsden CD. Extrapyramidal side-effects of metoclopramide. Lancet 1978; 2(8102):1254–1255.

112. Ahronheim JC. Metoclopramide and tremor. Ann Intern Med 1982; 97:621

113. Sethi KD, Patel B, Meador KJ. Metoclopramide-induced parkinsonism. South Med J 1989; 82:1581–1582.

114. Stacy M, Jankovic J. Tardive tremor. Mov Disord 1992; 7:53–57.

115. Tarsy D, Indorf G. Tardive tremor due to metoclopramide. Mov Disord 2002; 17:620–621.

116. Acharya SR, Kumar TN, Vasshadhara C. Metoclopramide—a cholinomimetic tremorogen? J Assoc Physicians India 1982; 30:119.

117. Bateman DN, Bevan P, Longley BP, Mastaglia F, Wandless I. Cimetidine induced postural and action tremor. J Neurol Neurosurg Psychiatry 1981; 44:94.

118. Gatti PJ, Gertner SB. Cardiovascular and behavioral actions of centrally administered cimetidine. J Cardiovasc Pharmacol 1984; 6:575–581.

119. Product information, Propulsid®, Janssen

120. Sempere AP, Duarte J, Cabezas C, Claveria LE, Coria F. Aggravation of parkinsonian tremor by cisapride. Clin Neuropharmacol 1995; 18:76–78.

121. Graber DJ, Meier KH. Acute Misoprostol toxicity. Ann Emerg Med 1991; 20:549–551.

122. Buge A, Rancurel G, Poisson M, Gazengel J, Dechy H, Freissinaud L, Emile J. 20 cases of acute encephalopathy with myoclonus during treatments with orally-administered bismuth salts. Ann Med Interne (Paris) 1974; 125:877–888.

123. Burns R, Thomas DW, Barron VJ. Reversible encephalopathy possibly associated with bismuth subgallate ingestion. Br Med J 1974; 1(901):220–223.

124. Gordon MF, Abrams RI, Rubin DB, Barr WB, Correa DD. Bismuth subsalicylate toxicity as a cause of prolonged encephalopathy with myoclonus. Mov Disord 1995; 10:220–222.

125. Ribadeau Dumas JL, Lechevalier B, Breteau M, Allain Y. The intracerebral distribution of bismuth in bismuth encephalopathy. Pathological and toxicological study of 3 cases (author's transl). Nouv Presse Med 1978; 7:4021–4025.

126. Escourelle R, Bourdon R, Galli A, Galle P, Jaudon MC, Hauw JJ, Gray F. Neuropathologic and toxicologic study of 12 cases of bismuth encephalopathy. Rev Neurol (Paris) 1977; 133:153–163.

127. Ross JF, Sahenk Z, Hyser C, Mendell JR, Alden CL. Characterization of a murine model for human bismuth encephalopathy. Neurotoxicology 1988; 9:581–586.

128. Minodier P, Pommier P, Moulene E, Retornaz K, Prost N, Deharo L. Star anise poisoning in infants. Arch Pediatr 2003; 10:619–621.

129. Ize-Ludlow D, Ragone S, Bernstein JN, Bruck IS, Duchowny M, Garcia Pena BM. Chemical composition of Chinese star anise (Illicium verum) and neurotoxicity in infants. JAMA 2004; 291:562–563.

130. Meseguer E, Taboada R, Sánchez V, Mena MA, Campos V, de Yébenes JG. Life-threatening parkinsonism induced by kava-kava. Mov Disord 2002; 17:195–196.

131. Schelosky L, Raffauf C, Jendroska K, Poewe W. Kava and dopamine antagonism. J Neurol Neurosurg Psychiatry 1995; 58:639–640.

132. Pfau W, Skog K. Exposure to β-carbolines norharman and Harman. J Chromatogr B Analyt Technol Biomed Life Sci 2004; 802:115–126.
133. Kuhn W, Muller T, Grosse H, Dierks T, Rommelspacher H. Plasma levels of beta-carbolines Harman and norharman in Parkinson's disease. Acta Neurol Scand 1995; 92:451–454.
134. Kuhn W, Muller T, Grosse H, Rommelspacher H. Elevated levels of Harman and norharman in cerebrospinal fluid of parkinsonian patients. J Neural Transm 1996; 103:1435–1440.
135. Louis ED, Zheng W, Jurewicz EC, Watner D, Chen J, Factor-Litvak P, Parides M. Elevation of blood beta-carboline alkaloids in essential tremor. Neurology 2002; 59:1940–1944.
136. Boniel T, Dannon P. The safety of herbal medicines in the psychiatric practice. Harefuah 2001; 140:780–783, 805.
137. Mattila M, Seppala T, Mattila MJ. Anxiogenic effect of yohimbine in healthy subjects: comparison with caffeine and antagonism by clonidine and diazepam. Int Clin Psychopharmacol 1988; 3:215–229.
138. Tibaldi JM, Barzel US, Albin J, Surks M. Thyrotoxicosis in the very old. Am J Med 1986; 81:619–622.
139. Burger AG, Philippe J. Thyroid emergencies. Baillieres Clin Endocrinol Metab 1992; 6:77–93.
140. Weber C, Scholz GH, Lamesch P, Paschke R. Thyroidectomy in iodine induced thyrotoxic storm. Exp Clin Endocrinol Diabetes 1999; 107:468–472.
141. Shaw PJ, Walls TJ, Newman PK, Cleland PG, Cartlidge NE. Hashimoto's encephalopathy: a steroid-responsive disorder associated with high anti-thyroid antibody titers—report of 5 cases. Neurology 1991; 41:228–233.
142. Erickson JC, Carrasco H, Grimes JB, Jabbari B, Cannard KR. Palatal tremor and myorhythmia in Hashimoto's encephalopathy. Neurology 2002; 58:504–505.
143. Gucuyener K, Serdaroglu A, Bideci A, Yazman Y. Soysal AS, Cinaz P. Tremor and myoclonus heralding Hashimoto's encephalopathy. J Pediatr Endocrinol Metab 2000; 13:1137–1141.
144. Mandel SH, Magnusson AR, Burton BT, Swanson JR, LaFranchi SH. Massive levothyroxine ingestion. Conservative management. Clin Pediatr (Phila) 1989; 28:374–376.
145. de Luis DA, Duenas A, Martin J, Abad L, Cuellar L, Aller R. Light symptoms following a high-dose intentional L-thyroxine ingestion treated with cholestyramine. Horm Res 2002; 57:61–63.
146. Bauer BA, Elkin PL, Erickson D, Klee GG, Brennan MD. Symptomatic hyperthyroidism in a patient taking the dietary supplement tiratricol. Mayo Clin Proc 2002; 77:587–590.
147. Marsden CD, Meadows JC. The effect of adrenaline on the contraction of human muscle—one mechanism whereby adrenaline increases the amplitude of physiological tremor. J Physiol 1968; 194:70–71P.
148. Abila B, Lazarus JH, Kingswood JC, Marshall RW, Wilson JF, Richens A. Tremor: an alternative approach for investigating adrenergic mechanisms in thyrotoxicosis. Clin Sci (Lond) 1985; 69:459–463.
149. Falkson G, Falkson HC. A phase II study of high-dose medroxyprogesterone acetate in advance breast cancer. Cancer Chemother Pharmacol 1983; 11:16–18.

150. Product Information, Depo-Provera®, Pharmacia & UpJohn.
151. Lance JW, Hinterberger H. Symptoms of pheochromocytoma, with particular reference to headache, correlated with catecholamine production. Arch Neurol 1976; 33:281–288.
152. Simons FE, Gu X, Silver NA, Simons KJ. EpiPen Jr vs. EpiPen in young children weighing 15 to 30 kg at risk for anaphylaxis. J Allergy Clin Immunol 2002; 109:171–175.
153. Conget JI, Vendrell J, Halperin I, Esmatjes E. Widespread tremor after injection of sodium calcitonin BMJ 1989; 298(6667):189.
154. Gijtenbeek JM, van den Bent MJ, Vecht CJ. Cyclosporine neurotoxicity: a review. J Neurol 1999; 246:339–346.
155. Trocha K, Winkler M, Haas J, Ringe B, Wurster U, Ehrenheim C. Neurological examinations after liver transplantation concerning patients under corticosteroids immunosuppression and either FK 506 or cyclosporine. Transpl Int 1994; 7(suppl 1):S43–S49.
156. Wijdicks EF, Wiesner RH, Dahlke LJ, Krom RA. FK 506-induced neurotoxicity in liver transplantation. Ann Neurol 1994; 35:498–501.
157. Uemoto S, Tanaka K, Honda K, Tokunaga Y, Sano K, Katoh H, Tamamoto E, Takada Y, Ozawa K. Experience with FK506 in living-related liver transplantation. Transplantation 1993; 55:288–292.
158. Yocum DE, Furst DE, Bensen WG, Burch FX, Borton MA, Mengle-Gaw LJ, Schwartz BD, Wisememandle W, Mekki QA. Safety of tacrolimus in patients with rheumatoid arthritis: Long-term experience. Rheumatology 2004; 43(8): 992–999.
159. Sandborn WJ, Present DH, Isaacs KL, Wolf DC, Greenberg E, Hanauer SB, Feagan BG, Mayer L, Johnson T, Galanko J, Martin C, Sandler RS. Tacrolimus for the treatment of fistulas in patients with Crohn's disease: a randomized, placebo-controlled trial. Gastroenterology 2003; 125:380–388.
160. Caraceni A, Gangeri L, Martini C, Belli F, Brunelli C, Baldini M, Mascheroni L, Lenisa L, Cascinelli N. Neurotoxicity of interferon-alpha in melanoma therapy: results from a randomized controlled trial. Cancer. 1998; 83:482–489.
161. Tan EK, Chan LL, Lo YL. "Myorhythmia" slow facial tremor from chronic interferon alpha-2a usage. Neurology 2003; 61:1302–1303.
162. Sarasombath P, Sumida K, Kaku DA. Parkinsonism associated with interferon alpha therapy for chronic myelogenous leukemia. Hawaii Med J 2002; 61:48, 57.
163. Shuto H, Kataoka Y, Horikawa T, Fujihara N, Oishi R. Repeated interferon-alpha administration inhibits dopaminergic neural activity in the mouse brain. Brain Res 1997; 747:348–351.
164. Barr RG, Rowe BH, Camrgo CA Jr. Methylxanthines for exacerbations of chronic obstructive pulmonary disease: meta-analysis of randomized trials. BMJ 2003; 327:643.
165. Buss DC, Marshall RW, Milligan N, McQueen I, Compston DA, Routledge PA. The effect of intravenous aminophylline on essential tremor. Br J Clin Pharmacol 1997; 43:119–121.
166. Mally J, Stone TW. Efficacy of an adenosine antagonist, theophylline, in essential tremor: comparison with placebo and propranolol. J Neurol Sci 1995; 132:129–132.

167. Mally J, Stone TW. The effect of theophylline on essential tremor: the possible role of GABA. Pharmacol Biochem Behav 1991; 39:345–349.
168. Koller W, Cone S, Herbster G. Caffeine and tremor. Neurology 1987; 37:169–172.
169. Wharrad HJ, Birmingham AT, Macdonald IA, Inch PJ, Mead JL. The influence of fasting and of caffeine intake on finger tremor. Eur J Clin Pharmacol 1985; 29:37–43.
170. Miller LS, Lombardo TW, Fowler SC. Caffeine, but not time of day, increases whole-arm physiological tremor in non-smoking moderate users. Clin Exp Pharmacol Physiol 1998; 25:131–133.
171. Ayd F. A survey of drug-induced extrapyramidal reactions. JAMA 1961; 175:1054–1060.
172. National Institute of Mental Health Psychopharmacology Service Center Collaborative Study Group. Phenothiazine treatment in acute schizophrenia. Arch Gen Psychiatry 1964; 10:246–261.
173. Friedman JH. Drug-induced parkinsonism. In: Lang AE, Weiner WJ, eds. Drug-Induced Movement Disorders. New York: Futura Publishing, 1992:41–84.
174. Sethi KD. Movement disorders induced by dopamine blocking agents. Semin Neurol 2001; 21:59–68.
175. Chaudhuri KR, Nott J. Drug-induced parkinsonism. In: Sethi KD, ed. Drug-Induced Movement Disorders. New York: Marcel Dekker, 2004:61–75.
176. Marti-Masso JF, Poza JJ. Cinnarizine-induced parkinsonism: ten years later. Mov Disord 1998; 13:453–456.
177. Calne DB, Webster RA. Tremor induced by tetrabenazine. Br J Pharmacol 1969; 37:468–475.
178. Gillman MA, Sandyk R. Parkinsonism induced by methyldopa. S Afr Med J 1984; 65:194.
179. Ross RT. Drug induced parkinsonism and other movement disorders. Can J Neurol Sci 1990; 17:155–162.
180. Louis ED. Etiology of essential tremor: should we be searching for environmental causes? Mov Disord 2001; 16:822–829.
181. Guzelian PS. Comparative toxicology of chlordecone (Kepone) in humans and experimental animals. Ann Rev Pharm Toxicol 1982; 22:89–113.
182. Taylor JR, Selhorst JB, Houff SA, Martinez AJ. Chlordecone intoxication in man. I. Clinical observations. Neurology 1978; 28:626–630.
183. Cannon SB, Veazey JE Jr, Jackson RS, Burse VW, Hayes C, Straub WE, Landrigan PJ, Liddle FA. Epidemic kepone poisoning in chemical workers. Am J Epidemiol 1978; 107:529–537.
184. Taylor JR. Neurological manifestations in humans exposed to chlordecone and follow-up results. Neurotoxicology 1982; 3:9–16.
185. Saad SF, El Tayeb IB, Mustafa A. Investigation of the effect of chloropenthane and certain chemically related compounds on the cerebral gama-aminobutyric acid contents in rats. Pol J Pharmacol Pharmacy 1978; 30:469–474.
186. Carr RL, Couch TA, Liu J, Coats JR, Chambers JE. The interaction of chlorinated alicyclic insecticides with brain GABA(A) receptors in channel catfish (Ictalurus punctatus). J Toxicol Environ Health 1999; 56:543–553.
187. Haymaker E, Ginzler AM. The toxic effects of prolonged ingestion of DDT on dogs with special reference to lesions in the brain. Am J Med Sci 1946; 212:423–431.

188. Andersen A, Ellingsen DG, Morland T, Kjuus H. A neurological and neurophysiological study of chloralkali workers previously exposed to mercury vapour. Acta Neurol Scan 1993; 88:427–433.
189. Netterstrom B, Guldager B, Heeboll J. Acute mercury intoxication examined with coordination ability and tremor. Neurotoxicol Teratol 1996; 18:505–509.
190. Clarkson TW. The toxicology of mercury. Crit Rev Clin Lab Sci 1997; 34:369–403.
191. Urban P, Lukas E, Benicky L, Moscovicova E. Neurological and electrophysiological examination on workers exposed to mercury vapors. Neurotoxicology 1996; 17:191–196.
192. Ehrenberg RL, Vogt RL, Smith AB, Brondum J, Brightwell WS, Hudson PJ, McManus KP, Hannon WH, Phipps FC. Effects of elemental mercury exposure at a thermometer plant. Am J Ind Med 1991; 19:495–507.
193. Cassano GB, Viola PL, Ghetti B, Amaducci L. The distribution of inhaled mercury (Hg^{203}) in the brain of rats and mice. J Neuropath Exp Neurol 1969; 28:308–320.
194. Coulehan JL, Hirsch W, Brillman J, Sanandria J, Welty TK, Colaiaco P, Koros A, Lober A. Gasoline sniffing and lead toxicity in Navajo adolescents. Pediatrics 1983; 71:113–117.
195. Seidman BC, Verity MA. Selective inhibition of synaptosomal γ-aminobutyric acid uptake by triethyllead: role of energy transduction and chloride ion. J Neurochem 1987; 48:1142–1149.
196. Walsh TJ, Tilson HA. Neurobehavioral toxicology of the organoleads. Neurotoxicology 1984; 5:67–86.
197. Michaelson IA. Effects of inorganic lead on RNA, DNA and protein content in the developing rat brain. Toxicol Appl Pharmacol 1973; 26:539–548.
198. Valpey R, Sumi SM, Copass MK, Goble GJ. Acute and chronic progressive encephalopathy due to gasoline sniffing. Neurology 1978; 28:507–510.
199. Wennberg A, Hagman M, Johansson L. Preclinical neurophysiological signs of parkinsonism in occupational manganese exposure. Neurotoxicol 1992; 21:122–124.
200. Roels H, Lauwrys R, Genet P et al. Relationship between external and internal parameters of exposure to manganese in workers from a manganese oxide and salt producing plant. Am J Ind Med 1987; 11:297–305.
201. Chia SE, Goh J, Lee G et al. Use of a computerized postural sway measurement system for assessing workers exposed to manganese. Clin Exp Pharm Physiol 1993; 20:549–553.
202. Komaki H, Maisawa S, Sugai K, Kobayashi Y, Hashimoto T. Tremor and seizures associated with chronic manganese intoxication. Brain Dev 1999; 21:122–124.
203. Pal PK, Samii A, Calne DB. Manganese neurotoxicity: a review of clinical features, imaging and pathology. Neurotoxicology 1999; 20:227–238.
204. Miyagi Y, Shima F, Ishido K, Yasutake T, Kamikaseda K. Tremor induced by toluene misuse successfully treated by a Vim thalamotomy. J Neurol Neurosurg Psychiatry 1999; 66:794–796.
205. Uchino A, Kato A, Yuzuriha T, Takashima Y, Hiejima S, Murakami M, Endoh K, Yoshikai T, Kudo S. Comparison between patient characteristics and cranial MR findings in chronic thinner intoxication. Eur Radiol 2002; 12:1338–1341.
206. McLean DR, Jacobs H, Mielke BW. Methanol poisoning: a clinical and pathological study. Ann Neurol 1980; 8:161–167.

207. Henzi H. Chronic methanol poisoning with the clinical and pathologic-anatomical features of multiple sclerosis. Med Hypotheses 1984; 13:63–75.

208. Peters HA, Levine RL, Matthews CG, Sauter SL, Rankin JH. Carbon disulfide-induced neuropsychiatric changes in grain storage workers. Am J Ind Med 1982; 3:373–391.

209. Chapman LJ, Sauter SL, Henning RA, Levine RL, Matthews CG, Peters HA. Finger tremor after carbon disulfide-based pesticide exposures. Arch Neurol 1991; 48:866–870.

210. Huang CC, Yen TC, Shih TS, Chang HY, Chu NS. Dopamine transporter binding study in differentiating carbon disulfide induced parkinsonism from idiopathic parkinsonism. Neurotoxicology 2004; 25:341–347.

211. Johnson JD, Meisenheimer TL, Isom GE. Cyanide-induced neurotoxicity: a role of neuronal calcium. Toxicol Appl Pharmacol 1986; 84:464–469.

212. Rosenow F, Herholz K, Lanfermann H, Weuthen G, Ebner R, Kessler J, Ghaemi M, Heiss WD. Neurological sequelae of cyanide intoxication—the patterns of clinical, magnetic resonance imaging, and positron emission tomography findings. Ann Neurol 1995; 38:825–828.

213. Blumenthal H, Vance D. Rest tremor associated with exposure to Monesin. J Neurol Neurosurg Psychiatry 1988; 51:729–730.

214. Klawans HL. Dystonia and tremor following exposure to 2,3,7,8-tetrachlorodibenzo-p-dioxin. Mov Disord 1987; 2:255–261.

215. Langston JW, Ballard P, Tetrud JW, Irwin I. Chronic parkinsonism in humans due to a product of meperidine-analog synthesis. Science 1983; 219:979–980.

216. Bergman H, Raz A, Feingold A, Nini A, Nelken I, Hansel D, Ben-Pazi H, Reches A. Physiology of MPTP tremor. Mov Disord 1998; 13(suppl 3):29–34.

217. Burnett JW, Weinrich D, Williamson JA, Fenner PJ, Lutz LL, Bloom DA. Autonomic neurotoxicity of jellyfish and marine animal venoms. Clin Auton Res 1998; 8:125–130.

218. Amitai Y. Clinical manifestations and management of scorpion envenomation. Public Health Rev 1998; 26:257–263.

219. Yoshimoto CM, Yanagihara AA. Cnidarian (coelenterate) envenomations in Hawai'I improve following heat application. Trans R Soc Trop Med Hyg 2002; 96:300–303.

220. Isbister GK, White J. Clinical consequences of spider bites: recent advances in our understanding. Toxicon 2004; 43:477–492.

221. Lira-da-Silva RM, Matos GB, Sampaio RO, Nunes TB. Retrospective study on Latrodectus stings in Bahia, Brazil. Rev Soc Bras Med Trop 1995; 28:205–210.

222. Nicholson GM, Graudins A. Spiders of medical importance in the Asia-Pacific: atracotoxin, latrotoxin and related spider neurotoxins. Clin Exp Pharmacol Physiol 2002; 29:785–794.

223. Boysen SR, Rozanski EA, Chan DL, Grobe TL, Fallon MJ, Rush JE. Tremorgenic mycotoxicosis in four dogs from a single household. J Am Vet Med Assoc 2002; 221:1441–1444, 1420.

224. Gordon KE, Masotti RE, Waddell WR. Tremorgenic encephalopathy: a role of mycotoxins in the production of CNS disease in humans? Can J Neurol Sci 1993; 20:237–239.

225. He S, Jiu Y, Bian H, Huang J, Ye S, Lan Z, Xin Y. An outbreak of poisoning from Penicillium cyclopium contaminated dried persimmon. Biomed Environ Sci 1992; 5:115–124.

226. Hod H, Har-Zahav J, Kaplinsky N, Frankl O. Pindolol-induced tremor. Postgrad Med J 1980; 56:346–347.

227. Koller W, Orebaugh C, Lawson L, Potempa K. Pindolol-induced tremor. Clin Neuropharmacol 1987; 10:449–452.

228. Teravainen R, Larsen A, Fogelholm R. Comparison between the effects of pindolol and propranolol on essential tremor. Neurology 1977; 27:439–442.

229. Malchow-Moller A, Larsen S, Hey H, Stokholm KH, Juhl E, Quaade F. Ephedrine as an anorectic: the story of the 'Elsinore pill.' Int J Obes 1981; 5:183–187.

230. Dietz AJ Jr. Amphetamine-like reactions to phenylpropanolamine. JAMA 1981; 245:601–602.

231. Supiyaphun P, Chochaipanichnon L, Kerekhanjanarong V, Saengpaniel S. A comparative study of the side effects between pseudoephedrine in Loratadine plus Psueudoephedrine Sulfate Repetabs Tablets and loratadine + pseudoephedrine tablet in treatment of allergic rhinitis in Thai Patients. J Med Assoc Thai 2002; 85:722–727.

232. Gonzalez Rodriguez JL, Mateos Arribas MT. Tremors, cramps, and myalgia after the use of ephedrine. Rev Esp Anestesiol Reanim 2002; 49:501–502.

233. Deuschl G, Bain P, Brin M, and an Ad Hoc Scientific Committee. Consensus statement of the Movement Disorder Society on tremor. Mov Disord 1998; 13(suppl 3):2–23.

24

Physiological Tremor

Neng Huang and James Tetrud

The Parkinson's Institute, Sunnyvale, California, USA

I. INTRODUCTION

Physiological tremor can be broadly defined as an involuntary and continuous oscillation of any limb segment occurring in otherwise normal subjects (1–3). This tremor type can be present when the limb segment is at rest, held against gravity, in motion, or under isometric contraction. The frequency of physiological tremor varies widely in different body parts, although 8–12 Hz oscillation has traditionally been evoked as the frequency range (4). The amplitudes of these oscillations are generally small such that normal finger tremor can barely be seen with the naked eye. However, by means of either optical magnification or mechanical-electrical transducers, such as accelerometers, physiological tremor can be recorded in any joint or muscle that can oscillate (3,4). Another type of tremor that can occur in normal subjects is enhanced physiological tremor, but unlike physiological tremor, this tremor type is easily visible to the naked eye, and can be quite symptomatic.

While physiological tremor may be of little clinical significance, understanding its physiological basis might provide insight into the mechanisms underlying other more clinically relevant tremor types such as enhanced physiological tremor, parkinsonian tremor, orthostatic tremor, and essential tremor. Furthermore, since there is increasing evidence suggesting that "central oscillator(s)" contribute to the generation of most tremor types, the study of physiological tremor could allow better understanding of these oscillators and their role in human motor control (5).

In this chapter, we provide an overview of physiological tremor, emphasizing its multifactorial origins and relationship to other tremor types.

II. ORIGINS OF PHYSIOLOGICAL TREMOR

A. Historical Note

Physiological tremor has been the subject of extensive study for over a century (6–11). In 1886, Schafter was the first to report the existence of rhythmic oscillations in muscles. He was able to record a 10 Hz tremulous twitch superimposed on regular muscle activity and suggested an underlying "neurogenic" origin of tremor (6). Over the past 50 years, studies of tremor have been greatly enhanced by the introduction of accelerometry and the application of spectral analysis (8). Linear piezoresistive accelerometers have provided a convenient method of measuring tremor frequency and amplitude since the weight of these sensors is only a few grams and they are small enough to be fixed to nearly any body part. Tremor has also been quantified using a device that senses changes in angular rate, utilizing a solid-state gyroscope (12). This device provides a sensitive and accurate measure of tremor frequency and amplitude that is independent of gravity (12). Recently, more sophisticated instruments have been used to study tremor. Brain electromagnetic activity and metabolism associated with tremor can be measured in real-time and with high spatial resolution by means of magnetoenecephalography (MEG) and functional magnetic resonance imaging (fMRI) (13,14). Electrical activity in various brain tissues can also be recorded directly during surgical procedures for certain movement disorders (15). Using these techniques, coherence analysis can be used to correlate brain electrical and metabolic function with peripherally measured tremor thus facilitating the identification and localization of putative central oscillators (16). Thus far, these studies suggest that the origin of physiological tremor is multifactorial, representing the combined output of a number of different oscillatory sources, but modified by the intrinsic resonant properties of limb segments (Fig. 24.1) (5).

B. Mechanical Factors in Physiological Tremor

The mechanical properties of a limb segment influence its intrinsic resonance frequency. As with any physical object, the resonance frequency of a limb segment is directly proportional to the square root of its stiffness and inversely proportional to the square root of its moment of inertia (17). For example, the resonant frequency around the elbow joint is 3–5 Hz, around the wrist joint 8–12 Hz, and around the metacarpal-phalangel joint 12–30 Hz (2). The effect of a limb's mechanical properties on tremor frequency can also be demonstrated by adding an external "load," such as a weight of 1000 mg to the dorsum of the hand, which increases inertia and causes resonance frequencies to decrease (17). The component of physiological tremor that results from the contribution of these mechanical properties is called *mechanical tremor* and a study of tremor in a large group of normal subjects has demonstrated that mechanical tremor is the main frequency component of physiological tremor in most individuals (18).

Another source of mechanical tremor derives from the thrust of heart contraction. This ballistocardiac impulse contributes to mechanical tremor in two ways: 1) It is the principle perturbation that drives body parts to oscillate at their own resonance frequency and 2) the cyclic ejection of blood from the heart provides a significant force to the entire body, creating oscillations that are occasionally visible to the naked eye. Although the ballistocardiac impulse

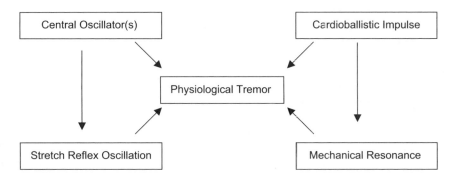

Figure 24.1   Simplified diagram depicting multifactorial origins of physiological tremor. Mechanical resonance frequency of limbs is the major determinant and is driven by the cardioballistic impulse. The cardioballistic impulse also contributes directly to physiological tremor. The stretch reflex-mediated oscillation plays a major role in enhanced physiological tremor. The central oscillator(s) contribute to the frequency-invariant component of physiological tremor, although their anatomical location is unknown.

may account for a large proportion of physiological tremor at rest, it appears to contribute very little to the tremor of limbs held against gravity (19). Supporting this notion is the observation that during space flight, when the effect of gravity has been eliminated, the ballistocardiac impulse becomes the dominant component of physiological tremor (20).

C. Stretch Reflex in Physiological Tremor

The spinal stretch reflex has been shown to contribute to oscillations of physiological tremor (1,21). For example, contraction in a flexor results in activation of the extensor muscle spindle, leading to a reflex contraction of the extensor through its segmental spinal α-motor neuron. The contraction in the extensor muscle group may in turn trigger a flexor muscle contraction, resulting in a feedback system analogous to a servo-loop. Oscillations will result when the reflex gain and conduction time through this feedback system are appropriate to cause synchronization of the spinal motor units. (17,22,23). There is also evidence that this synchronization may be modulated by central oscillator(s) (21). However, the contribution of this stretch-reflex-mediated oscillation to physiological tremor is believed to be relatively small, exerting its influence primarily by modulating the tremor amplitude (1,4). Marsden and colleagues have demonstrated that patients with tabes dorsalis or C5-T2 posterior root resection, in whom the reflex arc is impaired, exhibit preservation of the 8–12 Hz hand tremor (1). The addition of an external weight can lower the stretch reflex mediated oscillation frequency (5,17). This effect can be demonstrated by spectral analysis of accelerometry and electromyographic (EMG) recordings of tremor activity. In this paradigm, loading results in a downward shift of the synchronized frequency (17). Under certain circumstances, such as when large mechanical loads are applied to the limb or when there is unusual reflex enhancement such as fright and fatigue, the reflex mediated oscillation becomes dominant, as seen in enhanced physiological tremor (24,25).

D. Central Oscillators in Physiological Tremor

A central origin of physiological tremor has been proposed in a number of early studies (22,26,27). For example, preservation of postural physiological tremor has been demonstrated in patients with deafferented limbs who lack sensory feedback loops (26). Furthermore, many studies have demonstrated that normal subjects exhibit a component of 8–12 Hz physiological tremor that is not affected by external loading, as would be expected if the tremor was due primarily to mechanical factors (11). This component of 8–12 Hz tremor has been identified in muscle groups with widely varying mass, such as the soleus, biceps, extensor digitorum, and intrinsic hand muscles (11). Using tremor spectral analysis, this component can be identified as the frequency-invariant peak, irrespective of loading or unloading (17).

It is generally believed that the frequency-invariant component of physiological tremor is primarily the result of an oscillating system of neurons located within the central nervous system (5), although no correlation between electroencephalographic (EEG) activity and physiological tremor has been established. Presumably, the central oscillator(s) are located in sub-cortical nuclei such as the basal ganglia or thalamus, nuclei that are inaccessible to surface EEG or MEG (5).

McAuley and Marsden, in a review of physiological and pathological tremor, suggest that certain contradictions regarding the various proposed mechanisms of physiological tremor may be due to the variable conditions under which tremor has been recorded (5). They suggest that physiological tremor can be divided into different categories based on the relative contribution from peripheral and central processes. For example, physiological tremor registered at rest in normal subjects may be due primarily to cardioballistic (peripheral) effects, whereas postural physiological tremor may be more multifactorial in origin, having both peripheral and central contributions (5).

III. ENHANCED PHYSIOLOGICAL TREMOR

A. Description

While physiological tremor may be too subtle to produce clinical symptoms, enhanced physiological tremor is commonly encountered in clinical practice. The consensus statement on tremor from the Movement Disorder Society defines enhanced physiological tremor as: 1) an easily visible tremor that is mainly postural and of high frequency, 2) a tremor with no evidence of an underlying neurological disease, and 3) a tremor that usually has a reversible cause (3). Enhanced physiological tremor is relatively large in amplitude, with a single peak frequency between 8 and 12 Hz and symptomatic, often associated with fright, anxiety, fatigue, or a forceful muscle contraction. This tremor type can also be seen with certain metabolic disorders (e.g., hypoglycemia, hyperthyroidism) and treatment with certain drugs such as adrenergic agonists (e.g., bronchodilators in asthmatic patients), lithium, corticosteroids, and other "excitatory drugs" (Table 24.1).

B. Mechanism of Enhanced Physiological Tremor

The mechanism of enhanced physiological tremor is thought to be due to increased beta-adrenergic stimulation (1). As demonstrated by Marsden and colleagues, intravenous infusion of epinephrine or isoproterenol increases the amplitude of finger tremor and administration of the β-adrenergic blocker propranolol reduces the tremor amplitude (28). Because β-adrenergic stimulation sensitizes the group 1a muscle spindle afferents and enhances motor unit synchronization, it is believed that increased synchronization of the stretch reflex underlies the

Table 24.1   Common Conditions and Drugs Associated
with Enhanced Physiological Tremor

Nonpharmacological	Pharmacological
Anxiety	β-Adrenergic agonists
Exercise	Dopamine agonists
Hypoglycemia	Lithium, valproic acid
Thyrotoxicosis	Tricyclic antidepressants
Pheochromocytoma	Neuroleptics
Alcohol withdrawal	Caffeine, amphetamines
Fatigue	Theophylline
Fright	Steroids

neuronal mechanism of enhanced physiological tremor (1,4). A central mechanism in enhanced physiological tremor has also been proposed (29).

C.   Clinical Aspects of Enhanced Physiological Tremor

Differentiating enhanced physiological tremor from essential tremor can be clinically challenging requiring a comprehensive medical history to assess certain enhanced physiological tremor provoking factors. Past and current medications should be evaluated and a careful family history extracted. The lack of a family history of tremor, presence of an identifiable provoking factor, and reversibility of the tremor upon termination of the provoking factor, all support the diagnosis of enhanced physiological tremor. A basic metabolic profile that includes thyroid function testing and fasting blood glucose should also be sought. Clinically, both essential tremor and enhanced physiological tremor are absent or minimal at rest, appear and/or increase with limbs held against gravity, and are present, but not intensified, during volitional movement. Enhanced physiological tremor usually presents as a fine and rapid postural tremor, whereas classic essential tremor is of larger amplitude and lower frequency. When the diagnosis is questionable on clinical grounds, objective electrophysiological studies, such as quantitative computerized tremor analysis can be helpful (30). Also, Shahani and colleagues have reported that intravenous propranolol infusion can block enhanced physiological tremor, but has little effect on essential tremor (31).

   Many patients with enhanced physiological tremor require nothing more than simple reassurance when the cause of their tremor is identified. When pharmacological treatment is required, a β-adrenergic blocker such as propranolol can be beneficial. The drug can be taken as needed, such as during times of stress or anxiety. Benzodiazepines such as lorazepam, clonazepam, and diazepam can also be beneficial when β-blockers are contraindicated.

IV. CONCLUSION

Physiological tremor is universally present in every individual to varying degrees. The amplitude is usually subtle and clinically asymptomatic. The underlying cause of physiological tremor is multifactorial and likely related to both central and peripheral oscillatory mechanisms. The location of the central oscillator(s) has not been identified, and their functional significance is not well understood. Unlike physiological tremor, enhanced physiological tremor is usually visible and often symptomatic. This tremor type is thought to be mediated by increased spinal motor unit synchronization. A detailed history can usually help identify the underlying cause. Symptoms usually subside following termination of the provoking factors and, occasionally, a β-blocker or benzodiazepine may be needed for symptomatic relief.

REFERENCES

1. Marsden CD. Origins of normal and pathological tremor. In: Findley LJ, Capildeo R, eds. Movement Disorders: Tremor. New York: Oxford University Press, 1984:37–84.
2. Elble R, Koller W. Tremor. Baltimore: Johns Hopkins University Press, 1990.
3. Deuschl G, Bain PG, Brin M, Ad Hoc Scientific Committee. Consensus statement of the movement disorder society on tremor. Mov Disord 1998; 13(suppl 13):2–23.
4. Young RR. Physiological and enhanced physiological tremor. In: Findley LJ, Capildeo R, eds. Movement Disorders: Tremor. New York: Oxford University Press, 1984:127–134.
5. McAuley JH, Marsden CD. Physiological and pathological tremors and rhythmic central motor control. Brain 2000; 123:1545–1567.
6. Schafer EA, Canney HE, Tundsdall JO. On the rhythm of muscular response to volitional impulses in man. J Physiol (Lond) 1886; 7:111–117.
7. Friedlander W. Characteristics of postural tremor in normal and in various abnormal states. Neurology 1956; 6:716–724.
8. Halliday AM, Redfearn JW. An analysis of the frequencies of finger tremor in healthy subjects. J Physiol 1956; 134:600–611.
9. Marshall J, Walsh EG. Physiological tremor. J Neurochem 1956; 19:260–267.
10. Brumlik J. On the nature of normal tremor. Neurology 1962; 12:159–179.
11. Elble R. In: Findley LJ, Koller WC, eds. Mechanisms of Physiological Tremor and Relationship to Essential Tremor. New York: Marcel Dekker Inc., 1995:51–62.
12. Tetrud J, Felsing G, Sunnarborg D, Dellmeier W. Assessment of tremor using a solid-state angular rate sensor. 45th Annual Meeting of the American Academy of Neurology, New York, April 29, 1993.
13. Volkmann J. Oscillations of the human sensorimotor system as revealed by magnetoencephalography. Mov Disord 1998; 13(suppl 13):73–76.
14. Boecker H, Brooks DJ. Functional imaging of tremor. Mov Disord 1998; 13(suppl 3):64–72.
15. Benazzouz A, Breit S, Koudsie A, Pollak P, Krack P, Benabid AL. Intraoperative microrecordings of the subthalamic nucleus in Parkinson's disease. Mov Disord 2002; 17(suppl 3):145–149.

16. Raethjen J, Lindemann, Dumpelmann Matthias, Wenzelburger R, Stolze H, Pfister G, Elger CE, Timmer J, Deuschl G. Corticomuscular coherence in the 6–15 Hz band: is the cortex involved in the generation of physiologic tremor? Exp Brain Res 2002; 142:32–40.

17. Deuschl G, Raethjen J, Lindemann M, Krack P. The pathophysiology of tremor. Muscle Nerve 2001; 24:716–735.

18. Raethjen J, Pawlas F, Lindemann M, Wenzelburger R, Deuschl G. Determinants of physiologica tremor in a large normal population. Clinical Neurophysiology 2000; 111:1825–1827

19. Marsden CD, Meadows JC, Lange GW, Watson RS. The role of the ballistocardiac impulse in the genesis of physiological tremor. Brain 1969; 92:647–662.

20. Gallasch E, Moser M, Kozlovskaya IB, Kenner T, Noordergraaf A. Effects of an eight-day space flight on microvibration and physiological tremor. Am J Physiol 1997; 273:R86–R92.

21. Allum JHJ. Segmental reflex, muscle mechanical and central mechanisms underlying human physiological tremor. In: Findley LJ, Capildeo R, eds. Movement Disorders: Tremor. New York: Oxford University Press, 1984:135–155.

22. Elble R, Randall JE. Motor-unit activity responsible for 8- to 12-Hz component of human physiological finger tremor. J Neurophysiol 1976; 39:370–383.

23. Stein RB, Lee RG, Nichols TR. Modifications of ongoing tremors and locomotion by sensory feedback. Electromyogr Clin Neurophysiol 1978; 34:512–519.

24. Hagbarth KE, Young RR. Participation of the stretch reflex in human physiological tremor. Brain 1979; 102:509–526.

25. Brown TI, Rack PM, Ross HF. A range of different stretch reflex responses in the human thumb. J Physiol (Lond) 1982; 332:101–112.

26. Marsden CD, Meadows JC, Lange GW, Watson RS. Effect of deafferentation on human physiological tremor. Lancet 1967; 33:53–65.

27. Mori S. Entrainment of motor-unit discharges as a neuronal mechanism of synchronization. J Neurophysiol 1975; 38:859–870.

28. Marsden CD, Meadows JC. The effect of adrenaline on the contraction of human muscle—one mechanism whereby adrenaline increases the amplitude of physiological tremor. J Physiol 1968; 194:70P–71P.

29. Koster B, Lauk M, Timmer J, Winter T, Guschlbarer B, Glocker FX, Danek A, Deuscl G, Lucking CH. Central mechanisms in human enhanced physiological tremor. Neuroscience Letters 1998; 241:135–139.

30. Louis ED, Pullman SL. Comparison of clinical vs. electrophysiological methods of diagnosing of essential tremor. Mov Disord 2001; 16:668–673.

31. Shahani BT, Young RR. Physiological and pharmacological aids in the differential diagnosis of tremor. J Neurol Neurosurg Psychiatry 1976; 39:772–783.

25

Psychogenic Tremor

Nestor Galvez-Jimenez
The Cleveland Clinic Florida, Weston, Florida, USA

I. INTRODUCTION

Today, as in 1921, the words of Sir Henry Head resonate: "... Hysteria is sometimes said to imitate organic affections; but this is a highly misleading statement. The mimicry can only deceive an observer ignorant of the signs of hysteria or content with perfunctory examination" (1). In most cases of psychogenic movement disorders, especially tremor, the nature of the movement is quite obvious to the examiner but in some instances it may be quite challenging. The diagnosis requires careful review of the history and clinical examination as well as the phenomenology of the abnormal movements. Furthermore, prolonged periods of observations are necessary to clarify the nature of the movement. It is also quite helpful to carefully analyze the context or surrounding in which the movement disorder occurs or the circumstances that led to the onset of the abnormal movement. Psychiatry and legal issues may affect the evaluation, diagnosis and treatment of such patients; therefore, both should be carefully considered.

II. EPIDEMIOLOGY

Accurate data on the prevalence of psychogenic tremor is lacking and estimates are variable. At three movement disorders centers, (Columbia Presbyterian Medical Center, The Toronto Western Hospital, and Cleveland Clinic Florida), psychogenic tremor accounted for a quarter of all psychogenic movement disorders (Table 25.1) (2). Of a total of 272 patients with psychogenic movement disorders evaluated at the three centers, 22% had psychogenic tremor. Psychogenic dystonia was the most common psychogenic movement disorder (41.8%). Over a five year span, (1998–2002), a total of 56 cases of psychogenic movement disorders were evaluated at the Cleveland Clinic Florida's Movement Disorders program out of 2155 movement disorder cases. Of these, psychogenic tremor accounted for 32.1% (18/56) of all psychogenic movement disorders. Table 25.1 demonstrates that the Toronto Western Hospital and Cleveland Clinic Florida had more patients with psychogenic tremor, than any other psychogenic movement disorders, (39/120 total psychogenic patients for both centers) accounting for 64.9%. The New York group reported tremor (13%) as the second most common psychogenic movement disorder. Referral patterns and type of practice undoubtedly affects the prevalence of this disorder.

Table 25.1 Combined Data on Psychogenic Movement Disorders (PMDs) Seen at Three Movement Disorder Centers (2)

PMDs	CPMC	TWH	CCFla	Total
Dystonia	82 (53%)	16 (25%)	14 (25%)	112 (41.8%)
Tremor	21 (13%)	21 (32.8%)	18 (32.1%)	60 (22%)
Gait	14 (9%)	7 (10.9%)	1 (1.8%)	22 (8.1%)
Myoclonus	11 (7%)	16 (25%)	4 (7.1%)	31 (11.4%)
Blepharospasm/facial movements	4 (2%)	–	4 (7.1%)	8 (2.9%)
Parkinsonism	3 (1.9%)	4 (6.3%)	0	7 (2.6%)
Tics	2 (1.3%)	–	2 (3.6%)	4 (1.5%)
Stiff Person Syndrome	1 (0.6%)	–	–	1 (0.4%)
Other mixed/bizarre	14 (9%)	NL	13 (23.2%)	27 (9.9%)
Totals[a]	152	64	56	272

[a]Totals represent types of PMDs. Some patients have more than one pattern of PMDs.
Note: CPMC: Columbia-Presbyterian Medical Center (Listed all types of PMDs); TWH: Toronto Western Hospital (listed only the predominant PMDs); CCFla: Cleveland Clinic Florida (listed only the predominant PMDs); NL: not listed.

III. DIAGNOSTIC CATEGORIES OF PSYCHOGENIC MOVEMENT DISORDERS

Although the diagnostic categories for the diagnosis of psychogenic movement disorders were initially developed for psychogenic dystonia (3), these criteria may be applied to other psychogenic movement disorders including tremor.

1. *Documented psychogenic tremor or other psychogenic movement disorders.* The psychogenic movement disorders must be relieved by psychotherapy, administration of placebos or psychological suggestion including physiotherapy, or the patients must be witnessed as being free of symptoms when left alone supposedly unobserved.
2. *Clinically established psychogenic tremor or other psychogenic movement disorder.* When the phenomenology of tremor or other psychogenic movement disorder is inconsistent or incongruent with such movements over time, and one becomes suspicious that the movements are psychogenic and are associated with other neurological signs, such as false weakness, false sensory findings, and self-inflicted injuries. In addition multiple somatizations and obvious psychiatric disturbances are present.
3. *Probable psychogenic tremor or other psychogenic movement disorders.* There are three possibilities in this group: (1) Those in whom the tremor or other psychogenic movement disorders are inconsistent or incongruent with classic disease, and in whom there are not other features providing further support for such diagnosis or psychogenicity. (2) Those patients in whom the tremor or other psychogenic movement disorders are consistent and congruent with organic disease, but in whom other neurological signs are present that are definitively psychogenic such as false weakness, false sensory findings or self inflicted injuries. (3) Those patients in whom the tremor or other psychogenic movement disorders are consistent and congruent with organic disease, but in whom multiple somatizations are present.
4. *Possible psychogenic tremor and other psychogenic movement disorders.* The movements are consistent and congruent with organic disease but the examiner is suspicious that the tremor or other psychogenic movement disorders are psychogenic when an emotional disturbance is present, but these are not as compelling as the psychiatric features listed above for all other categories.

IV. CLINICAL FEATURES AND CLUES TO THE DIAGNOSIS

Psychogenic tremor is usually associated with a variety of co-morbidities and other features suggesting a "functional" etiology to their symptoms (Table 25.2) (3,4). In Charcot's clinic most patients were housed with the epileptics, where

Table 25.2 Features Suggestive of Psychogenic Tremor or Other Psychogenic Movement Disorders [Modified from (2,3)]

Historical
1. Abrupt onset
2. Static course
3. Spontaneous remissions or cures
4. Multiple somatizations
5. Multiple undiagnosed conditions
6. Negative family history of neurological diseases
7. Fibromyalgia
8. Presence of psychiatric disease
9. Previous functional disturbance
10. Employed in the health care profession
11. Pending litigation or compensation
12. Presence of secondary gain
13. Young woman

Clinical
1. Inconsistent character of the movement (amplitude, frequency, distribution, selective disability)
2. Presence of false weakness and/or sensory complaints
3. Paroxysmal movement disorder
4. Movement increase with attention or decrease with distraction
5. Suggestion; the ability to trigger or relieve the abnormal movement with unusual or nonphysiologic interventions such as pressure on trigger points, use of a tuning fork, etc.
6. Self-inflicted injuries
7. Deliberate slowness of movements
8. Functional disability out of proportion to examination findings
9. Movement disorder that is bizarre, multiple, or difficult to classify
10. No evidence of disease by laboratory or radiographic procedures

Treatment responses
1. Unresponsive to appropriate medications
2. Response to placebo therapy
3. Remission with psychotherapy

it is believed that many learned how to imitate movements (5). This lead to much criticism by Broca, Freud, and Gowers (6–8). They criticized Charcot's methods of hypnosis and suggestion using Augustine, Charcot's favorite subject, as an example to explain the weakness of such methods. Augustine was a young "impressionable" woman who suffered from all types of abnormal movements, convulsions, and catatonic behavior possibly reinforced by Charcot's methods. This led to continuous reinforcement of her movements, leading to the erroneous conclusion of perhaps real pathology (9). Although these observations were made more than a century ago, current observations of behavior and phenomenology of psychogenic movement disorders have not changed. Some cases of psychogenic tremor may be the result of imitation by patients who had witnessed similar symptoms in friends or family members. Therefore, the clinician should be aware of the possibility of malingering, factitious, conversion, or somatization disorders (Tables 25.3–25.5) (10). The most challenging aspect is distinguishing between malingering and conversion disorder (Table 25.6) (10). In some instances, serial careful observations over time or other observations made by well-trained personnel such as nurses, may prove helpful.

Historically there is a wealth of information provided by Charcot (5,9), Gowers (11), Wilson (12), and more recently by Fahn et al. (13) and Koller et al. (14) on the phenomenology and other characteristics of psychogenic tremor. Charcot described proximal tremors, affecting predominantly the shoulders or flexion extension at the elbow mimicking the use of a hammer as unique to hysteria. He used terms such as rhythmical and hammering "chorea" to describe such movements. Sir Henry Head (1) described hysterical tremors as a positive repetitive movement of a "high voluntary type," with variable velocity and ameliorating with distraction. He described a soldier with severe right arm and hand tremor who was able to play the banjo perfectly well. Gowers (11) described psychogenic or hysterical tremor in patients with hysterical paralysis. He noted the irregularity, coarse nature, influence of physical and emotional stimuli, and attention paid to the tremor by the sufferer. Wilson (12) described fluctuations and irregularity in such tremors. He noted that in persons who intentionally performed these movements fatigue became an early feature because the tremor was not part of their normal "programming."

Koller et al. (14) described 24 patients with clinically established or documented psychogenic tremor. The female to male ratio was 1.7:1, with patients having a mean age of 43.4 years ranging from 15–78 years. The duration of tremor ranged from one month to ten years. The onset of tremor was abrupt in 87.5% of cases and the majority (45%) showed no changes in their tremor over time. Complete resolution was seen in only 25% of cases, fluctuating course in 16% and worsening in 4%. The majority of patients (91%) had features

Table 25.3 Diagnostic Criteria for Somatization Disorders (10)

Somatization Disorder

1. History of many physical complaints beginning before age 30 years occurring over a period of many years resulting in medical treatment or significant impairment in social, occupational or other areas of functioning
2. The following criteria must have been met, with the symptoms occurring any time during the course of the disturbance:
   - Four pain symptoms in at least four different sites
   - Two gastrointestinal symptoms other than pain
   - One sexual symptom other than pain
   - One pseudoneurological symptom suggesting a neurological condition not limited to pain

---

Table 25.4 Diagnostic Criteria for Facititious Disorders (10)

Facititious Disorder
1. Intentional production or feigning of physical or psychological symptoms or signs (Munchausen syndrome)
2. The motivation for the behavior is to assume the sick role
3. External incentives for the behavior are absent (economic gain, avoidance of legal responsibilities, or improving physical well-being)

suggestive of a functional disorder such as nonphysiologic weakness, atypical gait, nonanatomical sensory loss, and a background of psychiatric diagnosis such as conversion disorder, depression, anxiety, and malingering. The phenomenology of the tremor was also congruent with psychogenicity such as reduction of tremor with distraction and variability of tremor frequency. Postural tremor was the most prominent feature, followed by rest and action tremors. Some patients had an associated head tremor (12%).

In a ten-year retrospective review (15) of 70 patients with clinically definite psychogenic tremor, 73% had an abrupt onset of symptoms in one limb with a rapid generalized spread of symptoms, and maximal disability at onset occurred in 46%. Symptoms remained static in 46% and took a fluctuating course in 17%. Spontaneous resolution and recurrence, easy distractibility, entrainment, and response to suggestion were features that supported such a diagnosis. Functional symptoms such as bizarre gait, give-way weakness, pseudoseizures, secondary gain, selective disability, and compensation or litigation issues were common. Most patients were refractory to conventional tremor therapy. The investigators found the "co-activation sign" on clinical examination and on electromyography to be quite helpful. They also emphasized the need for prolonged periods of observation in some patients, especially in those with an associated organic movement disorder. Psychogenic tremor may accompany many psychiatric

Table 25.5 Diagnostic Criteria for Malingering (10)

Malingering
1. The essential feature is the intentional production of false or grossly exaggerated physical or psychological symptoms, motivated by external incentives (i.e., avoiding work, obtaining financial compensation)
2. Malingering may represent adaptive behavior
3. Malingering should be suspected if there is a medicolegal issue (i.e., the person has been referred by his/her attorney)
4. Marked discrepancy between the person's claimed stress and disability and the objective findings
5. Lack of cooperation during the diagnostic evaluation and in complying with the prescribed treatment
6. Presence of antisocial personality disorder

Table 25.6 Diagnostic Criteria for Conversion Disorder (10)

1. One or more symptoms or deficits affecting voluntary motor or sensory functions that suggest a neurological or other general medical condition
2. Psychological factors judged to be associated with the symptom or deficit because the onset of symptoms is preceded by conflicts or other stressors
3. The symptom is not intentionally produced or feigned
4. The symptom cannot be explained by a general medical condition after a thorough medical and laboratory evaluation, or as a direct effect of a substance or culturally sanctioned behavior or experience
5. The symptom causes significant distress or impairment in social, occupational, or other important areas of functioning or warrants medical attention
6. The symptom is not limited to pain or sexual dysfunction, does not occur exclusively during the course of somatization disorder, and is not better accounted for by another mental disorder

disturbances such as anxiety, depression and post-traumatic stress disorder (16), and may be present in patients with organic movement disorders (2,17).

V. APPROACH TO TREATMENT

Although the concept of the treatment of psychogenic tremor as the treatment of the psychological or psychiatric condition sounds intuitively correct, the diagnosis and treatment of these tremors is quite difficult and often challenging even to the most experienced clinician. Extensive periods of observation are at times necessary for the correct diagnosis. An experienced neurologist should make the diagnosis, preferably a movement disorders specialist, as extensive experience in the diagnosis and phenomenology of psychogenic movement disorders is required. Some patients may benefit from video monitoring such as that used by epileptologists for the diagnosis of psychogenic seizures. A more convenient and economical assessment can be made in the office setting using videotaping using "induction" techniques or suggestion. The use of placebos or suggestion dates back to the days of Charcot, who used pressure points, pelvic pressure, and tuning forks among other techniques to induce "spells" in patients with hysteria.

The use of neuroimaging techniques and other laboratory testing are usually not necessary except when other conditions are suspected, such as Wilson's disease and thyroid disease. Electrophysiological studies may prove valuable, as tremor usually has specific patterns that can be easily discerned using appropriate techniques. Variability in tremor frequency, documentation of distractibility, persistence of tremor while there is ongoing muscle contraction, and abatement of tremor when the muscle contraction diminishes (co-activation sign) are helpful neurophysiologic observations when assessing a patient suspected of having psychogenic tremor (3,18). When assessing and treating patients with psychogenic tremor, it is important to emphasize the statement by Brown and Thompson "... a movement disorder should not be diagnosed as hysterical for no better reason that they are not yet officially described, ... a wait-and-see management policy is important in many of these cases as the phenotypes of confirmed organic movement disorders continue to increase" (19).

Many patients with psychogenic tremor have undergone a variety of treatments and at times expensive neurodiagnostic testing by the time they come for an expert opinion. The movement disorder specialist should make every effort to obtain a definitive diagnosis to avoid unnecessary testing and unrewarding and potentially unsafe treatments. The physician should approach the patient with empathy and present the diagnosis with a nonjudgmental attitude, yet avoiding uncertainty about the diagnosis. The use of a neurobiological explanation for the patient's symptoms helps in establishing trust, acceptance, and understanding of their diagnosis, and may help in the recovery (20). Using common symptom analogies such as the development of skin rashes and pruritus (neurodermatitis), dyspepsia and other epigastric symptoms, memory difficulties (pseudodementia) or labile hypertension in some patients with anxiety, somatization, and mood disorders may help present the symptoms to the patient and validate their presence. In addition, confirming the nature of the movement disorder but that the problem is not due to a structural lesion may help alleviate the anxiety that many patients have when the diagnosis is discussed. It is also important to emphasize the need for psychiatric consultation to assist in the long-term treatment plan. Therefore, the movement disorder specialist should have a good rapport and work closely with a psychiatrist interested in the evaluation and treatment of these patients. This is particularly important as many psychiatrists may have difficulty accepting the psychogenic nature of these symptoms.

REFERENCES

1. Head H. The diagnosis of hysteria. Br Med J 1922; 1:827–829.
2. Sa DS, Galvez-Jimenez N, Lang AE. Psychogenic movement disorders. In: Watts R, Koller W, eds. Movement Disorders, Neurologic Principles and Practice. 2nd ed. New York: McGraw-Hill, 2004.
3. Fahn S, Williams DT. Psychogenic dystonia. Adv Neurol 1988; 50:431–455.
4. Koller WC, Findley LJ. Psychogenic tremors. Adv Neurol 1990; 53:271–275.
5. Charcot J-M. Hystero-epilepsy: a young woman with a convulsive attack in the auditorium. In: Goetz CG, ed. Charcot The Clinician. The Tuesday lessons. New York: Raven Press, 1987:102–122.
6. Schiller F. Paul Broca: Founder of French Anthropology. Explorer of the Brain. New York: Oxford University Press, 1992.
7. Freud S. Hypnotism and suggestion (1888). In: Strachey J, ed. Collected Papers. London: Hogarth Press, 1957:11–24.
8. Gowers WR. Epilepsy and other chronic convulsive diseases: their causes, symptoms and treatment. New York: Dover Publication, 1964.

9. Didi-Huberman G. Invention of Hysteria. Charcot and the Photographic Iconography of the Salpetriere. Cambridge, Massachusetts: The MIT Press, 2003:85–174.
10. American Psychiatric Association. Diagnostic and Statistical Manual of Mental Disorders. 4th ed. (DSM IV). Washington: American Psychiatric Association, 1994.
11. Gowers WR. A Manual of disease of the Nervous System. Philadelphia: Blakston, 1888.
12. Wilson SAK. The approach to the study of hysteria. J Neurol Psychopathol 1931; 11:193–206.
13. Fahn S. Atypical tremor, rare tremor and unclassified tremors. In: Findley LJ, Capildeo R, eds. Movement Disorders. London: Macmillan Press, 1984:431–443.
14. Koller W, Lang AE, Vetere-Overfield B et al. Psychogenic tremors. Neurology 1989; 39:1094–1099.
15. Kim YJ, Pakiam A, Lang AE. Historical and clinical features of psychogenic tremor: A review of 70 cases. Can J Neurol Sci 1999; 26:190–195.
16. Walters AS, Henning WA. Noise-induced psychogenic tremor associated with posttraumatic stress disorders. Mov Disord 1992; 7:333–338.
17. Ranawaya R, Riley D, Lang A. Psychogenic dyskinesias in patients with organic movement disorders. Mov Disord 1990; 5:127–133.
18. Deuschl G, Koster B, Lucking CH, Scheidt C. Diagnostic and pathophysiological aspects of psychogenic tremors. Mov Disord 1998; 13:294–302.
19. Brown P, Thompson PD. Electrophysiological aids to the diagnosis of psychogenic jerks, spasms, and tremor. Mov Disord 2001; 16:595–599.
20. Ford B, Williams DT, Fahn S. Treatment of psychogenic movement disorders. In: Kurlan E, ed. Treatment of Movement Disorders. JB: Lippincott, 1995:475–485.

Index

Note: Italicized page numbers refer to illustrations and to tables